Do not remove from cardiac
Rehab. Room

Social Support and Cardiovascular Disease

THE PLENUM SERIES IN BEHAVIORAL PSYCHOPHYSIOLOGY AND MEDICINE

Series Editor: William J. Ray
                   Pennsylvania State University
                   University Park, Pennsylvania

A Continuation Order Plan is available for this series. A continuation order will bring delivery of each new volume immediately upon publication. Volumes are billed only upon actual shipment. For further information please contact the publisher.

Social Support and Cardiovascular Disease

Edited by

Sally A. Shumaker

Wake Forest University
Winston-Salem, North Carolina

and

Susan M. Czajkowski

National Heart, Lung, and Blood Institute
Bethesda, Maryland

PLENUM PRESS • *NEW YORK AND LONDON*

Library of Congress Cataloging-in-Publication Data

Social support and cardiovascular disease / edited by Sally A.
Shumaker and Susan M. Czajkowski.
    p.   cm. -- (The Plenum series in behavioral psychophysiology
and medicine)
    Includes bibliographical references and index.
    ISBN 0-306-43982-4
    1. Cardiovascular system--Diseases--Social aspects.
2. Cardiovascular system--Diseases--Psychological aspects.
I. Shumaker, Sally A.   II. Czajkowski, Susan M.   III. Series.
    [DNLM: 1. Cardiovascular Diseases--epidemiology.
2. Cardiovascular Diseases--etiology. 3. Cardiovascular Diseases-
-rehabilitation. 4. Social Environment.   WG 100 S6783 1993]
RA645.C34S67   1993
362.1'961--dc20
DNLM/DLC
for Library of Congress   93-20980
                                                               CIP

ISBN 0-306-43982-4

© 1994 Plenum Press, New York
A Division of Plenum Publishing Corporation
233 Spring Street, New York, N.Y. 10013

Printed in the United States of America

To our parents,
Lottie and Verl Shumaker
and
Agnes and Joseph Czajkowski,
who taught us the value of social support

Contributors

Terrence L. Amick, Donahue Institute for Governmental Services, University of Massachusetts, Amherst, Massachusetts 01003

Toni C. Antonucci, Institute for Social Research, University of Michigan, Ann Arbor, Michigan 48106

Sheldon Cohen, Department of Psychology, Carnegie-Mellon University, Pittsburgh, Pennsylvania 15213

Susan M. Czajkowski, Behavioral Medicine Branch, National Heart, Lung, and Blood Institute, National Institutes of Health, Bethesda, Maryland 20892

Dennis M. Davidson, University of California, San Francisco, School of Medicine, Cardiology Division, San Francisco General Hospital, San Francisco, California 94110

Kathleen Dracup, School of Nursing, University of California, Los Angeles, Los Angeles, California 90024

William W. Dressler, Department of Behavioral and Community Medicine, University of Alabama School of Medicine, Tuscaloosa, Alabama 35487

Christine Dunkel-Schetter, Department of Psychology, University of California, Los Angeles, Los Angeles, California 90024-1563

Kathleen Ell, School of Social Work, Hamovitch Social Research Center, University of Southern California, Los Angeles, California 90089-0411

Michael J. Follick, Institute for Behavioral Medicine, Cranston, Rhode Island 02920

Larry Gorkin, Institute for Behavioral Medicine, Cranston, Rhode Island 02920

Ellen M. Hall, Division of Behavioral Sciences and Health Education, Department of Health Policy and Management, Johns Hopkins School of Hygiene and Public Health, Baltimore, Maryland 21205

Helen P. Hazuda, Division of Clinical Epidemiology, Department of Medicine, University of Texas Health Science Center, San Antonio, Texas 78284-7873

Ernest H. Johnson, Department of Family Medicine, Morehouse School of Medicine, Atlanta, Georgia 30310-1495

Jeffrey V. Johnson, Division of Behavioral Sciences and Health Education, Department of Health Policy and Management, Johns Hopkins School of Hygiene and Public Health, Baltimore, Maryland 21205

Jay R. Kaplan, Bowman Gray School of Medicine, Wake Forest University, Winston-Salem, North Carolina 27157-1040

Robert M. Kaplan, Division of Health Care Sciences, Department of Family and Preventive Medicine, University of California, San Diego, La Jolla, California 92093-0622

Wendy Kliewer, Department of Psychology, Virginia Commonwealth University, Richmond, Virginia 23284

Stephen B. Manuck, Department of Psychology, University of Pittsburgh, Pittsburgh, Pennsylvania 15260

Raymond Niaura, Division of Behavioral Medicine, Miriam Hospital, Providence, Rhode Island 02906

Judith K. Ockene, Division of Preventive and Behavioral Medicine, University of Massachusetts Medical Center, Worcester, Massachusetts 01605

Kristina Orth-Gomér, National Institute for Psychosocial Factors and Health, 171 77 Stockholm, Sweden

Barbara R. Sarason, Department of Psychology, University of Washington, Seattle, Washington 98195

Irwin G. Sarason, Department of Psychology, University of Washington, Seattle, Washington 98195

Sally A. Shumaker, Department of Public Health Sciences, Bowman Gray School of Medicine, Wake Forest University, Winston-Salem, North Carolina 27103

Carol K. Whalen, Department of Psychology and Social Behavior, School of Social Ecology, University of California, Irvine, Irvine, California 92717

Dianne L. Wilkin, Institute for Behavioral Medicine, Cranston, Rhode Island 02920

Preface

The hypothesis that health can be affected by supportive interactions with individuals within one's social network has now been confirmed by a wealth of evidence that implicates the social environment in health status generally and in cardiovascular disease (CVD) risk specifically. The evidence includes an extensive epidemiological literature on the relationship between various measures of social support and morbidity, as well as all-cause and disease-specific mortality. This book represents an effort to examine comprehensively the existing research and theory in the area of social support and CVD and suggest priorities for future research. It is an outgrowth of the discussions and recommendations that took place at a working conference cosponsored by the National Heart, Lung, and Blood Institute and the University of California at Irvine, where a multidisciplinary group of researchers convened for several days to review critically the available evidence linking social support to CVD etiology, occurrence, and rehabilitation. Following a brief overview of some of the key concepts discussed in this book, we present some important issues to consider when examining the relationship of social support to disease, and we conclude with a synopsis of the individual chapters and considerations for future research in this area.

The term *social support* has been used to describe both the structure of a person's social environment and the resources (or functions) such environments provide. Structure includes the size, density, complexity, symmetry, and stability of an individual's family, friends, coworkers, and health professionals and community resources; it is usually referred to as one's "social network." The functional component of social support is defined as an individual's perception of the availability of support and of the resources provided, and it is labeled "social support"; however, the term *social support* is often used to describe both the structural and functional aspects of the social environment (e.g., the resources provided in a supportive exchange among network members; see Shumaker & Brownell, 1984).

In order to understand the role support plays in CVD, it is important to distinguish between various structures and functions of the social environment and to specify how each structure or function might increase or decrease the risk of CVD. A variety of measures have been used to assess social support from both a structural and functional perspective. Structural measures include items such as marital status, number and frequency of contacts with family and close friends, church membership, and involvement in community and other groups. Functional measures most often involve the perceived availability and quality of support. An example of a structural approach to the measurement of social support is the Social Activities Questionnaire (Donald & Ware, 1982), which contains 11 self-administered items that assess the number of supportive contacts available to and actually used by an individual. An example of a functional support measure, the Inventory of Socially Supportive Behaviors (Barrera, Sandler, & Ramsey, 1981) is a 40-item self-administered scale that focuses on the number and type of helping transactions received by an individual within a specific period of time. Another example of a functional measure of support is the Social Support Questionnaire (Sarason, Levine, Basham, & Sarason, 1983). This measure assesses both the perceived availability of and satisfaction with a number of functional aspects of support (e.g., informational support, tangible aid).

Several issues should be taken into account when developing models of the social support–CVD relationship. In terms of measurement, the viability of a given model depends on the measure used to assess social support; for example, a model suggesting that social support influences behavioral risk should use a definition of support that taps its social influence potential (e.g., social integration). A model proposing that support protects persons from the pathogenic influences of stress must operationalize support so as to reflect the availability of resources that aid in stress evaluation and coping (e.g., perceived availability of stress-reducing resources). The emphasis is on measures that are logically linked to proposed pathogenic processes.

Support–disease models can be classified in terms of whether the relationship between social support and disease represents a main effect or a stress-buffering effect. Main effect models suggest that support directly influences the pathogenic process irrespective of the level of stress a person is experiencing. In contrast, buffering models suggest that support affects health by decreasing the risks created by psychosocial stressors; thus it is effective only when a person is stressed (see Cohen & Wills, 1985). The definition and measure of support used influences the appropriateness of a main effect versus stress-buffering model. For example, there is evidence from the literature on psychological disorders that main effects are associated with a structural measure or the number of different roles a person has (social integration) and that buffering effects occur only when perceived availability of stress-buffering resources are assessed (Cohen & Wills, 1985; Kessler & McLeod, 1985).

The stability of the support characteristic under consideration is also an important issue in developing models of the relationship between support and CVD. Because atherosclerosis is a disease that develops over a long period of time, conceptions of social support that are stable over such periods make more sense in this context than conceptions that vary considerably over time. Also, the mechanisms proposed in models of support and CVD may be more or less important depending on the stage in the pathogenesis of the disease. For example, support-induced increases in neuroendocrine response may be more important for persons with severe atherosclerosis than for persons with minimal occlusion.

Finally, some of the proposed models allow for relationships between support and disease outcomes other than CVD. For example, a model may propose that support results in decreases (or, under some conditions, increases) in behaviors that put individuals at risk for CVD (e.g., smoking, poor diet, poor exercise habits). Because these behaviors are also risk factors for diseases other than CVD (e.g., cancer), such a model would be somewhat nonspecific in that regard. Similarly, models proposing that the neuroendocrine changes that may result from social support lead to the development of CVD also lack specificity, because these neuroendocrine changes may also suppress immune function and result in increased risk of infectious diseases and cancer.

Each of these issues is discussed in detail in this volume. The chapters in the first section address key concepts in social support and CVD; these chapters provide a basis for further discussion of the relationship between social support and CVD. In Chapter 1, Davidson presents a brief introduction to CVD, discussing the epidemiology, etiology, primary prevention, treatment, and prognosis for various cardiovascular disorders. Next, focusing on conceptual and methodological issues with regard to social support itself, Antonucci and Johnson overview concepts and methods used in social support research, and Sarason and Sarason provide a critical review of specific measures of support. Finally, Kaplan focuses on conceptual and operational aspects of health outcomes, another element in social support research. His chapter provides an overview of health status measures used in this area, as well as an elaboration of the decision theory approach to health status assessment.

Chapters in the second section focus on the empirical evidence for a relationship between social support and CVD. Orth-Gomér reviews the international epidemiological evidence for an association between social support and CVD, whereas Hazuda provides a critical evaluation of studies conducted in the United States.

In the following section, two chapters consider the individual, environmental, and cultural aspects of the relationship between social support and CVD. Johnson and Hall discuss the relationship of workplace social support to CVD and Dressler presents a cross-cultural perspective on the support–CVD relationship.

The last two sections address the role of social support in CVD etiology, progression, treatment, and recovery. Cohen, Kaplan, and Manuck describe models of the social support–CVD process and discuss potential psychological and biological underlying mechanisms. Whalen and Kliewer then present a developmental perspective, discussing social influences during childhood and adolescence that affect CVD risk. Finally, using Prochaska's stages-of-change model, Amick and Ockene consider the role of social support in modifying risk factors for CVD. In the final section, Gorkin, Follick, Wilkin, and Niaura review the evidence on the role of social support in CVD progression and treatment; Ell and Dunkel-Schetter present a review of research regarding social support during recovery from CVD; and Dracup discusses the relationship of social support to recovery and compliance within the context of formal CVD rehabilitation programs.

Thus this volume provides perspectives from the psychological, sociological, and medical communities in a critical review of the evidence linking social support to CVD. In addition to reviewing the relevant empirical and theoretical research, the chapters underscore a number of gaps in the literature and provide insights for the future direction of research in this area. Several key points are summarized below:

- Researchers need to identify the relative importance of different dimensions of social support (e.g., structural versus functional aspects of support) in the etiology of CVD, in CVD risk factors, and during the crisis and rehabilitative phases of CVD.
- The mechanisms through which social support affects the development of, occurrence of, and recovery from CVD should be examined.
- Research is severely limited on the influence of social support in the development of risk factors for CVD during childhood and adolescence.
- The influence of individual-difference variables (e.g., personality characteristics, hostility, coronary-prone behavior, social class), and environmental factors (e.g., control within work setting, economic

context) on the social support–CVD relationship warrants further exploration.

- The differential impact of social support on CVD at critical stages or transitions in life (e.g., marriage, death of spouse) need to be assessed.
- Research is needed that addresses the effects of stress on the social support–CVD relationship, especially in the development of risk factors.
- The process through which information concerning health is exchanged among support network members should be examined (e.g., sources of information exchanged, accuracy of information, effects of attitudinal similarity on health issues among network members, response of members to behavior change attempts, how resistance is encountered).
- The factors affecting the activation of social support in a crisis situation and the maintenance of this support over time need to be identified.
- Research is needed to explore the effects of social support on help-seeking behavior, decision making regarding treatment, immediate adjustment to a cardiovascular event, the adoption of and adherence to behaviors designed to reduce risk, and in maximizing recovery and rehabilitation of individuals experiencing a major cardiac event.
- The effects of the CVD process on social support and social networks should be considered.
- Researchers should focus on the ways interventions using social support can be designed to influence the impact of the CVD process on the individual and family members.

Researchers are just beginning to examine the role of social support systems in CVD etiology, incidence, and recovery. The empirical evidence reviewed in the volume—along with several untested but promising theoretical leads—suggest that social networks and social support may play a critical role in CVD. Only through future research, however, will we be able to understand what characteristics of the social environment are involved, how they influence the disease process, and under what conditions these effects occur.

References

Barrera, M. J., Sandler, I. N., & Ramsey, T. B. (1981). Preliminary development of a scale of social support: Studies of college students. *American Journal of Community Psychology, 9,* 435–447.

Cohen, S., & Wills, T. A. (1985). Stress, social support, and the buffering hypothesis. *Psychological Bulletin, 98,* 310–357.

Donald, C. A., & Ware, J. E., Jr. (1982). *The quantification of social contacts and resources.* Santa Monica, CA: RAND Corporation.

Kessler, R. C., & McLeod, J. D. (1985). Social support and mental health in community samples. In S. Cohen & S. L. Syme (Eds.), *Social support and health.* New York: Academic Press.

Sarason, I. G., Levine, H. M., Basham, R. B., & Sarason, B. R. (1983). Assessing social support: The Social Support Questionnaire. *Journal of Personality and Social Psychology, 44,* 127–139.

Shumaker, S. A., & Brownell, A. (1984). Toward a theory of social support: Closing conceptual gaps. *Journal of Social Issues, 40,* 11–36.

Contents

4. Measures of Health Outcome in Social Support Research ... 65

Robert M. Kaplan

II. ESTABLISHING A RELATIONSHIP BETWEEN SOCIAL SUPPORT AND CARDIOVASCULAR DISEASE

5. International Epidemiological Evidence for a Relationship between Social Support and Cardiovascular Disease 97

Kristina Orth-Gomér

6. A Critical Evaluation of U.S. Epidemiological Evidence and Ethnic Variation 119

Helen P. Hazuda

III. INDIVIDUAL, ENVIRONMENTAL, AND CULTURAL FACTORS IN SOCIAL SUPPORT AND CARDIOVASCULAR DISEASE

IV. THE DEVELOPMENT OF CARDIOVASCULAR DISEASE

V. THE CRISIS AND REHABILITATION
PHASES OF CARDIOVASCULAR DISEASE

13. **Social Support and Adjustment to Myocardial Infarction, Angioplasty, and Coronary Artery Bypass Surgery** 301

Kathleen Ell and Christine Dunkel-Schetter

14. **Cardiac Rehabilitation: The Role of Social Support in Recovery and Compliance** 333

Kathleen Dracup

PART I

Key Concepts

CHAPTER 1

An Introduction to Cardiovascular Disease

Dennis M. Davidson

The term *cardiovascular disease* refers to any disorder of the heart and blood vessels, including hypertension, coronary artery disease (CAD), cardiac dysrhythmias, cerebrovascular disease, valvular heart disease, cardiomyopathies, peripheral vascular disease, and congenital cardiac abnormalities. Each disorder has been characterized epidemiologically; incidence and prevalence rates vary widely by country and culture. Because hypertension, coronary artery disease, cardiac dysrhythmias, and cerebrovascular disease account for the majority of cardiovascular morbidity and mortality in developed countries, those topics are the focus of this chapter. For each of the disease categories, the epidemiology, etiology, risk indicators and primary prevention, diagnostic assessment, and treatment and prognosis are discussed.

Hypertension

Epidemiology

High blood pressure is the most common cardiovascular disease, with a prevalence exceeding 20% in most areas of Canada and the United States (Davidson, 1991). Hypertension is commonly defined as having a systolic

DENNIS M. DAVIDSON • University of California, San Francisco, School of Medicine, Cardiology Division, San Francisco General Hospital, San Francisco, California 94110.

Social Support and Cardiovascular Disease, edited by Sally A. Shumaker and Susan M. Czajkowski. Plenum Press, New York, 1994.

blood pressure (SBP) of 140 mm Hg or greater, a diastolic blood pressure (DBP) of 90 mm Hg or greater, or as taking antihypertensive medications. Prevalence rates are nearly equal in men and women, increase with age, and are higher in African Americans than in whites. The risk of coronary artery disease (CAD) and stroke increases directly with increasing levels of both SBP and DBP (Joint National Committee, 1993; Stamler, Stamler, & Neaton, 1993).

The Framingham Offspring Study prospectively determined the 8-year incidence of hypertension in 4,294 young women and men who were free of the disorder at baseline examination. Adiposity was the major contributor to changes in SBP and DBP in both genders during the follow-up period. Alcohol consumption was also a significant predictor of blood pressure elevation in women (Garrison, Kannel, Stokes, & Castelli, 1987).

Etiology

Fewer than 10% of cases of high blood pressure have surgically remediable causes; these include coarctation of the aorta, Cushing's syndrome, and pheochromocytoma, as well as structural abnormalities of the kidney or stenosis of the renal artery, which can alter renin-angiotensin-aldersterone relationships. Where an underlying etiology cannot be determined, the term *essential* (or *primary*) hypertension is applied, and the primary goal becomes control instead of cure.

Risk Indicators and Primary Prevention

In addition to obesity and heavy ethanol consumption, physiological indicators of risk for development of primary hypertension include aging, sodium intake and excretion imbalances, and a family history of hypertension. Ethnic and cultural differences in hypertension prevalence are attributable in part to differences in the above factors (Franco et al., 1985; Gorkin, 1987).

Approximately two thirds of all persons over the age of 65 have a SBP of 140 mm Hg or greater or a DBP of 90 mm Hg or greater (Joint National Committee, 1993). Elevations in SBP may be attributable in part to decreased compliance of the arterial walls, raising arterial resistance. The phenomenon of systolic hypertension in the elderly has been the subject of several long-term studies. When elevated DBP appears for the first time in this age group, a search for secondary causes is appropriate (Applegate, 1989).

The balance between sodium intake and excretion affects both normotensive and hypertensive individuals. In normals, decreases in total peripheral resistance counteract increases in sodium-induced rises in plasma volume, maintaining arterial pressure. Approximately half of all persons with hypertension respond to increased salt intake with rises in blood pressure. Such changes may relate to the renin-angiotensin-aldosterone and the sympathetic nervous systems (Schmieder, Messerli, Garavaglia, & Nunez, 1988).

Diagnostic Assessment

Blood pressure determinations in the same individual can vary widely with differences in environment and measurement technique. Optimally, at least two readings are taken from the individual in a resting state, using an appropriately sized cuff. If the mean value is elevated, readings should be taken in both arms and repeated at subsequent visits. Where significant lability in blood pressure readings are noted, ambulatory recordings for 24 or more hours may be indicated.

The medical history should be used to probe for factors contributing to hypertension, such as socioeconomic circumstances, emotional distress, and food preferences. A complete physical examination and laboratory tests may indicate a secondary cause for the elevated blood pressure.

Treatment and Prognosis

Nonpharmacological therapy is indicated in all hypertension patients. Modest long-term reductions of blood pressure have been documented with behavioral approaches, such as biofeedback and relaxation techniques, exercise, and smoking abstention. Dietary modifications (e.g., reduced intake of sodium, dietary fats, alcohol, and calories) can effectively lower blood pressure (Joint National Committee, 1993). If such efforts do not result in meeting blood pressure goals after a reasonable period of time, they should be continued in conjunction with pharmacological treatment. Figure 1 illustrates the current therapeutic approach.

Blood pressure reduction has resulted in a decrease in stroke mortality of 30% to 50%, as well as reductions in all-cause mortality, congestive heart failure, and progression to more severe hypertension. In treated persons with initial DBP greater than 104 mm Hg, coronary artery disease morbidity and mortality is also reduced (Davidson, 1991). Several studies of mild hypertension, however, have failed to show significant decreases in CAD morbidity and mortality. This may have resulted from a failure to reduce concurrently other CAD risk indicators either through potentially adverse effects (e.g., lipid elevations and serum potassium alterations with diuretic therapy) or through an exclusive focus of study design on

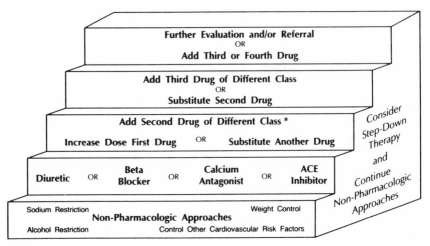

Figure 1. Individualized, step-care therapy for hypertension. ACE = angiotensin-converting enzyme. * = drugs such as diuretics, beta-adrenergic blockers, calcium channel antagonists, ACE inhibitors, alpha-adrenergic blockers, centrally acting alpha$_2$-adrenergic agonists, reserpine, and vasodilators. Source: From the Joint National Committee on Detection, Evaluation, and Treatment of High Blood Pressure (1988). The 1988 report of the Joint National Committee on Detection, Evaluation, and Treatment of High Blood Pressure. *Archives of Internal Medicine, 148,* 1023–1038. Reprinted by permission.

hypertension. Recognition of these factors and the availability of anti-hypertensive medications without adverse effects on lipids and electrolytes should result in clarification of these issues. When blood pressure and serum cholesterol have both been lowered, CAD mortality has been reduced (Samuelsson, Wilhelmsen, Andersson, Pennert, & Berglund, 1987).

Coronary Artery Disease (CAD)

Epidemiology

Since World War II, cardiovascular epidemiologists in many countries have cooperated to determine the incidence of CAD and stroke. Figure 2 illustrates the wide differences among countries and cultures; the excess risk of men is also evident (Davidson, 1991).

During the first two thirds of this century, CAD mortality rates rose in North America, but since the mid-1960s there has been a steady decline shared by most ethnic groups (Davidson, 1991). Several other economically

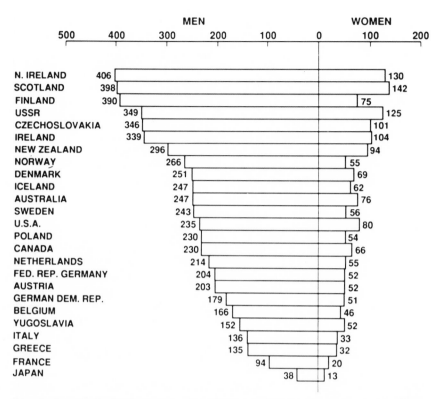

Figure 2. Age-standardized coronary artery disease mortality in men and women residents of selected countries in 1985. Source: D. M. Davidson (1991). *Preventive cardiology.* Baltimore: Williams & Wilkins. Reprinted by permission.

developed countries have exhibited similar reductions in CAD rates (Uemura & Pisa, 1988). In the United States, myocardial infarction is still the leading cause of death, claiming more than half a million lives annually (American Heart Association, 1992).

Etiology

To ensure the heart's survival and to maintain optimal function, the blood supplied through the coronary artery system must be adequate to meet the demands of the heart for oxygen. These demands have several determinants: heart rate, blood pressure, heart size, and the vigor of contraction (contractility). More oxygen is required when the heart is beating faster, is contracting more vigorously, or is developing more pressure in the left ventricle, or when the left ventricle is dilated; exercise, for example, results in increases in the first three factors. To meet the increased demand, nondiseased coronary arteries dilate to provide a greater cross-sectional area for blood flow. This dilation results from neural and hormonal signals to the richly innervated muscular layers of the arterial walls. Disease can limit this natural process in three major ways: atherosclerosis, thrombosis, and spasm.

Atherosclerosis encroaches on the cross-sectional area of the coronary artery lumen and can mechanically limit the mobility of arterial walls. If this process continues throughout one's lifetime, a point may ultimately be reached at which a sufficient flow cannot be generated through the obstructed coronary artery to meet the demands of the heart during exercise. When this supply-and-demand disparity occurs, the myocardial tissue contracts less well and the electrical conduction system embedded therein (which also needs oxygen) becomes less stable, leading to cardiac rhythm or conduction disorders. In some persons, pressurelike chest discomfort (termed *angina pectoris*) may occur. If oxygen demands are immediately lowered (e.g., by cessation of exercise), balance is restored, chest discomfort subsides, and the muscle and electrical tissue recover without permanent damage. If the disparity continues for several hours, permanent tissue damage is nearly certain, leading to myocardial infarction (MI).

Two other processes can affect the supply-demand balance, both acutely reducing supply. *Thrombosis*, or blood clotting, may occur at the site of atherosclerotic coronary artery narrowing. A clot ("thrombus") may be dislodged from the left atrium or left ventricle to enter and obstruct one of the coronary arteries. If the clot is not dissolved naturally or by drug treatment within a few hours, an MI will occur. The same outcome can result from a segment of a coronary artery going into *spasm* as a result of neural, hormonal, or local stimulation of the affected artery segment.

These three processes—atherosclerosis, thrombosis, and spasm—may interact. One such scenario involves an artery with 90% obstruction of its cross-sectional area from atherosclerosis. This disorder makes that segment of the artery more susceptible to spasm. If this occurs, and flow abruptly stops, a clot can form. Although the spasm may then subside, the clot may persist in blocking flow, eventually resulting in infarction.

Whereas the atherosclerotic process typically develops over many years, spasm and clot can be instantaneous. Because their etiologies are different, a multifaceted approach to prevention of MI is necessary when an individual is determined to be at high risk (Davidson, 1991).

Risk Indicators and Primary Prevention

Atherosclerosis has been clearly linked to several risk factors, including cigarette smoking, high blood pressure, high blood total cholesterol, low blood high-density lipoprotein (HDL) cholesterol, diabetes mellitus, male gender, and a family history of parental or sibling CAD at an early age. One's risk doubles with any of the following: 20 or more cigarettes per day, blood pressure of 170/100 or greater, a low-density lipoprotein (LDL) cholesterol of 170 mg/dl or greater, an HDL cholesterol below 35 mg/dl, diabetes mellitus, and a parent who had an MI before the age of 50 (Austin, King, Bawol, Hulley, & Friedman, 1987; Colditz et al., 1986; Stamler & Shekelle, 1988; Wingard & Barrett-Connor, 1987). If more than one risk indicator is present, the relative risks from each are multiplicative, not just additive. For example, a hypertensive diabetic smoker has an eightfold risk compared to a person of the same age and gender without those risks. Physical inactivity and obesity are also independently associated with CAD risk, but the relative CAD risk associated with these two conditions is usually less than two (Hubert, Feinleib, McNamara, & Castelli, 1983; Paffenbarger, Wing, & Hyde, 1978).

Oral contraceptive use concurrent with cigarette smoking can increase the risk of an MI more than twentyfold, whereas replacement estrogen therapy following menopause can lower MI risk (Baird, Tyroler, Heiss, Chambless, & Hames, 1985; Stadel, 1981; Wallace, Heiss, Burrows, & Graves, 1987). In addition, several social, psychological, and behavioral factors may contribute directly to the genesis and progression of atherosclerosis, whereas others are relevant to minimizing risk through alteration of the biological risk indicators mentioned above (Dimsdale, 1988; Manuck, Kaplan, & Matthews, 1986; Matthews & Haynes, 1986). These factors are considered more extensively in subsequent chapters.

The probability of thrombosis in a coronary artery is enhanced under any of several conditions: when flow is slowed, when the arterial wall is injured or in the process of repair, or when one or more alterations occurs in a cascade of clotting factors. The latter factor is subject to variation with time and can be influenced by cigarette smoking, alcohol, and a variety of medications (Imeson, Meade, & Stewart, 1987). Coronary artery spasm is more likely to occur under conditions of physiological or psychological stress, probably as a result of hormonal, sympathetic, and parasympathetic effects on the arterial wall musculature. Nitrates and calcium-channel blocking agents are effective in the prevention of coronary artery spasm (Winniford et al., 1987).

Changes in individual risk factors have been impressive in developed countries, notably in regard to the detection, treatment, and control of hypertension in the past two decades and similar efforts in hyper-cholesterolemia more recently (National Cholesterol Education Program Expert Panel, 1988). Although it remains the leading cause of death in North America, CAD has decreased in many regions since 1968 (Davis et al., 1985), in considerable measure because of changes in public awareness of CAD risk (Schucker et al., 1987).

Diagnostic Assessment

Many CAD patients will develop chest tightness (angina pectoris) when the heart's demand for coronary artery oxygen exceeds its rate of supply. The pain signals the individual to reduce physical activity level; heart rate and blood pressure then drop, balance is restored, and the pain recedes. Those individuals without this warning sign may be diagnosed from the electrocardiographic response to exercise testing on treadmill or bicycle. Changes in the ST segment of the exercise electrocardiogram (ECG) correlate well with a high probability of obstructive CAD. If femoral atherosclerosis is severe, however, lower extremity ischemia may restrict the patient's exercise duration and limit diagnostic inference from the test.

Better correlations are obtained with either of two radionuclide tests. The thallium exercise test involves injection of radioactive thallium at peak exercise. Imaging of the heart indicates areas of reduced blood perfusion, which can be compared with normal patterns at rest. With the technicium radionuclide ventriculogram, the radioisotope is added to the patient's red blood cells and reinjected intravenously. The blood pool then contains the diluted radioisotope tracer, and imaging can follow the blood flow through the heart. These indirect methods of assessing adequacy of coronary blood flow are often sufficient to guide management at this stage in CAD progression.

If hygienic and pharmacological means are inadequate to control the symptoms and signs of CAD, cardiac catheterization and coronary angio-gram procedures are done to determine directly the extent of coronary obstruction. Where high-grade arterial stenoses are present, balloon dila-tion (angioplasty) or coronary artery bypass surgery (CABS) may be indicated.

It should be noted that persons undergoing coronary angiography do not represent a random sample of the general population. Recently, several studies have attempted to correlate personality characteristics with the degree of coronary atherosclerosis on angiogram. Because the decision to undertake angiography depends primarily on chest pain, modified by the individual's level of pain tolerance and willingness to report this symptom to the physician, it appears that a variety of factors other than personality type may account for differences noted (Fried & Pearson, 1987; Pickering, 1985).

Treatment and Prognosis

In noncritical situations, changes in health behaviors are the first step in treatment. These include developing physical (aerobic) fitness, which lowers heart rate and blood pressure (and thus oxygen demand); modifying nutritional intake (which can lower blood pressure, blood cholesterol, and body weight); and smoking abstention.

Pharmacological therapy employs three main categories of agents: nitrates, beta-adrenergic blocking agents, and calcium-channel blocking agents. Nitrates improve oxygen supply through dilation of coronary arteries and prevention of spasm; they reduce demand by lowering arterial pressure. Beta-adrenergic blocking agents work exclusively on the demand side by lowering heart rate, blood pressure, and cardiac contractility. Calcium-channel blockers improve supply by preventing spasm and by dilating coronary arteries, while lowering demand through reductions in blood pressure. The success of these agents can be monitored by frequency of angina pectoris (when present) or through prolonged exercise time before the appearance of ischemic signs. Anticoagulants and agents that minimize platelet aggregation can be employed in a prophylactic mode to minimize the risks of thrombosis, particularly following bypass surgery and coronary angioplasty.

Following an MI or bypass surgery, there are four distinct phases in the recovery of the cardiac patient (Davidson, 1983). In an uncomplicated MI or CABS, the *hospital phase* typically lasts from 5 to 7 days. Most hospitals use a multistep plan that integrates electronic monitoring, gradual ambulation, and exercise with education and consultation in nutrition, stress reduction, and occupational planning. Patients progress from the coronary care unit (CCU) to a cardiac surveillance unit during their transition to hospital discharge. An *early home phase* follows discharge and is reported by patients and their families to be the most stressful time in their recovery.

A third phase (if available and elected) is *outpatient cardiac rehabilitation* participation. This typically begins 4 to 10 weeks after hospital discharge and lasts between 10 and 12 weeks. Three times weekly, patients exercise for 20 to 40 minutes under the supervision of CCU-trained nurses. Participation in such programs is often accompanied by psychosocial improvement, particularly reduction of depression (Dracup, Moser, Marsden, Taylor, & Guzy, 1991). The *maintenance phase* follows, encompassing the remainder of the patient's life. Continued cigarette smoking after MI represents the biggest modifiable risk; mortality is halved with abstention. Smoking cessation can also delay the onset of recurrent angina after an MI (Daly, Graham, Hickey, & Mulcahy, 1985) and retard progressive vessel occlusion in patients after bypass surgery (Hermanson et al., 1988) and coronary angioplasty (Blackshear, O'Callaghan, & Califf, 1987), as well as in individuals with angiographically documented CAD who did not have bypass surgery (Hermanson et al., 1988).

Cardiac Dysrhythmias and Sudden Death

Epidemiology

In economically developed countries, sudden cardiac death (SCD) accounts for approximately 15% of fatalities; of all cardiovascular deaths, two thirds are sudden. SCD usually occurs in the present of significant CAD, but it may occur in those whose only indication of risk is the presence of ventricular dysrhythmias (Lown, 1987).

Etiology

Timing of contraction of the cardiac chambers is furnished by the electrical system of the heart. Cells in the heart's natural pacemaker, the sinoatrial (S-A) node, spontaneously depolarize approximately 60 to 70 times per minute in a person at rest. A wave of depolarization spreads through the two atria nearly simultaneously, causing right and left atrial contraction. The electrical impulse converges on the atrioventricular (A-V) node, where it pauses briefly while blood flows from the atria into the ventricles. The depolarization impulse then travels through a specialized conduction system that causes the right and left ventricles to contract in a pattern that optimizes ejection of blood into the pulmonary artery and aorta, respectively. In the event of S-A node failure, the A-V node will spontaneously depolarize at approximately 45 to 50 times per minute. If the A-V node fails, certain cells in the ventricles may spontaneously depolarize at approximately 35 to 40 times per minute. If no cells spontaneously depolarize, cardiac arrest occurs.

Spontaneous depolarization of isolated ventricular cells in the presence of normal S-A and A-V nodal function results in a ventricular premature contraction (VPC). Three or more consecutive VPCs are defined as ventricular tachycardia. Ventricular tachycardia or VPCs arising from more than one focus increase the risk of electrical instability in the heart. Either condition can lead to ventricular fibrillation, which provides no effective ejection of blood, leading to cardiac arrest.

Risk Indicators and Primary Prevention

Ventricular fibrillation may be triggered by behavioral and neural factors, as documented in animal studies. Differing psychological stressors may alter the electrical threshold at which ventricular fibrillation can be induced, particularly those that involve recall of emotionally charged experiences. This may explain such diverse phenomena as voodoo death, the increased rates of sudden death in the Hmong tribespeople who migrated from Laos to North America, and an excessive proportion of SCDs on Mondays. Ventricular dysrhythmias are also related to neural and humoral inputs to the heart and are often modified during exercise or sleep (Lown, 1987).

Diagnostic Assessment

Ambulatory ECG monitoring for 24 hours has become standard for assessment of ventricular dysrhythmias. Such monitoring has confirmed that the rhythm immediately preceding cardiac arrest is usually ventricular fibrillation. Computer programs use waveform recognition algorithms to categorize ventricular complexes and, subject to human confirmation, diagnose rhythm disorders.

Survivors of ventricular fibrillation and cardiac arrest frequently undergo electrophysiological studies in the cardiac catheterization suite, during which ventricular dysrhythmias are deliberately introduced and terminated. Intravenous medications are introduced, followed by repeat induction of the dysrhythmias, allowing testing of the effectiveness of various pharmacological preparations (Wilber et al., 1988).

Treatment and Prognosis

After a first cardiac arrest, the recurrence rate may be as high as 30% during the first year (Myerburg et al., 1984). Coupling a wide variety of drugs with electrophysiological ventricular fibrillation induction studies, the risk of SCD has been reduced to between 5% and 10% per year (Lampert, Lown, Graboys, Podrid, & Blatt, 1988). The automatic implantable cardiac defibrillator has reduced the risk of SCD even further (Weaver, Hill, & Fahrenbruch, 1988).

Cerebrovascular Disease

Epidemiology

The incidence of stroke in the United States exceeds 400,000 annually and is negatively related to socioeconomic status (Wing et al., 1988). Rates are similar or greater in other economically developed countries (Aho et al., 1980; American Heart Association, 1992).

Within the past ten years, mortality from stroke has been halved in Japan (Uemura, 1988); in the United States, rates have decreased by one third in the last 20 years (Wing et al., 1988). Although survival following stroke has improved (Garraway, Whisnant, & Drury, 1983), stroke incidence has decreased even more dramatically (Wolf, 1986). These gains may be attributed in part to enhanced detection and treatment of hypertension and hypercholesterolemia and through reductions in smoking (Klag, Whelton, & Seidler, 1989).

Etiology

An acute stroke may result from (a) obstruction of the cerebral arterial system by atherosclerosis, thrombus, or embolus, with consequent diminished blood flow to cerebral tissues, or (b) spontaneous rupture of cerebral arteries with consequent hemorrhage into, and compression of, cerebral tissues. A brief period of insufficient blood flow to cerebral tissue is termed a transient ischemic attack (TIA). If the lack of flow persists, or if hemorrhage occurs, cerebral tissue dies, resulting in loss of peripheral function controlled by the affected area of the brain.

The survival rate in hemorrhagic stroke patients in the United States is approximately 30% at 6 months, whereas approximately 60% of individuals experiencing thrombotic or embolic strokes are alive 6 months thereafter. Five-year figures are approximately 20% and 30%, respectively (Baum & Robins, 1981).

Risk Indicators and Primary Prevention

Risk factors for thrombotic cerebrovascular disease are similar to those for coronary artery disease, including age, gender, smoking, SBP, diabetes, and blood cholesterol (Kaste & Koivisto, 1988). Embolic stroke is more frequent in the presence of atrial fibrillation (Dyken et al., 1987).

The major modifiable risk factors for hemorrhagic cerebrovascular disease are hypertension and coagulation abnormalities, including those induced by alcohol (Weisberg, 1988). In the Systolic Hypertension in the

Elderly Program (SHEP) trial, active treatment of blood pressure of persons having systolic but not diastolic hypertension reduced the incidence of stroke by 35% (SHEP Cooperative Research Group, 1991). In a study of U.S. physicians who were taking every-other-day doses of either one aspirin tablet or placebo, hemorrhagic strokes were doubled in the aspirin group, although the incidence of fatal and nonfatal MI was sufficiently lower to warrant termination of that component of the trial (Steering Committee, 1989).

Diagnostic Assessment

Discovery of the atherosclerotic process prior to a stroke is facilitated by the accessibility of the carotid arteries to auscultation by stethoscope and to ultrasound Doppler examination. Unfortunately, cerebral vessels can only be examined by angiography.

CAD frequently coexists with atherosclerotic cerebrovascular disease; the leading cause of death in persons with cerebrovascular disease is MI. These observations have led to the recommendation for coronary angiography in individuals with documented extracranial atherosclerosis (Graor & Hetzer, 1988).

Treatment and Prognosis

Atherosclerotic plaques in carotid arteries can be surgically removed by an endarterectomy, and angiographically documented cerebral artery aneurysms can be repaired surgically. Programs for the rehabilitation of stroke patients are usually the province of physiatrists (specialists in physical medicine and rehabilitation). Prognosis after a stroke depends on the residual function of motor, somatic sensory, and visual systems (Reding & Potes, 1988). Reduction of recurrent stroke risk can be facilitated with smoking abstention and careful BP monitoring as well as surgical intervention when feasible.

Conclusion

Epidemiological studies of hypertension, coronary artery disease, cardiac dysrhythmias, sudden cardiac death, and stroke have identified physiological and demographic indicators of risk. In the past decade, considerable advances have been made in the behavioral and pharmacological treatment of persons at risk, substantially improving their prognosis.

A considerable amount of variance in CAD occurrence and recurrence remains to be explained, however, indicating the necessity of further exploration of social and psychological factors. Subsequent chapters examine social support as an important contributor to cardiovascular health and disease.

ACKNOWLEDGMENTS. Supported in part by National Heart, Lung, and Blood Institute Preventive Cardiology Academic Award HL 01243.

References

Aho, K., Harmsen, P., Hatano, S., Marquardsen, J., Smirnov, V. E., & Strasser, T. (1980). Cerebrovascular disease in the community: Results of a WHO collaborative study. *Bulletin of the World Health Organization, 58,* 113–130.

American Heart Association. (1992). *1993 Heart and Stroke Facts.* Dallas, TX: Author.

Applegate, W. B. (1989). Hypertension in elderly patients. *Annals of Internal Medicine, 110,* 901–905.

Austin, M. A., King, M.-C., Bawol, R. D., Hulley, S. B., & Friedman, G. D. (1987). Risk factors for coronary heart disease in adult female twins: Genetic heredility and shared environmental influences. *American Journal of Epidemiology, 125,* 308–318.

Baird, D. D., Tyroler, H. A., Heiss, G., Chambless, L. E., & Hames, C. G. (1985). Menopausal change in serum cholesterol: Black/white differences in Evans County, Georgia. *American Journal of Epidemiology, 122,* 982–993.

Baum, H. M., & Robins, M. (1981). The National Survey of Stroke. Survival and prevalence. *Stroke, 12*(Suppl. 1), I59–I68.

Blackshear, J. L., O'Callaghan, W. G., & Califf, R. M. (1987). Medical approaches to prevention of restenosis after coronary angioplasty. *Journal of the American College of Cardiology, 9,* 834–848.

Colditz, G. A., Stampfer, M. J., Willett, W. C., Rosner, B., Speizer, F. E., & Hennekens, C. H. (1986). A prospective study of parental history of myocardial infarction and coronary heart disease in women. *American Journal of Epidemiology, 123,* 48–58.

Daly, L. E., Graham, I. M., Hickey, N., & Mulcahy, R. (1985). Does stopping smoking delay onset of angina after infarction? *British Medical Journal, 291,* 935–937.

Davidson, D. M. (1983). Recovery after cardiac events. In R. L. Frye (Ed.), *Clinical Medicine, vol. 20* (chap. 6). Philadelphia: J.B. Lippincott.

Davidson, D. M. (1991). *Preventive cardiology.* Baltimore: Williams & Wilkins.

Davis, W. B., Hayes, C. G., Knowles, M., Riggan, W. B., Van Bruggen, J., & Tyroler, H. A. (1985). Geographic variation in declining ischemic heart disease mortality in the United States, 1968–1978, I. Rates and change, whites aged 35–74 years. *American Journal of Epidemiology, 122,* 657–672.

Dimsdale, J. E. (1988). A perspective on type A behavior and coronary disease. *New England Journal of Medicine, 318,* 110–112.

Dracup, K., Moser, D. K., Marsden, C., Taylor, S. E., & Guzy, P. M. (1991). Effects of a multidimensional cardiopulmonary rehabilitation program on psychosocial function. *American Journal of Cardiology, 68,* 31–34.

Dyken, M. L., Wolf, P. A., Barnett, H. J. M., Bergan, J. J., Hass, W. K., Kannel, W. B., Kuller,

L., Kurtzke, J. F., & Sundt, T. M. (1987). Risk factors for stroke: A statement for physicians by the Subcommittee on Risk Factors and Stroke of the Stroke Council. *Stroke, 18,* 9–15.

Franco, L. J., Stern, M. P., Rosenthal, M., Haffner, S. M., Hazuda, H. P., & Comeaux, P. J. (1985). Prevalence, detection and control of hypertension in a biethnic community: The San Antonio Heart Study. *American Journal of Epidemiology, 121,* 684–696.

Fried, L., & Pearson, T. A. (1987). The association of risk factors with arteriographically defined coronary artery disease: What is the appropriate control group? *American Journal of Epidemiology, 125,* 844–853.

Garraway, W. M., Whisnant, J. P., & Drury, I. (1983). The changing pattern of survival following stroke. *Stroke, 14,* 699–703.

Garrison, R. J., Kannel, W. B., Stokes, J., III, & Castelli, W. P. (1987). Incidence and precursors of hypertension in young adults: The Framingham Offspring Study. *Preventive Medicine, 16,* 235–251.

Gorkin, L. (1987). Behavioral medicine research in the etiology of essential hypertension: Bridging the cardiovascular reactivity and renal dysfunction paradigms. *Behavioral Medicine Abstracts, 8,* 159–162.

Graor, R. A., & Hetzer, N. R. (1988). Management of coexistent carotid artery and coronary artery disease. *Current Concepts of Cardiovascular Disease, 23,* 19–23.

Hermanson, B., Omenn, G. S., Kronmal, R. A., Gersh, B. J., & Participants in the Coronary Artery Surgery Study. (1988). Beneficial six-year outcome of smoking cessation in older men and women with coronary artery disease. *New England Journal of Medicine, 319,* 1365–1369.

Hubert, H. B., Feinleib, M., McNamara, P. M., & Castelli, W. P. (1983). Obesity as an independent risk factor for cardiovascular disease: A 26-year followup of participants in the Framingham Heart Study. *Circulation, 67,* 968–977.

Imeson, J. D., Meade, T. W., & Stewart, G. M. (1987). Day-by-day variation in fibrinolytic activity and mortality from ischaemic heart disease. *International Journal of Epidemiology, 16,* 626–627.

Joint National Committee on the Detection, Evaluation, and Treatment of High Blood Pressure (1993). Fifth report of the Joint National Committee on the Detection, Evaluation, and Treatment of High Blood Pressure. *Archives of Internal Medicine, 153,* 154–183.

Kannel, W. B., Skinner, J. J., Schwartz, M. J., & Shurtleff, D. (1970). Intermittent claudication: Incidence in the Framingham Study. *Circulation, 41,* 875–883.

Kaste, M., & Koivisto, P. (1988). Risk of brain infarction in familial hypercholesterolemia. *Stroke, 19,* 1097–1100.

Klag, M. J., Whelton, P. K., & Seidler, A. J. (1989). Decline in U.S. stroke mortality. Demographic trends and antihypertensive treatment. *Stroke, 20,* 14–21.

Lampert, S., Lown, B., Graboys, T. B., Podrid, P. J., & Blatt, C. (1988). Determinants of survival in patients with malignant ventricular arrhythmia associated with coronary artery disease. *American Journal of Cardiology, 61,* 791–797.

Lown, B. (1987). Sudden cardiac death: Biobehavioral perspective. *Circulation, 76*(Suppl. 1), 186–196.

Manuck, S. B., Kaplan, J. R., & Matthews, K. A. (1986). Behavioral antecedents of coronary heart disease and atherosclerosis. *Arteriosclerosis, 6,* 2–14.

Matthews, K. A., & Haynes, S. G. (1986). Type A behavior pattern and coronary disease risk: Update and critical evaluation. *American Journal of Epidemiology, 123,* 923–960.

Myerburg, R. J., Kessler, K. M., Estes, D., Conde, C. A., Luceri, R. M., Zaman, L., Kozlouslis, P. L., & Castellanos, A. (1984). Long term survival after prehospital cardiac arrest: Analysis of outcome during an 8 year study. *Circulation, 70,* 538–546.

National Cholesterol Education Program Expert Panel. (1988). Report of the National Cholesterol Education Program Expert Panel on detection, evaluation, and treatment of high blood cholesterol in adults. *Archives of Internal Medicine, 148*, 36–69.

Paffenbarger, R. S., Wing, A. L., & Hyde, R. T. (1978). Physical activity as an index of heart attack risk in college alumni. *American Journal of Epidemiology, 108*, 161–175.

Pickering, T. G. (1985). Should studies of patients undergoing coronary angiography be used to evaluate the role of behavioral risk factors for coronary heart disease? *Journal of Behavioral Medicine, 85*, 203–213.

Reding, M. J., & Potes, E. (1988). Rehabilitation outcome following initial unilateral hemispheric stroke: Life table analysis approach. *Stroke, 19*, 1354–1358.

Samuelsson, O., Wilhelmsen, L., Andersson, O. K., Pennert, K., & Berglund, G. (1987). Cardiovascular morbidity in relation to change in blood pressure and serum cholesterol levels in treated hypertension. *Journal of the American Medical Association, 258*, 1768–1776.

Schmieder, R. E., Messerli, F. H., Garavaglia, G. E., & Nunez, B. D. (1988). Dietary salt intake: A determinant of cardiac involvement in essential hypertension. *Circulation, 78*, 951–956.

Schucker, B., Bailey, K., Heimbach, J. T., Mattson, M. E., Wittes, J. T., Haines, C. M., Gordon, D. J., Cutler, J. A., Keating, V. S., Goor, R. S., & Rifkind, B. M. (1987). Change in public perspective on cholesterol and heart disease: Results from two national surveys. *Journal of the American Medical Association, 258*, 3527–3531.

SHEP Cooperative Research Group. (1991). Prevention of stroke by antihypertensive drug treatment in older persons with isolated systolic hypertension: Final results of the Systolic Hypertension in the Elderly Program. *Journal of the American Medical Association, 265*, 3255–3264.

Stadel, B. V. (1981). Oral contraceptives and cardiovascular disease. *New England Journal of Medicine, 305*, 612–618, 672–682.

Stamler, J., & Shekelle, R. (1988). Dietary cholesterol and human coronary heart disease. *Archives of Pathology and Laboratory Medicine, 112*, 1032–1040.

Stamler, J., Stamler, R., & Neaton, J. D. (1993). Blood pressure, systolic and diastolic, and cardiovascular risks. US population data. *Archives of Internal Medicine, 153*, 598–615.

Steering Committee of the Physicians' Health Study Research Group. (1989). Final report on the aspirin component of the ongoing Physicians' Health Study. *New England Journal of Medicine, 321*, 129–135.

Uemura, K. (1988). International trends in cardiovascular diseases in the elderly. *European Heart Journal, 9*(Suppl. D), 1–8.

Uemura, K., & Pisa, Z. (1988). Trends in cardiovascular mortality in industrialized countries since 1950. *World Health Statistics Quarterly, 41*, 155–178.

Wallace, R., B., Heiss, G., Burrows, B., & Graves, K. (1987). Contrasting diet and body mass among users and nonusers of oral contraceptives and exogenous estrogens: The Lipid Research Clinics Program Prevalence Study. *American Journal of Epidemiology, 125*, 854–859.

Weaver, W. D., Hill, D., & Fahrenbruch, C. E. (1988). Use of the automatic external defibrillator in the management of out-of-hospital cardiac arrest. *New England Journal of Medicine, 319*, 661–666.

Weisberg, L. A. (1988). Alcoholic intracranial hemorrhage. *Stroke, 29*, 1565–1569.

Wilber, D. J., Garan, H., Finkelstein, D., Kelly, E., Newell, J., McGovern, B., & Ruskin, J. N. (1988). Out-of-hospital cardiac arrest: Use of electrophysiologic testing in the prediction of long-term outcome. *New England Journal of Medicine, 318*, 19–24.

Wing, S., Casper, M., Davis, W. B., Pellum, A., Riggan, W., & Tyroler, H. A. (1988). Stroke mortality maps: United States whites aged 35–74 years, 1962–1982. *Stroke, 19*, 1507–1513.

Wingard, D. L., & Barrett-Connor, E. (1987). Family history of diabetes and cardiovascular disease risk factors and mortality among euglycemic, borderline hyperglycemic, and diabetic adults. *American Journal of Epidemiology, 25*, 948–958.

Winniford, M. D., Jansen, D. E., Reynolds, G. A., Apprill, P., Black, W. H., & Hillis, L. D. (1987). Cigarette smoking-induced coronary vasoconstriction on atherosclerotic coronary artery disease and prevention by calcium antagonists and nitroglycerin. *American Journal of Cardiology, 59*, 203–207.

Wolf, P. A. (1986). Cigarettes, alcohol, and stroke. *New England Journal of Medicine, 315*, 1087–1089.

CHAPTER **2**

Conceptualization and Methods in Social Support Theory and Research as Related to Cardiovascular Disease

Toni C. Antonucci and Ernest H. Johnson

The purpose of this chapter is to consider the conceptual and methodological issues of current importance in the study of social support, especially as they pertain to the study of cardiovascular diseases. A main goal of the chapter is to provide the reader with a broad perspective on the usefulness of social support in the study of psychosocial risk factors for cardiovascular disease. The life-span developmental nature of psychosocial relationships generally, and social support specifically, is emphasized. Although the data are generally suggestive of important links between social support and cardiovascular disease, the limited number of studies militate against drawing firm conclusions about the role of social support as either a predictor of cardiovascular disease onset or a modifier of the severity of such disease. The final goal of this chapter is to present a framework for future studies of the relationship between social support and cardiovascular disease. Ideally, future research should be designed to capitalize on both the life-span nature of psychosocial relationships and the developmental nature of the progression of the various cardiovascular diseases.

TONI C. ANTONUCCI • Institute for Social Research, University of Michigan, Ann Arbor, Michigan 48106.   ERNEST H. JOHNSON • Department of Family Medicine, Morehouse School of Medicine, Atlanta, Georgia 30310-1495.

Social Support and Cardiovascular Disease, edited by Sally A. Shumaker and Susan M. Czajkowski. Plenum Press, New York, 1994.

Concepts and Measures in the Study of Social Support

Social support benefits and suffers from the fact that it has colloquial meaning to both disciplinary scholars and the lay public. As a result, this research has benefitted from skyrocketing attention, but has suffered from a certain lack of definitional specificity. In part, this lack accurately reflects the concept itself, but it also reflects a lack of scholarly precision (Antonucci, 1985; Shumaker & Brownell, 1984).

There are several different approaches to defining the concept of social support. It can be defined by one's feelings about the relationship or the person with whom one has the relationship; by the existence of a relationship; or by the number, type, and nature of interactions one has with significant or supportive others. These definitions range from clinical or qualitative (some might say nebulous or intrapsychic) to more specific and objectifiable (some might say scientific or quantitative) assessments of activities, people, or exchanges. To understand this definitional quagmire, it is useful to review the recent history of the concept, especially with respect to its hypothesized relationship to health and well-being.

Interest in the concept of social support can be traced to two seminal publications by Cassel and Cobb, who emphasized the role of social relationships in establishing host resistance. Cobb (1976), as a physician, and Cassel (1976) as an epidemiologist, highlighted the emotional aspects of relationships and defined social support as providing the supported other with a feeling of belongingness, of being part of a larger group. These early definitions were based on predominantly clinical observations suggesting that people who were socially connected were likely to have a better prognosis with respect to both maintaining health and recovering from illness.

Because this hypothesized relationship was based on clinical observations, epidemiologists next tried to establish this relationship using a more scientific and empirical approach. To do this, they began to apply the concept of social support, broadly defined, to epidemiological data already available. Berkman and Syme (1979), using morbidity and mortality data from Alameda County, California, and constructing their Social Network Index, were able to corroborate these earlier clinical observations. Specifically, Berkman and Syme showed lower levels of mortality and, to some degree, morbidity 9 years later among individuals who had earlier reported themselves to be "better connected." This finding has been replicated in several samples (Blazer, 1982; House, Robbins, & Metzner, 1982; House, Umberson, & Landis, 1988; Orth-Gomér, this volume; Orth-Goér & Johnson, 1987; Schoenbach, Kaplan, Fredman, & Kleinbaum, 1986).

Most of the earlier studies were based on secondary analyses of data; as a result, the support data tended to be of the factual, demographic type. Berkman and Syme (1979) translated their "feeling of belongingness" into variables best described as support network measures or measures of social integration. They included objective assessments of the existence of social ties as indicated, for example, by marital status or the frequency of interactions with friends and relatives. Other measurement advances also attempted to maintain objectivity and did so by assessing such things as number of people in the network (size), gender and age of network members, years network members were known, number of network members who knew each other (density), and number of different roles or different activities related to each network member (multiplexity). These types of assessments have been labeled structural or quantitative measures of support relationships, or social support network assessments. They are nonevaluative assessments of the existence or quantity of relationships (Israel, 1982). With large data sets, this type of measure has shown low but consistent associations with all-cause mortality and morbidity, and specifically with that related to cardiovascular disease. Although there has been a tremendous effort to establish the beneficial effects of social support on health and well-being, relatively little work has focused on how social support *influences* health (Antonucci & Jackson, 1987; House, Landis, & Umberson, 1988).

Researchers suggest that quantitative measures such as those used in epidemiological research do not directly assess the critical characteristics of support relationships, which both Cassel and Cobb proposed influence host resistance or health more generally. For example, these measures do not directly assess the individual's sense of belongingness. By asking individuals to list the number of people with whom they have relationships, it may be possible to obtain an indirect assessment of such feelings. To measure feelings of belongingness directly, and thus to be in keeping with the original presumed causal link between social relationships and health, it is assumed that the *quality* of these relationships, not just their quantity or existence, must be assessed. It may be that the large epidemiological studies have been able to show a relationship between the existence of social relationships and health because such studies include a relatively large subgroup of qualitatively superior social relationships. These relationships then produce or "carry" the low, but consistent, statistical association between quantitative support measures and health.

The early epidemiological population-based studies sought to achieve a degree of scientific objectivity. The modern scientific method requires that any experiment achieve a sufficient degree of objectivity to permit replication. Some have argued that the spirit of Cassel's and Cobb's original observations were lost when these "objective" or "quantitative" assessment techniques were used. Others tried to achieve a respectable amount of objectivity by developing a specific definition of social support while also remaining close to Cassel and Cobb's original sense of the term. Thus, for example, Kahn and Antonucci (1980) proposed that social support could be defined as interpersonal transactions including one or more of the following: affect (expressions of liking, admiration, respect, or love); affirmation (expressions of agreement with or acknowledgement of the appropriateness of some act or statement of another person); and aid (transactions in which direct aid or assistance is given, including things, money, information, advice, time, and/or entitlement). This definition maintains the spirit of the original concept but allows more specificity; although not totally objective, it has demonstrated a respectable degree of test-retest reliability. A more detailed report of the reliability and validity of social support assessment scales has been published by Heitzmann and Kaplan (1988).

Another approach to the objective assessment of support is to assess or count the frequency of certain types of interactions or, more specifically, the kinds of "support" exchanged. The actual entity of support has been labeled *function* in the support literature. Functions have the advantage of at least some degree of objectivity; for example, one can ask if the supportive other lends you money, takes care of you when you are sick, or helps you with chores around the house. This has been called instrumental or tangible aid.

Another type of function that can be assessed, but which must be considered less objective than instrumental support, is affective or emotional support. This has been defined as whether the support person makes you feel loved or cares for you. An assessment of this type of support clearly implies a high level of subjectivity or evaluation of the relationship. In between aid and affect on this objective–subjective continuum is the type of support labeled affirmation, information, or advice. This is not quite as subjective as affective or emotional support but is considerably less objective than tangible aid. A number of social support researchers, particularly psychologists, suggest that the quantitative assessment of neither structural nor functional variables taps the psychological concept of interest to those who wish to understand the processes and mechanisms through which social support has its effects (Antonucci & Jackson, 1987; Berkman, 1985; House, Umberson, & Landis, 1988; Pearlin, 1985).

One additional point should be noted, especially when considering measures of social support: The decision of which measurement technique is the best to measure social support is not a simple one. First, a number of conceptual issues, as outlined above, must be considered. Some "simple" questions include whether the researcher is interested in the subjects' *perception* of support or if they have actually been the *recipient* of certain supportive behaviors (e.g., sick care). This issue might be labeled actual versus potential support. For example, when asking about sick care, one can ask if care was provided when sick or if this person presumably would take care of you if you were sick. Of course the former question is more objective than the latter question because it asks for a report of behavior already exhibited. But if the individual either has not been sick or has not asked for help when sick, it may be necessary to access the perception that support would be provided if requested. A second issue is that different measurement techniques require and allow the use of different types of questions and tools. Social support has been measured through face-to-face interviews, in-depth questionnaires, telephone interviews, direct observations, and third-party informants. Although many may argue that face-to-face interviewing is the technique with the most potential, each of the other measurement techniques has been used with varied success (Jackson & Antonucci, in press).

Social Support and Cardiovascular Disease

A great deal of recent research focuses on the relationship between health/illness/well-being and social support. A central focus of this chapter is to emphasize the integration of the two different concepts, each of which is complex in its own right. The social support literature is advancing at an incredible pace; books, book chapters, and journal articles are accumulating steadily (examples of recent books on this topic include Cohen & Syme, 1985; Litwak, 1985; Sarason, Sarason, & Pierce, 1990; Sauer & Coward, 1985; Whittaker & Garbarino, 1983). Similarly, there is a tremendous amount of recent research on the relationship between psychosocial factors (e.g., Type A behavior, anger-hostility, depression, and anxiety) and cardiovascular disease, especially coronary heart disease (CHD) and essential hypertension (Berkman, Leo-Summers, & Horwitz, 1992; Chesney & Rosenman, 1985; Cohen & Mathews, 1987; Diamond, 1982; Johnson, 1987; Johnson & Broman, 1987; Johnson & Julius, 1990; Julius & Johnson, 1985). The study of the relationship between social support and cardiovascular disease, however, is a relatively new venture that continues to struggle with conceptual and methodological issues concerning how social support should be defined and measured (Davidson & Shumaker, 1987). The longitudinal and developmental nature of both social support and cardiovascular disease requires special conceptual and methodological attention.

The view of social support within an attachment across the life-span framework, as suggested previously (see Antonucci, 1976; Kahn & Antonucci, 1980; Lerner & Ryff, 1978; Levitt, in press; Parkes & Stevenson-Hinde, 1982; Parkes, Stevenson-Hinde, & Marris, 1991), most readily approximates the life-span developmental perspective of social relationships. Viewing an individual's support environment as a convoy that develops and changes, but accompanies the individual as he or she moves through events and age best captures this notion of social support. Similarly, cardiovascular disease is an evolving condition that is influenced by both developmental and environmental changes. Much like that of social support, the development of cardiovascular disease evolves across the life span. It is highly conceivable, for example, that the biological/psychological factors involved in the onset or initiation of cardiovascular disease are not the same ones responsible for its maintenance or progression (Julius & Johnson, 1985).

Therefore it would appear that a major research and methodological difficulty is in knowing *where* in the progression of the disease *which* social support components (i.e., measures) are most important for predicting outcome measures reflective of the state of the disease. For example, the dimensions of social support that are of importance for a person who has suffered a second myocardial infarction (MI) and is attempting to return to work may be considerably different from those of an obese child or an adolescent with hypertension. Although there may be critical underlying psychological processes and mechanisms that are the same (e.g., the supportive exchange may involve the supportive other communicating to the supported individual the belief that she or he can achieve a particular goal), specific details will probably vary considerably. The support structure of the adult who has suffered a near-fatal MI is likely to be strongly influenced by the degree of satisfaction and happiness in marriage and at work, as well as supportive bonds with friends. In contrast, the obese adolescent with hypertension may be more likely to focus on the quality (and quantity) of supportive relationships with peers and secondarily on the relationships with parents. There is a strong need for future research to focus on these types of similarities and differences.

Adolescents whose obesity is causing hypertension must have social networks that believe in their ability to lose weight and that will make every effort to help them achieve that goal. Similarly, as Bandura's (1986) and Ewart's (1992) work on recovering MI patients have shown, the beliefs of social network members in the patient's recovery is critical. Appropriate developmental differences suggest that for adolescents the relevant supportive others are likely to be peer group members, whereas for adults, the most important supportive others are likely to be family members, especially the spouse.

The individual is a social and developing human being. At each age, specific characteristics emerge or are particularly relevant. The child experiences interactions with significant others, most often the parents; certain qualities of these interactions have been documented as better, others worse. For example, it is better if interactions with significant others tend to be contingent, that is, if the adult individual responds to the directed (and sometimes nondirected) utterances of the child. In behavioral terms this might mean that the smiling infant learns that adults will smile back, or that the gurgling, preverbal infant learns that adults will respond verbally to these nonsensical sounds. Early theorists (Ainsworth, Blehar, Waters, & Wall, 1978; Lewis & Goldberg, 1969) argued that as a result of such interactive sequences, infants begin to view the world as a place that is responsive, that can be influenced (some have used stronger language, such as controlled). The ethologists (Ainsworth et al., 1978; Bowlby, 1969) argued that good early social relationships provide the infant with a secure base from which to explore the world and thereby influence other areas of development in addition to social development.

To extend this view of social relationships, one would consider the parent–infant interaction model and the importance of these social relationships for the child's social and general development. This base of relationships is extended in numbers (i.e., the child may have more relationships with more individuals) and in the domains of influence (interactions will be social, exploratory, cognitive, or personal). Thus, one can assume that on the basis of both intra- and interindividual development and experiences, individuals develop predispositions or expectations about the nature of social relationships.

To extend this scenario by example, individuals develop contingent responsive interactions with close and important others. Individuals come to expect the world to be responsive to their actions. Children come to expect that they can influence their external environment because they have been able to do so in the case of early attachment figures. As children grow, develop, and mature, they are exposed to more people, and, (under optimal conditions) if the environment is consistent with that provided by early attachment figures, they learn that there are more people or things in the world whom they can influence. The network of people, things, and expectations expands. As children become adults, the contingencies become more complicated. They benefit from increased abilities and capabilities and also from increased complexities of their individual environment. Thus, children and adolescents optimally extend their networks from mother to parents to extended family to peers. They learn to view themselves as persons who can influence others and have some control over events. For the obese child coping with hypertension this may translate into a desire and belief in his or her own ability to control caloric intake as well as an ability to both seek and maintain sound relationships with appropriately supportive peers.

Antonucci and Jackson (1987) present an adult version of this continuum of interactive sequences. They suggest that contingent interaction sequences between individuals have important and long-lasting effects. Not only does the individual's personal behavior affect that of another, but with each interactive sequence the generalizability of this influence is learned. The building up of this type of contingent interactive sequence develops interpersonal efficacy (Antonucci & Jackson, 1987). This can be seen as directly parallel to the infant literature. As the securely attached infant benefits from a secure base from which to explore the world, the adult benefits from a buildup of a contingent interactive sequence with important others that develops in the individual a sense of personal efficacy. Individuals with higher levels of interpersonal efficacy are more likely to view themselves as people who can accomplish things on their own, can influence others, can help others when they choose to, and can achieve the goals they set for themselves.

It may be that this same higher level of interpersonal efficacy enables the individual to influence his or her own health, be it by staying healthy (e.g., through the maintenance of a healthy life-style), by providing the ability to withstand a life-threatening event (e.g., a myocardial infarction), or by participation in one's own recovery (e.g., through rehabilitation programs). Bandura (1986) found that perceived self-efficacy of recovering MI patients was predictive of their recovery, but their wives' perceptions of their efficacy was even more predictive! In fact, the longitudinal analyses suggested that the wife's beliefs influenced her husband's beliefs, rather than vice versa. This appears to be an interesting and somewhat unique example of social support affecting the health (in this case, the recovery) of an individual.

The next question has to do with the influence of these ongoing and developing social relationships on health and disease (see Chapter 9 for a further discussion of this issue). The evolution of social relationships was viewed above as continuing and life-long in nature; the same can be said for cardiovascular diseases. For the purpose of this chapter, which focuses specifically on social relationships and cardiovascular disease, it is useful to look at the continuum of cardiovascular disease. It has been argued that there are certain traditional risk factors (e.g., family background of cardiovascular disease, cholesterol, alcohol and tobacco usage, lack of exercise, and poor diet) that increase the relative risk of developing cardiovascular disease (see Chapter 8). Focusing now on the continuum of cardiovascular disease, two questions arise: do social relationships influence the disease, and do they differentially influence the disease continuum (e.g., onset, progression of disease, established or chronic phase, recovery from a potentially fatal event such as MI, mortality from cardiovascular disease). Another important question is, does social support directly effect certain predisposing or traditional risk factors (e.g., alcohol intake, dietary changes, weight gain) that in turn affect the cardiovascular disease continuum? We assume that the answer to this question is yes, but major methodological limitations inherent in the published research (most of which pertain to mortality outcome studies) make it impossible to justify and defend our answer at this time.

As indicated above, the majority of studies linking various conceptions of social support to cardiovascular disease focus on total mortality (see Cohen, 1988, for a review). Very few systematic attempts have been made to determine if and how the various conceptions of social support are associated with other facets of the continuum of cardiovascular disease. Moreover, of the various indexes of social support available, only the structural index of social ties—often termed social integration (SI)—has been used often enough in research in these areas to permit a reasonable evaluation of its relationship to cardiovascular disease. A prototypic SI index includes marital status, close family and friends, participation in group activities, and church and religious affiliations.

The overall pattern of findings from the mortality studies indicates that healthy persons with higher SI scores are at lower risk for mortality than their counterparts with lower SI scores (Berkman & Syme, 1979; House et al., 1982; Schoenbach et al., 1986). Moreover, this pattern persists after controlling for such traditional cardiovascular disease risk factors as cigarette smoking, alcohol usage, relative weight, and hypertension. Whereas high SI scores appear to decrease total mortality risk for males only (House et al., 1982; Schoenbach et al., 1986), some studies have found that SI scores affect total mortality for both males and females (Orth-Gomér & Johnson, 1987). The findings from the more detailed analyses of the mortality studies show that women with lower SI scores were at higher risk of death from ischemic heart disease (House et al., 1982). A study reported by Ruberman, Weinblatt, Goldberg, and Chaudhary (1984) shows that lower SI scores predict mortality for male survivors of acute myocardial infarctions over a 1- to 3-year follow-up period. In addition to social integration, a few studies examine the relationship between mortality and the degree of satisfaction with social networks (Berkman & Syme, 1979; Blazer, 1982; House et al., 1982). For the most part, marital satisfaction and satisfaction with social activities are unrelated to total mortality.

From a life-span developmental perspective, the findings from the mortality studies do not clearly identify the stage(s) of the disease process (e.g., onset of the disease, increased severity of disease, faster progression of disease, prolonged recovery from disease) upon which social support has an impact. Equally important is the failure to describe the process by which social support affects mortality. In a general sense, the etiological significance of social support as a relevant psychosocial risk factor for cardiovascular disease is weak. It would appear that the etiological significance of social support would be best demonstrated in studies of cardiovascular morbidity rather than mortality investigations. Although these studies are more difficult to interpret, the evidence implicating a role of social support in cardiovascular disease would be enhanced by the demonstration of a significant relationship between social support and morbid events (e.g., hypertension, EKG abnormalities reflective of distortions in the structure or functioning of the heart, coronary heart disease) before the eventual mortality from cardiovascular disease.

A small number of studies (Blumenthal et al., 1987; Haynes, Feinleib, & Kannel, 1980; Joseph, 1980; Medalie & Goldbourt, 1976; Reed, McGee, & Yano, 1984; Reed, McGee, Yano, & Feinleib, 1983; Seeman & Syme, 1987) have examined the association of social support to coronary heart disease (CHD). Medalie and Goldbourt (1976) showed that men reporting being loved and supported by their wives were buffered from the effect of high anxiety on the incidence of angina pectoria. Similarly, Johnson (1987) found that supportive interactions with coworkers buffered the effect of work stress on CHD prevalence for both men and women. In the Honolulu Heart Study (Reed et al., 1984), there was no significant stress-buffering effect of any measure of social support for males in predicting CHD incidence.

Two recent studies have looked at income, living alone, marital status, and the possession of a confidante as predictors of survival in patients with coronary artery disease (Case, Moss, Case, McDermott, & Eberly, 1992; Williams, Barefoot, & Califf, 1992). Both studies demonstrated clearly that, independent of clinical and angiographic indicators of disease extent, being married, having fewer economic resources, and being socially isolated predict poor survival even for those who undergo revascularization. In fact, the association with low levels of social support persists among patients with equal assess to medical care (Ruberman, 1992). Fiebach, Viscoli, and Horwitz (1990) found that gender should not be considered an independent risk factor, but that, in this patient population, women were far more likely than men to be unmarried (50% versus 83%). A part of this is related to the fact that women outlive men by 7 years (Wenger, 1990) and, as a consequence, a woman is more likely to serve as caretaker for her husband during a prolonged terminal illness than vice versa. Because women are often unwilling to relinquish their caretaking role when manifestations of coronary artery disease set in, they tend to postpone invasive investigation and treatment. When they are at last free to have themselves attended to, they are in a poor functional class—elderly, usually living alone, and possible in economic difficulty.

In the studies by Seeman and Syme (1987) and Blumenthal et al. (1987), social support was significantly related to coronary artery disease in both men and women undergoing diagnostic angiography. Seeman and Syme (1987) reported that the availability of greater instrumental support and perceived love from significant others was related to lower atherosclerosis. It should be noted that atherosclerosis was not significantly related to SI, its structural components, or the level of emotional support from family and friends. Similarly, Blumenthal et al. (1987) found no main effect of emotional support on atherosclerosis. They did, however, find an interaction between the Type A behavior pattern and emotional support; greater occlusion of coronary arteries was significantly related to lower emotional support among Type A individuals but to more emotional support among Type Bs. This finding provides a hint of how complex the relationships between social support and cardiovascular disease might be.

Another critical methodological issue is one of sampling bias. For example, one of the major difficulties in interpreting the role of social support in angiographic studies is the sample bias inherent in examining symptomatic patients (Cohen & Mathews, 1987). These studies generally attempt to discriminate between patients with symptoms who have coronary artery disease and those who do not; no normal or nonsymptomatic patients are studied. Therefore, no information is available concerning the relationships between coronary artery disease in nonsymptomatic individuals and social support.

To understand the influence of social support and cardiovascular disease on each other, it is useful to begin with early or predisposing traditional risk factors. The first question to be asked is, do social support and social relationships influence the predisposing and traditional factors known to be associated with cardiovascular disease? Here, it is useful to limit the question in reasonable ways. Gender (being male) and race (being black) are risk factors for cardiovascular disease. Obviously, though, the type of social relationships one has does not influence whether one is either male or black and, in turn, one's predisposition to develop cardiovascular disease on these grounds. It is possible, however, that there are unique aspects of the social relationships of men and women, and blacks and whites, that might contribute to the known gender and race differences in susceptibility to cardiovascular disease.

Some suggestive evidence of the relationship between social support and cardiovascular disease can be garnered from what is known about the relationship between Type A behavior and cardiovascular disease. Individuals with Type A personalities are more likely to develop cardiovascular disease, although gender and age mediate the relationship (Chesney & Rosenman, 1985; Matthews, 1982; Rosenman, 1987). Are Type A individuals more likely to have what the attachment theorists would call insecure attachment relationships (i.e., poor social relationships)? Another way of phrasing this question is, are Type A individuals who have poor levels of social support more at risk for cardiovascular disease than Type B individuals or Type A individuals with strong social supportive relationships? Similarly, work on suppressed hostility and anger (Chesney & Rosenman, 1985; Johnson & Julius, 1990) suggests that these individuals are predisposed toward hypertension. Is this because of specific characteristics of their social relationships and supportive environment? Or does the hypertensive patient's poor management of anger and hostility disrupt important relationships with family and friends thus increasing the relative risk for hypertension?

These examples, as well as the reports by Seeman and Syme (1987) and Blumenthal et al. (1987), suggests several ways in which social support and social relationships can affect the individual's propensity to develop cardiovascular disease. Whereas much of the literature concerning the relationships between social support and cardiovascular disease focuses on mortality studies, recent studies concentrate on rehabilitation and long-term recovery (see Chapter 12 for a review). The extent to which an individual feels comfortable with or supported by his or her supportive others may influence how that individual weathers the storm of a crisis event. For example, individuals with chest pain who feel that family members or friends would be willing to help them seek medical care may be significantly more likely to decide to seek such care (Antonucci, Kahn & Akiyama, 1989). In the case of crisis events (e.g., myocardial infarction) when time is critical, such a perspective can be lifesaving. But in many ways, the perception of social support may be more important than the specific supportive behavior emitted by the supportive other. Thus, although it is critical that there be someone who is willing to help with such physical necessities as driving to the hospital or doctor, it is equally, if not more, important that individuals believe in their ability to cope with crises. Examples from the literature include the early social support work of Nuckolls, Cassel, and Kaplan (1972) and Norbeck and Tilden (1981), who showed that pregnant women under stress experienced fewer labor and delivery complications if they felt supported. The work of Sosa, Kennel, and Klaus (1980) showed that women who had a supportive, nonexpert companion with them during labor and delivery also had fewer perinatal problems.

Finally, and perhaps most importantly from a practical perspective, these findings provide some insights about how the concept of social support can be applied to the treatment of cardiovascular disease. Thus, we may be able to develop models that help define those characteristics of supportive relationships that help the individual cope with crises and maximize the potential for rehabilitation. In this latter regard, two types of research and theoretical work are particularly interesting and important. The general issue is the negative influence of social relationships. Earlier we discussed some of the circumstances when social relationships might be seen to be a negative predisposing factor (e.g., when infants are insecurely attached they might lack a secure base from which to explore the environment). Early work on maternal deprivation clearly indicates that social deprivation could lead to problems in a broad array of developmental arenas. Of particular interest is the post–World War II finding that children who were separated from parents showed numerous effects of the separation above and beyond what might be labeled as social or emotional consequences (Bowlby, 1969). The presence of positive social relationships has been shown to have a positive affect on health and well-being. The absence of such relationships can also be seen as influential, although in a negative way. People who lack important and secure social relationships may be at greater risk for cardiovascular disease and other health-related problems (Davidson & Shumaker, 1987).

In addition to the lack of positive social relationships (and thus of the positive impact of social support), there has been some speculation that negative support may operate under certain circumstances. In these cases, the individual has an accumulated assortment of relationships that can only be described as influencing the individual negatively. This may practically translate into interactions that support such counterproductive behaviors as smoking, drinking, poor diet, or lack of exercise. Although social support is most often thought of as having a positive influence on cardiovascular disease, the possibility that support has a negative influence on pre-, peri-, or post-cardiovascular disease should not be overlooked. Because social relationships are complex phenomena, it is also likely that the same individuals who provide positive supports also provide negative supports. Teenagers may receive peer support for the positive development of age-appropriate independence from friends who also provide support for negative behaviors such as smoking (see, e.g., Antonucci, 1985; Ingersoll-Dayton & Antonucci, 1988; Rook, 1984).

It may also be the case that some supportive environments can address certain aspects of a health–illness continuum better than others. For example, it has been documented that dense networks can be assets with normative life events or crises but can be a detriment and less helpful than nondense networks when the individual is facing a nonnormative life event (Hirsch, 1980). The same may be true for social support and health; some support relationships may be an asset at one point in the disease continuum but not another. Being warm and loving may shelter or insulate an individual with predisposing factors to cardiovascular disease, because it minimizes the impact of stress. It may also be very helpful post-cardiac event. On the other hand, such a network may be detrimental to the long-term rehabilitation of an individual if it encourages dependency. Similarly, multifaceted, extended networks may be more helpful when one is recovering from a cardiac event by connecting the patient with others who have experienced similar health crises or who can help facilitate life style changes.

Methodological Issues and Future Research Agenda

If the complex perspective on interrelationships outlined above is adopted, the next critical issue is one of the appropriate method for future research. It is virtually impossible to design a realistic study that will be capable of addressing all of the theoretical and conceptual issues outlined above; however, it is useful to be aware of the kind of data that would be optimal. Ideally one would wish for a longitudinal, in-depth study of both social relationships and the health-related variables of interest using reliable and valid instruments. In the case of social relationships one would want to examine the developing infant's social relationships and how they mature and expand over time.

As stated earlier, there appears to be much confusion and conceptual ambiguity regarding how the dimensions of social support should be defined, and considerably more disagreement as to how these dimensions should be measured. To develop appropriate and valid measures that take into consideration life-span developmental changes will require intense effort. Future studies are also needed to examine the processes by which social support affects cardiovascular disease. It might be that social support has no direct effect on cardiovascular disease onset or its severity, but a strong impact on such chronic disease risk factors as weight gain and obesity, smoking, alcohol intake, exercise and leisure-time activities that affect the progression of the disease. A related question is whether age, gender, or ethnic origin modify relationships between social support, chronic disease risk factors, and cardiovascular disease. A basic thesis that needs to be examined is as follows: If social support has a role or involvement in the development (or onset or severity) of cardiovascular diseases such as CHD or hypertension, then this is most likely secondary to excessive perception of (or exposure to) mental stress or through an excessive activation of the autonomic nervous system. In either case, the primary link between social support (or any psychosocial factors) and the physiological/biochemical abnormalities we refer to as cardiovascular disease are probably the effect-mediated neuroendocrine responses.

Future investigations of these complex issues will undoubtedly require a multidisciplinary approach to assess the quality and quantity of both social support and biochemical/physiological activity reflective of the pathogenic processes involved in specific cardiovascular diseases. One would wish for a longitudinal study of those variables thought to reflect the continuum from poor to excellent cardiovascular health. In the case of cardiovascular disease, this would include assessment and follow-up of known traditional risk factors (e.g., family history of disease, cholesterol, sodium intake, alcohol and tobacco use, weight gain, obesity) as well as factors reflective of the state of cardiovascular health (e.g., blood pressure level, cardiovascular reactivity to stress, EKG and other heart function measures as determined from ultrasound echo dappler). The interrelationship between the two sets of data should be studied continuously, with special attention to any changes resulting from alterations in the structural or functional aspects of social support. This ideal may be impossible to achieve, although some ongoing prospective, population-based studies may be able to provide relevant, if partial, data. In the interim, cross-sectional studies should and can be conducted that attempt to develop more practical short-term designs to acquire information using pragmatic approximations of the ideal outlined above. A few examples of this type of study are the angiographic studies reported by Seeman and Syme (1987) and Blumenthal et al. (1987).

Summary and Conclusions

In this chapter we outline a life-span view of social relationships and a long-term view of the health–illness continuum. The goal of the chapter is to propose a new way of thinking about the link between social support and cardiovascular disease. The link is neither singular nor simple. It is not simply a matter of counting the number of friends and relatives who visit an individual after he or she has suffered a myocardial infarction. Rather, it is a complex array of interrelationships that develop over the individual's lifetime and influence each point of the continuum of health and illness which includes both predisease health states, crisis events, and postevent recovery and rehabilitation. These theoretical and conceptual issues serve to inform the measurement techniques best employed to address the specific questions of interest.

ACKNOWLEDGMENTS. This chapter was written while the first author held a Research Career Development Award from the National Institute on Aging and was a visiting scholar at the Institute Nationale Santé de Education et Recherche Medicale in Paris, France.

References

Ainsworth, M.D.S., Blehar, M.C., Waters, E., & Wall, S. (1978). *Patterns of attachment*. Hillsdale, NJ: Erlbaum.

Antonucci, T. C. (1976). Attachment: A life-span concept. *Human Development*, (19) (3), 135–142.

Antonucci, T. C. (1985). Personal characteristics, social networks and social behavior. In R. H. Binstock & E. Shanas (Eds.), *Handbook of aging and the social sciences* (2nd ed., pp. 94–128). New York: Van Nostrand Reinhold.

Antonucci, T. C. & Jackson, J. S. (1987). Social support, interpersonal efficacy, and health. In L. Carstensen & B. A. Edelstein (Eds.), *Handbook of clinical gerontology* (pp. 291–311). New York: Pergamon.

Antonucci, T. C., Kahn, R. L., & Akiyama, H. (1989). Psychosocial factors and the response to cancer symptoms. In R. Yancik & J. Yates (Eds.), *Cancer in the elderly: Approaches to early detection and treatment* (pp. 40–52). New York: Springer.

Bandura, A. (1986). *Social foundations of thought and actions*. Englewood Cliffs, NJ: Prentice Hall.

Berkman, L. F. (1985). The relationship of social networks and social support to morbidity and mortality. In S. Cohen & S. L. Syme (Eds.), *Social support and health* (pp. 241–252). New York: Academic Press.

Berkman, L. F., Leo-Summers, L., & Horwitz, R. I. (1992). Emotional support and survival after myocardial infarction. *Annals of Internal Medicine, 117*, 1003–1009.

Berkman, L. F., & Syme, S. L. (1979). Social networks, host resistance, and mortality: A nine year follow-up study of Alameda County residents. *American Journal of Epidemiology, 109*(2), 186–204.

Blazer, D. G. (1982). Social support and mortality in an elderly population. *American Journal of Epidemiology, 115*, 684–694.

Blumenthal, J. A., Burg, M. M., Barefoot, J., Williams, R. B., Haney, T., & Zimet, G. (1987). Social support, Type A behavior and coronary artery disease. *Psychosomatic Medicine, 49*, 331–339.

Bowlby, J. (1969). *Attachment and loss, vol. 1: Attachment*. New York: Basic Books.

Case, R. B., Moss, A. J., Case, N., McDermott, M., & Eberly, S. (1992). Living alone after myocardial infarction: Impact on prognosis. *Journal of the American Medical Association, 267*, 515–519.

Cassel, J. (1976). The contribution of the social environment to host resistance. *American Journal of Epidemiology, 104*(3), 253–286.

Chesney, M. A., & Rosenman, R. H. (1985). *Anger and hostility in cardiovascular and behavioral disorders*. Washington, DC: Hemisphere.

Cobb, S. (1976). Social support as a moderator of life stress. *Psychosomatic Medicine, 38*, 300–314.

Cohen, S. (1988). Psychosocial models of the role of social support in the etiology of physical disease. *Health Psychology, 7*(3), 269–297.

Cohen, S., & Mathews, S. (1987). Social support, Type A behavior, and coronary artery disease, *Psychosomatic Medicine, 49*, 325–330.

Cohen, S., & Syme, S. L. (Eds.). (1985). *Social support and health*. New York: Academic Press.

Davidson, D., & Shumaker, S. (1987). Workshop summary: Social support and cardiovascular disease. *Arteriosclerosis, 7*, 101–104.

Diamond, E. L. (1982). The role of anger and hostility in essential hypertension and coronary heart disease. *Psychological Bulletin, 92*, 410–433.

Ewart, C. K. (1992). Role of physical self-efficacy in recovery from heart attach. In R. S. Schwarzer (Ed.), *Self-efficacy: Thought control of actions.* Washington, DC: Hemisphere.

Fiebach, N. H., Viscoli, C. M., Horwitz, R. I. (1990). Differences between women and men in survival after myocardial infarction: Biology or methodology? *Journal of the American Medical Association, 263*, 1092–1096.

Haynes, S. G., Feinleib, M., & Kannel, W. B. (1980). The relationship of psychosocial factors to coronary heart disease in the Framingham Study: Eight year incidence of coronary heart disease. *American Journal of Epidemiology, 111*, 37–58.

Heitzmann, C. A., & Kaplan, R. M. (1988). Assessment of methods for measuring social support. *Health Psychology, 7*(1), 75–109.

Hirsch, B. (1980). Natural support systems and coping with major life changes. *American Journal of Community Psychology, 8*, 159–172.

House, J. S., Landis, K. R., & Umberson, D. (1988). Social relationships and health. *Science, 241*, 540–544.

House, J. S., Robbins, C., & Metzner, H. C. (1982). The association of social relationships and activities with mortality: Perspective evidence from the Tecumseh community health study. *American Journal of Epidemiology, 116*(1), 123–140.

House, J. S., Umberson, D., & Landis, K. R. (1988). Structures and processes of social support. *Annual Review of Sociology, 14*, 293–318.

Ingersoll-Dayton, B., & Antonucci, T. C. (1988). Non-reciprocal social support: Another side of intimate relationships. *Journal of Gerontology: Social Sciences, 43*(3), 65–73.

Israel, B. A. (1982). Social networks and health status: Linking theory, research and practice. *Patient Counseling and Health Education, 4*(2), 65–79.

Jackson, J. S., & Antonucci, T. C. (in press). Survey methodology in life-span human development research. In S. H. Cohen & H. W. Reese (Eds.), *Life-span developmental psychology: Methodological innovations* (pp. 1–52). Hillsdale, NJ: Erlbaum.

Johnson, E. H. (1987). Behavioral factors associated with hypertension in black Americans. In S. Julius & D. R. Bassett (Eds.), *Handbook of Hypertension, vol. 9: Behavioral factors in hypertension* (pp. 181–197). Amsterdam: Elsevier Sciences.

Johnson, E. H., & Broman, C. L. (1987). The relationship of anger expression to health problems among black Americans in a national survey. *Journal of Behavioral Medicine, 10*(2), 103–116.

Johnson, E. H., & Julius, S. (1990). Is there a hypertensive coronary-prone personality? In F. Buhler & J. Farosh (Eds.), *Handbook of Hypertension, vol. 10: Management of hypertension* (pp. 33–41). Amsterdam: Elsevier Sciences.

Joseph, J. (1980). *Social affiliation, risk factor status, and coronary heart disease: A cross sectional study of Japanese-American men.* Unpublished doctoral dissertation, University of California, Berkeley.

Julius, S., & Johnson, E. H. (1985). Stress, autonomic hyperactivity, and essential hypertension: An enigma. *Journal of Hypertension, 3*, 11–17.

Kahn, R. L., & Antonucci, T. C. (1980). Convoys over the lifecourse: Attachment, roles, and social support. In P. B. Baltes & O. Brim (Eds.), *Life-span development and behavior, vol. 3* (pp. 253–286). New York: Academic Press.

Lerner, R., & Ryff, C. (1978). Implementation of the life-span view of human development: The sample case of attachment. In P. B. Baltes (Ed.), *Life-span development and behavior, vol. 1* (pp. 1–43). New York: Plenum Press.

Levitt, M. J. (1991). Attachment and close relationships: A life span perspective. In J. L. Gewirtz & W. F. Kurtines (Eds.), *Intersections with attachment* (pp. 183–205). Hillsdale, NJ: Erlbaum.

Lewis, M., & Goldberg, S. (1969). Perceptual-cognitive development in infancy: A generalized expectancy model as a function of mother-infant interaction. *Merrill-Palmer Quarterly, 15,* 81–100.

Litwak, E. (1985). *Helping the elderly.* New York: Guilford.

Matthews, K. (1982). Psychological perspectives on the Type A behavior pattern. *Psychology Bulletin, 91,* 293–323.

Medalie, J. H., & Goldbourt, U. (1976). Angina pectoris among 10,000 men: Psychosocial and other factors as evidenced by a multivariate analysis of a 5 year incidence study. *American Journal of Medicine, 60,* 910–921.

Norbeck, J. S., & Tilden, V. (1981). Life stress, social support, and emotional equilibrium in complications of pregnancy: A prospective multivariate study. *Journal of Health and Social Behavior, 24,* 30–46.

Nuckolls, K. B., Cassel, J., & Kaplan, B. H. (1972). Psychosocial assets, life crisis and the prognosis of pregnancy. *American Journal of Epidemiology, 95,* 431–441.

Orth-Gomér, K., & Johnson, J. V. (1987). Social network interaction and mortality: A six year follow-up study of a random sample of the Swedish population. *Journal of Chronic Disease, 40*(10), 949–957.

Parkes, C. M., & Stevenson-Hinde, J. (1982). *The place of attachment in human behavior.* New York: Basic Books.

Parkes, C. M., Stevenson-Hinde, J., & Marris, P. (Eds.). (1991). *Attachment across the life cycle,* New York: Routledge.

Pearlin, L. I. (1985). Social structure and processes of social support. In S. Cohen & S. L. Syme (Eds.), *Social Support and Health* (pp. 13–60). New York: Academic Press.

Reed, D., McGee, D., Yano, K., & Feinleib, M. (1983). Social networks and coronary heart disease among Japanese men in Hawaii. *American Journal of Epidemiology, 117,* 384–396.

Reed, D., McGee, D., & Yano, K. (1984). Psychosocial processes and general susceptibility to chronic disease. *American Journal of Epidemiology, 119,* 356–370.

Rook, K. S. (1984). The negative side of social interaction: Impact on psychological well-being. *Journal of Personality and Social Psychology, 46,* 1097–1108.

Rosenman, R. H. (1987). Type A behavior and hypertension. In S. Julius & D. R. Bassett (Eds.), *Handbook of hypertension, vol. 9: Behavioral factors in hypertension* (pp. 141–149). Amsterdam: Elsevier Science.

Ruberman, W. (1992). Psychosocial influences on mortality of patients with coronary heart disease. *Journal of the American Medical Association, 267,* 559–560.

Ruberman, W., Weinblatt, E., Goldberg, J. D., & Chaudhary, B. S. (1984). Psychosocial influences on mortality after myocardial infarction. *New England Journal of Medicine, 311,* 552–559.

Sarason, B. R., Sarason, I. G., & Pierce, G. R. (Eds.). (1990). *Social support: An interactional view.* New York: John Wiley.

Sauer, W. J., & Coward, R. T. (Eds.). (1985). *Social support networks and care of the elderly.* New York: Springer.

Schoenbach, V. J., Kaplan, B. H., Freman, L., & Kleinbaum, D. G. (1986). Social ties and mortality in Evans County, Georgia. *American Journal of Epidemiology, 123,* 577–591.

Seeman, T. E., & Syme, S. L. (1987). Social networks and coronary artery disease: A comparison of the structure and function of social relations as predictors of disease. *Psychosomatic Medicine, 49,* 340–353.

Shumaker, S. A., & Brownell, A. (1984). Toward a theory of social support: Closing conceptual gaps. *Journal of Social Issues, 40*, 11–36.

Sosa, R., Kennel, J., & Klaus, M. (1980). The effect of a supportive companion on perinatal problems, length of labor, and mother-infant interactions. *New England Journal of Medicine, 305*, 597–600.

Wenger, N. K. (1990). Gender, coronary artery disease, and coronary bypass surgery. *Annals of Internal Medicine, 112*, 557–558.

Whittaker, J. K., & Garbarino, J. (1983). *Social support networks: Informal helping in the human services.* New York: Aldine.

Williams, R. B., Barefoot, J. C., Califf, R. M. (1992). Prognostic importance of social and economic resources among medically treated patients with angiographically documented coronary artery disease. *Journal of the American Medical Association, 267*, 520–524.

CHAPTER 3

Assessment of Social Support

Barbara R. Sarason and Irwin G. Sarason

Social support is a concept that, because of its pervasive role in human affairs, needs operationalization and assessment. One of the primary confusions about social support is that the term is linked both to objective events (actual availability of others) and to subjective estimates (perceptions of others' willingness to help). The clarification of the social support concept and its measurement are important because there is growing evidence that personal adjustment and social behavior, as well as health maintenance and recovery from illness, can be influenced significantly by a person's access to supportive others. If social support deficits (however they might be defined) are related to negative outcomes, and if it is important to identify people who vary along the social support continuum, a method is needed for accurately measuring the relevant social resources.

During the past decade many attempts have been made to quantify social support, and a large number of instruments are available. It is important for researchers to recognize that social support instruments that differ in their conceptual bases may also differ in which aspects of social relationships they assess and in their adequacy as measurement tools. In this chapter we are concerned primarily with the methods of measurement used in social support research, but the underlying conceptualizations that led to specific measurement approaches will also be discussed.

This chapter deals with both theoretical and practical issues. First, it will highlight the theoretical roots of the different approaches to the

BARBARA R. SARASON AND IRWIN G. SARASON • Department of Psychology, University of Washington, Seattle, Washington 98195.

Social Support and Cardiovascular Disease, edited by Sally A. Shumaker and Susan M. Czajkowski. Plenum Press, New York, 1994.

assessment of social support. Second, it will provide as much practical information as possible about how a researcher might choose the most appropriate measure depending on the focus of the research. Topics dealt with include how to fit the choice of an instrument to the research question, the effects of psychometric characteristics of the assessment instruments on the potential research findings, and general guidelines for the measurement of the social support construct. We also discuss what is known about the comparability of instruments based not only on their psychometric characteristics, but also on their conceptualization.

Origins of Social Support Research

The formal history of research on social support is a relatively brief one, going back only a little over a decade, although the concept has a much longer history. Durkheim's (1951) development of the idea of anomie, Cooley's (1909) concept of the primary group, Bowlby's (1969) ideas on attachment, Rogers's (1942) conception of the therapeutic process, and Likert's (1961) focus on support as the core of the supervisory process are all examples of important theoretical perspectives that have contributed to present thinking about the role of social support in people's lives.

In addition to the work of these theorists and others, clinical observations, research findings, and political and social changes have provided impetus for work on social support. Clinicians first observed anecdotally and then through formalized studies that support (defined by the existence of a social network or a confidant) helped prevent illness, reduce birth complications, and speeded recovery (e.g., Gore, 1978; Nuckolls, Cassel, & Kaplan, 1972). Administration of emotional support by health care personnel or others was shown in several studies to be beneficial to health (Auerbach & Kilmann, 1977; Whitcher & Fisher, 1979). Epidemiological research also provided data from large population samples indicating the effect of supportive relationships on mortality (Berkman & Syme, 1979; House, Robbins, & Metzner, 1982; see also Chapters 5 and 6).

The common focus of much early work on social support involved the concept of support as a resource that moderated stress. Sociological studies suggested that stressors were more common in certain groups, such as the economically disadvantaged. During the 1960s in the United States, the War on Poverty resulted in large-scale intervention attempts focused on prevention, including preschool programs for children at risk, an emphasis on maternal health and well-child programs, community mental health centers, and a proliferation of support groups of various types, many agency sponsored. In all these areas, effort was directed at providing a variety of types of support—services as well as practical help and provision of associations with others—that might help compensate for a deficiency in personal relationships (Pilisuk & Parks, 1986).

As this brief history indicates, there was interest in social support on the part of many different disciplines. As a result of this multidisciplinary interest, however, the definitions of social support reflect a wide variety of viewpoints. Perhaps one of the most urgent exhortations for anyone planning a research project involving social support is to look carefully at the definitions used in prior research efforts upon which the current project is built. Later in this chapter we will discuss what is known about the relationships among measures based on some of these definitions.

In the initial work that sparked interest in the role of social support in health, its presence was operationalized in a simplistic way, usually as the presence of a spouse or possibly a confidant. Although this definition is appealing because of its ease of measurement, it may be misleading because it lumps together emotionally satisfying and conflictful relationships. Early researchers in the field of social support also used other measures of social relationships, including the frequency of contacts with friends and relatives, the number of such relationships, and membership in and attendance at meetings of organized groups. Like marital status, this information is relatively easy for subjects to report and easy to quantify, although these measures are not as high as marital status in reliability of report. A combined measure that includes these questions is often referred to as a measure of social integration; the Social Network index, developed by Berkman and Syme (1979) for the Alameda County study, represents a formalization of this approach.

A forward step in measuring social support came from attempts to understand the meaning of the association between the presence of a close relationship to health. A number of theorists in the fields of epidemiology and sociology began to conceptualize social support in terms of the various functions relationships fulfill (Cobb, 1976; Kaplan, Cassel, & Gore, 1977; Weiss, 1974). More recently, interest in social support as a personality variable has surfaced (Henderson, 1984; Sarason, Pierce, & Sarason, 1990; Sarason, Sarason, & Shearin, 1986).

Current Assessment Approaches as a Function of Their Origins

Social support measures may be divided into three general categories: network measures, measures of support actually received or reported to have been received, and measures of the degree of support the person perceives to be available.

Network Measures

Network measures focus on the embeddedness of the person within a group and the interrelationships within the network matrix. The unique features of this approach are that (a) it extends the range of social relationships examined, (b) it provides a method for describing the structural pattern of relationships and makes possible an analysis of the impact of different patterns, and (c) it can help to clarify the multiple aspects and effects, both positive and negative, of the relationships recorded (Wellman, 1981; Wilcox, 1981). The face validity of the network approach to mapping the social world of the person is clear; in contrast, its usefulness in understanding the causal relationships between social relationships and health has not as yet been established (House & Kahn, 1985). Despite this limitation, the network approach can yield unique information that may be helpful in understanding the role of social support.

Network characteristics commonly assessed include structural and interactional properties (e.g., size, density or linkage among the network members, and reciprocity) or qualitative aspects (the content and quality of the relationships; Israel, 1982). Conflicting associations with well-being have been found for the structural and interactional characteristics of network measures. For example, Hirsch (1980) studied the effect of different patterns of social networks on mental health for a group of women in transition: recent, relatively young widows and mature women returning to college full-time. He found that the structure of ties among family and friends was a major factor related to level of symptoms, mood, and self-esteem. For example, the higher the network density (i.e., the higher the proportion of actual to potential ties that existed among the women's family members and friends), the more likely the women were to have a high level of symptoms, depressed mood, and low self-esteem. In contrast, Gallo (1982) reported a positive association between network density and well-being. Although seemingly contradictory, these results make intuitive sense. Hirsch's findings may reflect the women's ability to utilize less connected members of their network in making a role transition. Gallo's results were based on a community sample of subjects aged 60 and over, for whom the role transition was not a factor. This interpretation of the divergent findings in the two studies is consistent with Vaux and Harrison's (1984) suggestion that low-density networks may be most effective in facilitating transitions and adjustment to new circumstances, whereas high-density networks may be helpful when "retrenchment, recuperation, and validation are the appropriate response" to a stressor (p. 19).

Network analysis can also focus on the reciprocity of relationships. In general, relationships in which both the focal person and the network person initiate contact are conducive to health. In contrast, those in which the initiation is one-sided are not health promotive, although in close relationships this notion of reciprocity is based upon an extended time period and not on a series of immediately reciprocated interchanges (Levitt, 1991).

The size of the network can also affect satisfaction with support. Stokes (1983) found a curvilinear relationship between number of confidants and satisfaction with support among college students. The demands and responsibilities of maintaining numerous relationships may not be offset by the benefits that accrue from them; neither network size nor the size of the group of persons with whom the respondent feels close is predictive of support reported to be received (Stokes & Wilson, 1984). In contrast to density and reciprocity, which are often clarified by the network technique, the number of supporters can be determined in simpler ways than through a complex network analysis.

Although network measures have provided some promising leads, there is little empirical evidence of their utility in the study of health and social support (House & Kahn, 1985). Another caution to the investigator is that only a small number of studies using the term *network* actually assessed the kinds of structural properties emphasized by network analysts. Careful mapping of social networks in large samples is costly. As a result, most studies report findings based on small and idiosyncratic samples. House and Kahn (1985) recommend that gathering data on more than 5 to 10 persons in a network yields rapidly diminishing returns.

Received Support

Social support can be viewed as what has been received or what is perceived to be available should the need arise. Recent research findings, however, suggest little comparability between the two definitions. For example, Ward, Sherman, and LaGory (1984) found that subjective network assessments are only partly a function of actual network availability and involvement and that the perceived sufficiency of social ties is more important in determining a sense of well-being of older adults than the subjects' assessment of the actual availability of those in the network. Antonucci and Israel (1986) found that perception of available support is a better predictor of well-being than the report of what is actually obtained from the support giver. McCormick, Siegert, and Walkey (1987) compared a perceived support measure and a received support measure and showed that these assessed empirically distinct constructs.

In a study of examination stress experienced by dental students, Cooper (1986) found that perceived functional support and supportive transactions both play potentially important, though quite distinct, roles; the two are only weakly related. Perceived support plays a role in the stress appraisal process and serves as a coping resource. Supportive transactions, in contrast, serve as coping assistance that facilitates or hinders adjustment as a complex factor of the fit between the demands of the stressor, the type of support given, and the characteristics of the individual. Rosenberg (1985) compared the effects of perceived and received support in dealing with a stressor and found that well-being was enhanced by perceived support but not by support received as a result of specific desires. Received support has also been found to be related positively to stress, whereas most measures of perceived social support and stress are inversely related (Cummins, 1987).

Perceived Available Support

Perceived available support emphasizes the role of the subjective appraisal of the individual in the association between social support and health. A considerable body of research has demonstrated a relationship between both support satisfaction and perceived available support and psychological status (Procidano & Heller, 1983; Sandler & Barrera, 1984; Sarason, Levine, Basham, & Sarason, 1983). In general, low support satisfaction is associated with increased psychological distress. A number of research efforts have concluded that it is the perceived aspect of social support, rather than actual support received, that is health protective (Antonucci & Israel, 1986; Wethington & Kessler, 1986).

Received support and perceived available support may play somewhat different roles in moderating the effects of stress on health or adjustment. The amount of received support is directly influenced by the existence of a stressful situation. It is also affected by the presence of relationships that provide the potential for support and the perception of these other persons that the individual is distressed and/or incapable of dealing with a situation. Received support may have a positive effect on health or adjustment because it decreases the impact of the stressor, or a negative effect on these outcomes because it adversely affects the person's coping efforts or personal appraisal of coping effectiveness. In contrast, perceived social support as a stable characteristic that develops as a function of both earlier and present-day relationships may serve to enhance adjustment or health by producing feelings of self-worth and efficacy that may lessen the amount of perceived stress. Both these consequences tend to enhance coping efforts and thus increase the changes of a positive outcome.

Perceived social support can be looked at in terms of *aggregate* and *functional* support. The aggregate view includes the person's appraisal of the support that would be available if needed and his or her satisfaction with the appraisal of available support. The functional view is concerned with the importance of matching the support available to the person's need.

The Aggregate View

The aggregate view of social support emphasizes the importance of feeling loved and cared about by others as the central element in the protective effect of social support. Proponents of this position argue that if the person has close and caring relationships, these individuals can be counted on to provide support; if that is not possible, they will assist the person to find others to provide the necessary support. Basic to this view is the idea that feeling loved and cared about will enhance the person's own self-efficacy, threat appraisal, and coping repertoire (Sarason, Shearin, Pierce, & Sarason, 1987).

Some evidence suggests that social support defined in this way may best be conceptualized as a personality variable. Sarason et al. (1986) have shown that both perceived available social support and satisfaction with that support are quite stable over several years, even if those years encompass a significant developmental transition with consequent changes in network membership.

This view of social support stems, in part, from Bowlby's (1969, 1979, 1980) work on attachment and deals with the working models people develop about themselves and about relationships as a result of early experience. A number of studies have demonstrated a relationship between perceived social support and both an individual's perceptions of others and his or her evaluation of their own experiences. For a more complete discussion of this view of perceived social support see Sarason et al. (1990).

When support is investigated as a protection against the negative effects of stress, the source of the stress as well as the sources of support must be considered. For instance, resistance to stress in the workplace is associated to a greater degree with support perceived to be available from those associated with the work environment than that from family or friends (Holahan & Moos, 1982).

Functional Support

Early in the history of work on social support, a number of influential papers delineated the functions that social support provides as a contributor to well-being or health (Cobb, 1976; Kaplan et al., 1977; Weiss, 1974).

The idea of investigating the effects of social support in terms of the specific needs would appear to be useful not only in understanding how support functions promote health and prevent disorder, but in clarifying how effective interventions might be carried out. A number of researchers have espoused this point of view and have constructed instruments designed to measure the functional components of support. Among these measures that are focused on perceived support are the Interpersonal Support Evaluation List (ISEL; Cohen, Mermelstein, Karmack, & Hoberman, 1985) and the Social Provisions Scale (SPS; Cutrona & Russell, 1987). Cohen and Wills (1985) have theorized that the buffering effect of social support, in which it serves to insulate or partially protect those who are vulnerable from the effects of stress, is a function of the match between the need engendered by the stressor and the type of support given. They believe that mismatched support is the reason that many research efforts have produced conflicting findings concerning buffering. Cutrona and Russell (1987) have presented the results of programmatic research with the SPS that they believe demonstrates how the support functions needed differ with developmental status and life situation.

Other researchers have not been as satisfied with the functional approach, at least as these and other current instruments measure the different functions (House & Kahn, 1985; Orth-Gomér & Undén, 1987; Sarason et al., 1987; Stokes, 1983). The problem with existing functional instruments is that the scales measuring the different functions are usually very highly correlated. At times, the intercorrelations among the functional subscales of these instruments are as high as the subscale reliabilities, which suggests that the subscales may not be assessing distinct measures. Even if the measure's subscales have been derived through a factor analytic procedure, the high intercorrelations among factors suggest the possibility that a general social support factor underlies the different components of social support. At best, what seems to emerge is that most of the scales measure emotional support and that this may sometimes be differentiated from tangible support.

Some researchers take a different point of view of highly correlated subscales. For instance, Brookings and Bolton (1988) argue for the ISEL (a measure constructed rationally rather than empirically) that although the intercorrelations of the subscales suggest a common factor of general support, the use of this instrument as a undimensional scale results in the loss of unique information from the subscales. This view, while appealing, should be adopted with caution. As yet these researchers have not demonstrated that the unique variance associated with each scale has a *meaningful* relationship with other variables. In addition, demonstrating that each subscale has unique, reliable variance is insufficient to establish the construct validity of these scales. Further research is needed to indicate that each subscale measures the unique aspects of the functional support construct it is intended to assess.

Measures of functional support and measures that describe the structural and qualitative aspects of support were found by Broadhead et al. (1983) to have a minimal correlation. Unlike functional measures, structural measures have been convincingly demonstrated to predict adverse health outcomes, generally defined as all-cause mortality (Orth-Gomér & Undén, 1987). Thus, at present, the functional approach to the assessment of social support remains an intriguing possibility that has yet to be realized. (See Chapter 9 for further discussion of this issue.)

Psychometric Qualities of Measures and Research Outcomes

Questionnaires and other assessment tools devised to measure social support differ not only in theoretical viewpoint and in the nature of the support evaluated, but also in length, format, and sensitivity to different portions of the distributions of scores. Even more important, these measurement instruments vary greatly in the amount and type of validity and reliability information available. Although researchers may appreciate, in the abstract, the importance of the reliability and validity of instruments they use, often these factors are not adequately attended to when assessment tools are chosen. In addition, it is important to evaluate the format of the measures to be used in light of the research questions to be answered. In this section we will briefly comment on each of these issues.

Reliability

In any research project, selection of reliable instruments should be of primary concern. This is specially true when the relationships among variables are expected to be in the moderate range, so that at most about one quarter of the variability will be explained. When error is involved in the measurement of either or both variables of interest, the correlation between them is attenuated. This means that the chances of observing a significant relationship between two variables, even if one actually exists, are greatly diminished when either of the measures is of low reliability. The observed correlation between two measures is equal to the true correlation between the measures (if there were no error in measurement) multiplied by the square root of the product of the reliabilities of the two measures:

$$\text{observed correlation}_{ab} = \text{true correlation}_{ab} \sqrt{\text{reliability}_a \times \text{reliability}_b}$$

The impact of this relationship can be seen in Table 1, which was developed by Heitzmann and Kaplan (1988) for a review of social support measures. For purposes of demonstration of the effects of reliability or correlational relationships, they assumed that the maximum true correlation between a social support measure and various outcome measures of interest to health researchers would not exceed .5. This is a conservative assumption, because a variety of sources of variability contribute to most health outcomes. Table 1 illustrates how selected social support measures ranging from high to low in reliability might be expected to correlate with a variety of criterion measures for which estimates of reliability are available. It clearly shows the effect of test reliability on the expected observed correlation and on the expected significance for a study with 50 subjects. For instance, the table shows that if the true correlation were .5, the correlation of the outcome measures with the SSQN (with a reliability of .97) would be significant in all but one case. At the other extreme, the SSS measure (with a reliability of .28) would produce no significant observed correlations with the criterion measures. A review of Table 1 clearly demonstrates how investigators may set themselves on an almost

Table 1.   Correlations between Selected Social Support
and Health-Related Criterion Measures Differing in Reliability

	Health-related measure				
Social support measures	OARS Mental Health Questionnaire (.32)	Clinical ratings (.41)	Schedule of recent events (.55)	Blood pressure (.65)	Sickness Impact Profile (.97)
SSQ-N (.97)	.278	.32[a]	.37[a]	.40[a]	.48[a]
SSSS short form (.69)	.24	.27	.31[a]	.33[a]	.41[a]
ASSIS support need measure (.52)	.20	.23	.27	.29[a]	.36[a]
SSS (1968 items; .28)	.15	.17	.20	.21	.26

[a]If $r \geq .2818$, then $p < .05$.
Note: Measures of social support—SSQ-N-Social Support Questionnaire = Number (Sarason, Levine, Basham, & Sarason, 1983); SSSS short form = Social Support Satisfaction Scale (Blaik & Genser, 1980); ASSIS = Arizona Social Support Interview Schedule (Barrera, Sandler, & Ramsey, 1981); SSS = Social Support Scales (Dean, Lin, & Ensel, 1981). Reliability estimates for health measures—OARS (Mental Health Questionnaire of the Older American Research and Service Center Instrument; Fillenbaum, 1978); clinical ratings (Bergner, Bobbit, Carter, & Gilson, 1981); Schedule of Recent Events (Holmes & Rahe, 1967); blood pressure (Hypertension Detection and Follow-Up Program Cooperative Group, 1979); Sickness Impact Profile (Bergner et al., 1981).
Source: "Assessment of Methods for Measuring Social Support," by C. A. Heitzmann and R. M. Kaplan, 1988, Health Psychology, 7, p. 102. Copyright 1988 by Lawrence Erlbaum Associates. Adapted by permission.

inevitable course toward a lack of results if they fail to select measures with adequate reliability.

Because the true relationship of variables cannot usually be estimated closely in the early stages of research on a particular problem, lack of attention to the reliability of assessment instruments can lead researchers to conclude that little relationship exists between variables, not as a function of the true relationship, but because of inadequate measurement. As Heitzmann and Kaplan point out many standard medical measurements are actually not highly reliable so that it is even more important that the psychological assessment measures be of high reliability.

As a general rule, a measure of social support should have a reliability coefficient of at least .80; at that level, random error does not severely effect the correlations obtained. At times an investigator may wish, for reasons of ease of administration or other considerations, to select an instrument of lower reliability. If this is done, however, it should be borne in mind that the outcome measure must have a high reliability to be able to detect relationships. The important thing to remember is that the reliability of the measures used should be known and the data interpreted with the reliabilities in mind.

The most useful method of computing reliability is the coefficient alpha, which assesses the internal consistency of a measure. It is easy to compute and requires only one test administration; the minimal effort necessary for its computation is far outweighed by the information it gives about the reliability of the scale. Not only should the internal reliability of existing instruments selected for assessment be known, but alphas also should be computed for any groups of questions that the investigator may intend to sum together.

Another form of reliability, stability of scores over time (most often termed test-retest reliability) may also be important. Clearly stability over time is important in the short term, but whether this characteristic is desirable in a measure over the longer term is less clear. For instance, the issue arises as to whether social support should be viewed as an enduring characteristic of a person. Until we know more about the answer to this question, measures that have some sensitivity to changes over time should be sought in some research situations.

Validity

Validity serves to define what inferences can be made as a result of the score on a measure. It is important to remember strictly speaking, it is not the test that is validated, but rather the test in relation to the purpose for which it is being used (Cronbach, 1971). It is possible to have a measurement instrument that is valid for assessing one type of variable but not at all valid for another. Several types of validity are often discussed, but not all are equally relevant in the social sciences and in particular for the assessment of social support. *Criterion* or *predictive validity* refers to how well the instrument can be used to predict a particular behavioral outcome. Predictive validity can be completely atheoretical; if college grades were predicted well by speed of finger tapping, that measure would have criterion validity. In the social sciences, criterion validity is often not a useful construct because no useful criterion variables exist. For example, what is the criterion for social support? There is likely to be no specific type of behavior in the subject that can be used to validate a measure of social support. Instead, it is necessary to formulate a set of items that reflect the content of the specific theoretical construct. Like criterion validity, however, the concept of *content validity* is not particularly useful in the social sciences because the concepts of interest are abstract phenomena for which it is difficult to agree on a definition of the universe of content. Clear agreement on content validity may be possible in measuring a particular reading or arithmetic skill (e.g., comprehension or addition), but not in the case of an abstract, theoretically derived variable such as social support.

Because of the limited usefulness of both criterion and content validity in assessing the theoretical constructs of the social sciences, primary attention has been focused on *construct validity*. Construct validity demands a theoretical basis because it rests on making theoretical predictions that lead to empirical tests of the relatedness of operationally defined measures of the construct involved. First, the researcher must define the construct and operationalize it in terms of an assessment instrument. Establishing construct validity for the instrument then involves three steps: (a) specification of theoretical relationships between the constructs of interest, (b) examination of the empirical relationship between the assessment instrument and a measure (or measures) of one or more of the theoretically related concepts, and (c) interpretation of the empirical evidence to determine whether it supports the theoretical predictions. If the measures relate in a theoretically predictable way, the next step is to gather both convergent and discriminant evidence about the instrument.

Convergent validity is demonstrated by establishing the dimensions of the relationship between the measure and a variety of other measures that are hypothesized to be similar. Discriminant validity is established by showing that the scores produced by the measure differ from those of other measures defined by a different set of criteria. Discriminant validity is crucial because it provides evidence that the measure of social support is not confounded with other factors such as neuroticism, depression, or social desirability. Developers of some social support instruments have provided evidence of convergent and construct validity for these measures, but only a few have dealt with discriminant validity (Cutrona & Russell, 1987; Heitzmann & Kaplan, 1988).

Issues Related to Test Format

In the selection of an instrument to measure social support, the researcher is always faced with conflicting demands for efficiency, practicality, and psychometric soundness. For many uses the measure should be brief, simple, and easily administered; however, for each of these virtues a price may have to be paid. For example a measure consisting of only one or a few items is likely to lack adequate test-retest reliability.

Measures that have a yes-no format rather than allowing for more gradations of response may produce data that are not normally distributed, thus making data analysis difficult. A yes-no format is likely to produce a skewed distribution that reduces the sensitivity of the measure in either the high or low group. Even if the researcher can meet the assumptions of the necessary statistical tests through transformations or can afford to ignore some of the requirements because of the use of a very large sample, it is important that any lack of sensitivity not fall in the part of the distribution of greatest research interest. For example, if the study is focused on those generally lacking in social support, then if the scale lacks sensitivity at the high end because the distribution is negatively skewed, the situation is not too serious. But if the researcher is interested in the possible deleterious effects of the receipt of a great deal of support, this same lack of sensitivity in a measure of received support would greatly affect the chance of answering the research question.

Another format issue is the use of open-ended response measures. Although these may enrich the interpretation of the data, without an effective scoring system not only is the data analysis cumbersome, but the reliability with which the responses are classified may be a concern.

It is important to assess instruments under consideration in terms of the educational background, age, and gender of the potential respondents, as well as the cultural context in which the assessment will be carried out. The respondents should perceive the questions as clear, easily interpretable, and appropriate in terms of the stated purpose of the research; the instructions should be easily understood, and the response alternatives should be clear and unambiguous. Another important factor, especially in large epidemiological surveys, is that some types of items—particularly those found in instruments that assess the functions of support—may be inapplicable to some cultural contexts (Orth-Gomér & Undén, 1987). For example, an item such as "If I need to get to the airport, I can count on

someone to give me a ride" may be inappropriate for many rural populations or areas outside of the United States.

Relationship among Social Support Instruments

There is little information about the relationships among scores on
different types of measures of social support. Sarason et al. (1987) carried
out a series of three studies in an attempt to clarify the overlap in the wide
variety of definitions of social support. They compared the scores of the
same individuals on several measures derived from the various viewpoints
described above. These studies also assessed the similarity or dissimilarity
of relationships of each of these social support measures with a variety of
other variables. Table 2 lists the social support instruments used and
briefly describes the perspective of each as well as its general format.

The first of the three studies compared measures of received support
as measured by the Inventory of Socially Supportive Behaviors (ISSB;
Barrera, Sandler, & Ramsey, 1981), perceived support as measured by the
Social Support Questionnaire (SSQ; Sarason et al., 1983), and a social
network measure, the Social Network List (SNL; Stokes, 1983). There was
very little relationship between the ISSB and the SNL, but a moderate
correlation of each with the SSQ. Table 3 shows the interrelationships of
some of the scales of these measures. The ISSB and the SNL also tended to
have quite small correlations with individual-difference measures for
attachment, social anxiety, social desirability, shyness, and loneliness
compared to the relationships of those variables to the SSQ.

The second study compared several measures of perceived support.
These included the SSQ, the Interpersonal Support Evaluation List (ISEL;
Cohen et al., 1985), and the Perceived Social Support from Friends and
Family instrument (PSS; Procidano & Heller, 1983). There were generally
high correlations among the scales of these measures. Although the
measures have much in common, a multivariate analysis of the relations
among them demonstrated they are differentially sensitive to parts of the
continuum defined by the satisfaction score of the SSQ. This difference
seemed attributable to the format differences among the three questionnaires and to gender differences in response patterns. In general, these
three measures of perceived support related quite similarly to individual-
difference variables of depression and anxiety, although the similarity was
greater for men than for women.

In the third study, two methodologically different data-gathering
techniques—a questionnaire (SSQ) and a structured interview, the Interview Schedule for Social Interaction (ISSI; Henderson, Byrne, Duncan-

Table 2. Social Support Instruments Compared in Three Studies

Instrument	Type of support assessed	Assessment procedure
Interpersonal Support Evaluation List (Cohen et al., 1985)	Measures the perceived availability of tangible support, appraisal support, self-esteem support, and belonging support	48-item questionnaire (12 items per scale) that uses yes/no format[a]
Inventory Schedule for Social Interation (Henderson et al., 1980)	Assesses both the perceived availability and perceived adequacy for each of two dimensions: attachment and social integration	52-item structured interview that codes subjects' responses on a variety of scales
Inventory of Socially Supportive Behaviors (Barrera et al., 1981)	Measures the frequency of received supportive behaviors in the past month	40-item questionnaire using scale (from "not at all" to "every day")
Perceived Social Support from Friends and Family (Procidano & Heller, 1983)	Measures the subject's perceptions of the extent to which family and friends fulfill the individual's need for support, information, and feedback	Two 20-item scales that use yes/no/don't know format
Social Network List (Stokes, 1983)	Assesses the subject's perceived social network on characteristics including size, density, and number (and percentage) of friends, relatives, and confidants	Subjects complete a matrix for up to 20 network members, indicating the member's relationship to the subject and to the other members
Social Support Questionnaire (Sarason et al., 1983)	Measures the number (N) of perceived available supports and satisfaction (S) with perceived available support	Questionnaire format, subjects list up to 9 available supports for each of 27 items on a 6-point scale[b]

[a]A revised form of the ISEL with a 4-point Likert scale response mode is now available.
[b]A short form of the SSQ with a 6-item format is now available (Sarason, Sarason, Shearin, & Pierce, 1987).

Jones, & Scott, 1980)—were compared. Table 4 shows the relationships among the scales of these measures. The ISSI availability scales correlated reasonably well with the SSQ scales. The ISSI adequacy scales, which had been expected to have a relationship with the satisfaction scale of the SSQ, showed little correlation with that scale. As in the prior study, characteristics of the test may have had an effect on the outcome. The adequacy

Table 3.   Intercorrelations of Social
Support Measures in Study 1

	Variable				
	1	2	3	4	5
SSQ					
1. Number of supports		$.51^b$	$.28^b$	$.43^b$	.08
2. Satisfaction with support			$.24^b$	$.15^a$	$.16^a$
ISSB					
3. Total score				$.17^a$	.13
SNL					
4. Network size					$-.02$
5. Network density					

$^a p < .05$, two tailed
$^b p < .001$, two tailed
Note: $N = 194$ to 206; SSQ = Social Support Questionnaire; ISSB = Inventory of Socially Supportive Behaviors; SNL = Social Network Test
Source: "Interrelations of Social Support Measures: Theoretical and Practical Implications," by B. R. Sarason, E. N. Shearin, G. R. Pierce, & I. G. Sarason, 1987, Journal of Personality and Social Psychology, 52, p. 817. Copyright 1987 by American Psychological Association. Adapted by permission.

Table 4.   Intercorrelations of Questionnaire (SSQ)
and Interview (ISSI) Measures of Social Support

	Variable					
	1	2	3	4	5	6
ISSI						
1. Attachment availability		$.44^b$	$.48^c$	.13	$.52^c$	.23
2. Attachment adequacy			.20	$.65^c$	.17	.04
3. Social integration availability				.14	$.63^c$	$.36^a$
4. Social integration adequacy					.15	$.32^a$
SSQ						
5. Number of supports						$.45^b$
6. Satisfaction with supports						

$^a p < .05$, two tailed
$^b p < .01$, two tailed
$^c p < .001$, two tailed
Note: $N = 40$ to 42; ISSI = Interview Schedule for Social Interaction; SSQ = Social Support Questionnaire.
Source: "Interrelations of Social Support Measures: Theoretical and Practical Implications," by B. R. Sarason, E. N. Shearin, G. R. Pierce, & I. G. Sarason, 1987, Journal of Personality and Social Psychology, 52, p. 828. Copyright 1987 by American Psychological Association. Adapted by permission.

measures of the ISSI are focused on a single individual for each type of support situation. In the SSQ the satisfaction score is derived from the general satisfaction with the support perceived to be available from all persons mentioned in response to each item.

Clearly, any one study can compare only a small number of social support measures. Some researchers have compared two different instruments in the course of a study (see Sandler & Barrera, 1984; Stokes & Wilson, 1984). As in the studies reported above, the general finding in these latter studies has been moderate to low correlation between measures, depending on the similarity of the definition of social support and of the format of the measures.

Perhaps the most useful way to integrate what is presently known is to view social support as a complex construct that involves several components. These components include at least three subconstructs: (a) the degree of embeddedness in a supportive network and the characteristics of that network, (b) actual interactions that are at least intended by the originator to be supportive, and (c) the beliefs and perceptions of support held by the individual. Each of these definitions provides a legitimate basis for measuring social support. At present, however, the links between them and the relationship of each to physical and mental well-being are not clearly elucidated. The problem is not the choice between these definitions; the error that some researchers have made is a failure to recognize these distinctions and to separate them clearly in their empirical work. This confusion has contributed to many of the disparities in research findings. One of the most valuable contributions this chapter might make is to encourage researchers first to clarify which aspects of social support are relevant to the questions they are asking and then to select a measure that reflects these. At some time in the future, each of these views of social support may be given a distinctive label, but until that time a clear definition of what is measured may help to make clear the meaning of the findings reported.

What Should Govern the Choice of a Social Support Measure

As the study comparing social support measures suggests, instruments derived from the different perspectives of social support do not measure the same thing. Even instruments derived from the same perspective may produce different results depending upon the format of each. Based on this knowledge, researchers need to do several things. First, they need to make themselves aware of the variety of social support measures available and to learn as much as possible about the psychometric characteristics of those instruments. Although the number of existing social support measures is large, only a relatively few measures have sufficient psychometric information available. Several reviews of instruments for which some psychometric data exist are available (Bruhn & Phillips, 1984; Heitzmann & Kaplan, 1988; House & Kahn, 1985; O'Reilly, 1988; Orth-Gomér & Undén, 1987; Rock, Green, Wise, & Rock, 1984; Tardy, 1985). Of these, Heitzmann and Kaplan (1988) present a particularly valuable discussion of the implications of the psychometric characteristics of the instruments, and Orth-Gomer and Unden focus on the measures they review in terms of their potentially applicability to population surveys. (See Chapter 9 for a discussion of these issues with regard to cardiovascular disease studies.)

How social support is conceptualized and measured may be highly relevant to the particular end point of interest to the researchers. For example, Blazer (1982) found that the magnitude of the relationship between social support and risk of mortality over a 30-month period depended on the definition of support. A measure of perceived support was more strongly related to mortality than support defined either as frequency of interaction with friends and family or in terms of availability of roles and attachment (i.e., number of living children and siblings, marital status). Antonucci and Israel (1986) also found that people's appraisal of the support available to them may be even more important than their actual interpersonal contacts. For certain end points, though, actual support might be as pertinent or more pertinent than perceived support. A homebound elderly person might need both a general feeling of being loved and valued by children who live in another city and actual help with chores twice a week.

A final decision about which measure of social support is most appropriate for a particular project requires thinking through which aspects of social support fit most logically with particular indices of health, well-being, and personal adjustment. When theory does not dictate selection of the measure of social support most appropriate for a given study, pilot work comparing different types of measures will often prove useful in making the selection. The important point is that work on social support has developed sufficiently so that researchers cannot be satisfied using just any index.

The framing of the researcher question has important implications for the choice of measure of social support in cardiovascular research. Some relationships or lack of relationships that are already found in the literature should be helpful in determining the definition of social support that may be most relevant. For instance, measures of network size seem in general to be unrelated to health outcome. Measures of social integration predict white male mortality from all causes, but weaker relationships between this measure and mortality have been found for nonwhite groups (for summaries, see Berkman & Seeman, 1986; House, Landis, & Umberson, 1988). The relationships between mortality risk and social integration that have been found are most robust in the most socially isolated segment of the male group. Mortality risk among men who have had at least one myocardial infarction is also predicted by measures of social integration (Rubberman, Weinblatt, Goldberg, & Chaudhary, 1984). A clear relationship for women between social integration and mortality has only been found in one of the three large epidemiological studies that allowed comparison of risks for men and women (the Alameda County Study; Berkman & Syme, 1979). Measures of social integration may be less valid not only for women but also for rural and small-town environments as opposed to urban settings (House et al., 1988).

When the chosen end point is morbidity, a measure of social integration does not appear to be a useful predictor; measures of perceived social support have a better chance of showing associations with the development of disorder. For instance, Seeman and Syme (1987) found that the feeling of being loved (despite its measurement by a single item and thus its lessened reliability) was the most significant predictor of coronary artery disease among three social support measures when all other risk factors were taken into account. Network instrumental support was somewhat less strong as a predictor, and problem-oriented emotional support had no significant relationship with the outcome measure. This study illustrates the value of using several different definitions of social support in attempting to clarify its relationship with cardiovascular disease.

Measures of received support are confounded with stressful life events, because people who experience such events generally receive more support on that account. If a measure of received support is used, a measure of life events should also be included. It may also be wide to include measures of personality variables that are or may be related to increased risk. For example, a measure of Type A tendencies might be important in understanding what is often a complex relationship between social support and coronary artery disease (Blumenthal et al., 1987).

In addition to the importance of developing a theoretical basis for selection of a social support instrument, the use of a measure with adequate reliability is clearly essential. Both Heitzmann and Kaplan (1988) and O'Reilly (1988) provide conveniently organized information on reliability and also aspects of validity for a wide variety of social support measures. If at all possible, researchers should avoid creating their own ad hoc measures and also should attempt to go beyond single items in a questionnaire as a way to establish level of social support. Finally, although proof of the relationship between coronary heart disease and social relationships is probably stronger than the evidence was for Type A behavior when it was certified as a risk factor—and is approaching the level that established cigarette smoking as a risk factor for a range of diseases (House et al., 1988)—better theory and data are needed to establish the links in this relationship. One of the best ways to improve this situation, in addition to following the guidelines on reliable instruments above, is to utilize a variety of definitions of social support contemporaneously in order to understand better which are related to coronary heart disease and under what circumstances. The most beneficial aspect of this approach will be to develop a broader theory of the role of social support by clearly distinguishing which aspects of the omnibus concept are relevant in the linking of social relationships and heart disease, and to provide clues as to what the mechanisms might be that are responsible for this link.

References

Antonucci, T. C., & Israel, B. (1986). Veridicality of social support: A comparison of principal and network members' responses. *Journal of Consulting and Clinical Psychology 54*, 432–437.

Auerbach, S. M., & Kilmann, P. R. (1977). Crisis intervention: A review of outcome research. *Psychological Bulletin, 84*, 1189–1217.

Barrera, M. J., Sandler, I. N., & Ramsey, T. B. (1981). Preliminary development of a scale of social support: Studies of college students. *American Journal of Community Psychology, 9*, 435–447.

Bergner, M., Bobbit, R. A., Carter, W. B., & Gilson, B. S. (1981). The Sickness Impact Profile: Development and final revision of a health status measure. *Medical Care, 19*, 898–806.

Berkman, L. F., & Seeman, T. (1986). The influence of social relationships on aging and the development of cardiovascular disease—a review. *Postgraduate Medical Journal, 62*, 805–807.

Berkman, L. F., & Syme, S. L. (1979). Social networks, host resistance, and mortality: A nine-year follow-up study of Alameda County residents. *American Journal of Epidemiology, 109*, 186–204.

Blaik, R., & Genser, S. G. (1980). Perception of social support satisfaction: Scale development. *Personality and Social Psychology Bulletin, 6*, 172.

Blazer, D. G. (1982). Social support and mortality in an elderly community population. *American Journal of Epidemiology, 115*, 684–694.

Blumenthal, J. A., Burg, M. M., Barefoot, J., Williams, R. G., Haney, T., & Zimet, G. (1987). Social support, Type A behavior, and coronary artery disease. *Psychosomatic Medicine, 49*, 331–339.

Bowlby, J. (1969). *Attachment and loss; vol. 1: Attachment*. New York: Basic Books.

Bowlby, J. (1979). The making and breaking of affectional bonds. *British Journal of Psychiatry, 130*, 201–210.

Bowlby, J. (1980). *Attachment and loss; vol 3: Loss, sadness and depression*. New York: Basic Books.

Broadhead, W. E., Kaplan, B. H., James, S. A., Wagner, E. H., Schoenbach, V. S., Grimson, R., Heyden, S., Tibblin, G., & Gehlbach, S. (1983). The epidemiologic evidence for a relationship between social support and health. *American Journal of Epidemiology, 117*, 521–537.

Brookings, J. B., & Bolton, B. (1988). Confirmatory factor analysis of the Interpersonal Support Evaluation List. *American Journal of Community Psychology, 16*, 137–147.

Bruhn, J. G., & Phillips, B. U. (1984). Measuring social support: A synthesis of current approaches. *Journal of Behavioral Medicine, 7*, 151–169.

Cobb, S. (1976). Social support as a moderator of life stress. *Psychosomatic Medicine, 38*, 300–314.

Cohen, S., Mermelstein, R., Karmack, T., & Hoberman, H. N. (1985). Measuring the functional components of social support. In I. G. Sarason & B. R. Sarason (Eds.), *Social support: Theory, research and applications*. Dordrecht, Netherlands: Martinus Nijhoff.

Cohen, S., & Wills, T. A. (1985). Stress, social support, and the buffering hypothesis. *Psychological Bulletin, 98*, 310–357.

Cooley, C. H. (1909). *Social organization: A study of the larger mind*. New York: Scribner.

Cooper, M. L. (1986). *The role of supportive transactions and perceived functional support as stress buffers*. Unpublished doctoral dissertation, University of California, Santa Cruz.

Cronbach, L. J. (1971). Test validation. In R. L. Thorndike (Ed.), *Educational measurement*. Washington, DC: American Council on Education.

Cummins, R. C. (1987). Perceptions of social support, receipt of supportive behaviors and locus of control as moderators of chronic stress, *American Journal of Community Psychology, 16*, 685–700.

Cutrona, C. E., & Russell, D. W. (1987). The provisions of social relationships and adaptation to stress. *Advances in Personal Relationships, 1*, 37–67.

Dean, A., Lin, N., & Ensel, W. M. (1981). The epidemiological significance of social support systems in depression. *Research in Community Mental Health, 2*, 77–109.

Durkheim, E. (1951). *Suicide: A study in sociology* (J. A. Spaulding & G. Simpson, Trans.). New York: Free Press.

Fillenbaum, G. G. (1978). Validity and reliability of the Multidimensional Functional Assessment Questionnaire. In E. Pfeiffer (Ed.), *Multidimensional functional assessment: The OARS methodology*. Durham, NC: Duke University, Center of the Study of Aging and Human Development.

Gallo, F. (1982). The effects of social support network on the health of the elderly. *Social Work in Health Care, 8*(2), 65–74.

Gore, S. (1978). The effects of social support in moderating the health consequences of unemployment. *Journal of Health and Social Behavior, 19*, 157–165.

Heitzmann, C. A., & Kaplan, R. M. (1988). Assessment of methods for measuring social support. *Health Psychology, 7*, 75–109.

Henderson, S. (1984). Interpreting the evidence on social support. *Social Psychiatry, 19*, 49–52.

Henderson, S., Byrne, D. G., Duncan-Jones, P., & Scott, R. (1980). Measuring social relationships: The Interview Schedule for Social Interactions. *Psychological Medicine, 10*, 723–734.

Hirsch, B. (1980). Natural support systems and coping with major life changes. *American Journal of Community Psychology, 8*, 159–172.

Holahan, C. J., & Moos, R. H. (1982). Social support and adjustment: Predictive benefits of social class indices. *American Journal of Community Psychology, 10*, 403–413.

Holmes, T. H., & Rahe, R. H. (1967). The Social Readjustment Rating Scale. *Journal of Psychosomatic Research, 11*, 213–218.

House, J. S., & Kahn, R. L. (1985). Measures and concepts of social support. In S. Cohen & S. L. Syme (Eds.), *Social support and health*. Orlando: Academic Press.

House, J. S., Landis, K. R., & Umberson, D. (1988). Social relationships and health. *Science, 241*, 540–545.

House, J. S., Robbins, C., & Metzner, H. L. (1982). The association of social relationships and activities with mortality: Prospective evidence from the Tecumseh Community Health Study. *American Journal of Epidemiology, 116*, 123–140.

Hypertension Detection and Follow-Up Program Cooperative Group. (1979). Five year find-ings of the Hypertension Detection and Follow-up Program: I. Reduction in mortality of persons with high blood pressure, including mild hypertension. *Journal of the American Medical Association, 242,* 2562–2571.

Israel, B. A. (1982). Social networks and health status: Linking theory, research and practice. *Patient Counseling and Health Education, 4,* 65–79.

Kaplan, B. H., Cassel, J., & Gore, S. (1977). Social support and health. *Medical Care, 15,* 47–58.

Levitt, M. J. (1991). Attachment and close relationships: A life span perspective. In J. L. Gewirtz & W. F. Kurtines (Eds.), *Intersections with attachment.* Hillsdale, NJ: Erlbaum.

Likert, R. (1961). *New patterns of management.* New York: McGraw-Hill.

Lin, N., Dean, A., & Ensel, W. (Eds.). (1986). *Social support, life events, and depression.* Orlando, FL: Academic Press.

McCormick, I. A., Siegert, R. J., & Walkey, F. H. (1987). Dimensions of social support: A factorial confirmation. *American Journal of Community Psychology, 15,* 73–77.

Nuckolls, K. G., Cassell, J., & Kaplan, B. H. (1972). Psychosocial assets, life crises, and the prognosis of pregnancy. *American Journal of Epidemiology, 95,* 431–441.

O'Reilly, P. (1988). Methodological issues in social support and social network research. *Social Science and Medicine, 8,* 863–873.

Orth-Gomér, K., & Undén, A. L. (1987). The measurement of social support in population surveys. *Social Science and Medicine, 24,* 83–94.

Pilisuk, M., & Parks, S. H. (1986). *The healing web.* Hanover, NH: University Press of New England.

Procidano, M. E., & Heller, K. (1983). Measures of perceived social support from friends and from family: Three validation studies. *American Journal of Community Psychology, 11,* 1–24.

Rock, D. L., Green, K. E., Wise, B. K., & Rock, R. D. (1984). Social support and social network scales: A psychometric review. *Research in Nursing and Health, 7,* 325–332.

Rogers, C. R. (1942). *Counseling and psychotherapy.* Boston: Houghton-Mifflin.

Rosenberg, M. R. (1985). *Social support: Mechanisms of action and stressor-support specificity.* Doctoral dissertation, Southern Illinois University, Carbondale.

Rubberman, W., Weinblatt, E., Goldberg, J. D., & Chaudhary, B. S. (1984). Psychosocial influences on mortality after myocardial infarction. *New England Journal of Medicine, 311,* 522–559.

Sandler, I. N., & Barrera, M., Jr. (1984). Toward a multimethod approach to assessing the effects of social support. *American Journal of Community Psychology, 12,* 37–52.

Sarason, B. R., Pierce, G. R., & Sarason, I. G. (1990). Social support: The sense of acceptance and the role of relationships. In B. R. Sarason, I. G. Sarason, & G. R. Pierce (Eds.), *Social support: An interactive view.* New York: Wiley.

Sarason, B. R., Shearin, E. N., Pierce, G. R., & Sarason, I. G. (1987). Interrelations of social support measures: Theoretical and practical implications. *Journal of Personality and Social Psychology, 52,* 813–832.

Sarason, I. G., Sarason, B. R., & Shearin, E. N. (1986). Social support as an individual difference variable: Its stability, origins, and relational aspects. *Journal of Personality and Social Psychology, 50,* 845–855.

Sarason, I. G., Levine, H. M., Basham, R. B., & Sarason, B. R. (1983). Assessing social support: The Social Support Questionnaire. *Journal of Personality and Social Psychology, 44,* 127–139.

Sarason, I. G., Sarason, B. R., Shearin, E. N., & Pierce, G. R. (1987). A brief measure of social support: Practical and theoretical implications. *Journal of Social and Personal Relationships, 4,* 497–510.

Seeman, T. E., & Syme, S. L. (1987). Social networks and coronary artery disease: A comparison of the structure and function of social relations as predictors of disease. *Psychosomatic Medicine, 49,* 341–354.

Stokes, J. P. (1983). Predicting satisfaction with social support from social network structure. *American Journal of Community Psychology, 11,* 141–152.

Stokes, J. P., & Wilson, D. G. (1984). The Inventory of Socially Supportive Behaviors: Dimensionality, prediction, and gender differences. *American Journal of Community Psychology, 12,* 53–69.

Tardy, C. H. (1985). Social support measurement. *American Journal of Community Psychology, 13,* 187–202.

Vaux, A., & Harrison, D. (1985). Support network characteristics associated with support satisfaction and perceived support. *American Journal of Community Psychology, 13,* 245–267.

Ward, R. A., Sherman, S. R., & LaGory, M. (1984). Subjective network assessments and subjective well-being. *Journal of Gerontology, 39,* 93–101.

Weiss, R. S. (1974). The provisions of social relationships. In Z. Rubin (Ed.), *Doing unto others.* Englewood Cliffs, NJ: Prentice-Hall.

Wellman, B. (1981). Applying network analysis to the study of support. In B. Gottlieb (Ed.), *Social networks and social support.* Beverly Hills, CA: Sage.

Wethington, E., & Kessler, R. C. (1986). Perceived support, received support, and adjustment to stressful life events. *Journal of Health and Social Behavior, 27,* 78–89.

Whitcher, S. J., & Fisher, J. D. (1979). Multidimensional reaction to therapeutic touch in a hospital setting. *Journal of Personality and Social Psychology, 36,* 87–96.

Wilcox, B. L. (1981). Social support, life stress, and psychological adjustment: A test of the buffering hypothesis. *American Journal of Community Psychology, 9,* 371–386.

CHAPTER 4

Measures of Health Outcome in Social Support Research

Robert M. Kaplan

A wide variety of papers link social support to health outcomes (see Berkman, 1984; Broadhead et al., 1983; Wallston, Alagna, DeVellis, & DeVellis, 1983). Stressful life events in the personal, social, occupational, or marital realms may have important consequences, and social support may soften the impact of these events. Wallston et al. (1983) suggest that social support is a crucial factor in coping with physical disability and illness. Family, friends, and other social contacts aid in the reduction of emotional distress and problems resulting from illness or injury (Davidson, Bowden, & Tholen, 1979; Porrit, 1979).

The notion that social support enhances health outcomes is widely embraced in the medical, public health, and psychological literatures (Cohen & Syme, 1985). Systematic investigation of this problem, however, is hampered for several reasons. First, measures of social support have varied from study to study; even the definition of social support has been quite inconsistent (Heitzmann & Kaplan, 1988). A second and perhaps more disturbing problem is that few studies relating social support to health have considered the complex issues in assessing health status. This chapter reviews some of the measurement issues that complicate studies relating social support to health outcome. First, I consider issues in the measurement of social support, and then review the measures that social support scales have been validated against. Consideration is also given to

ROBERT M. KAPLAN • Division of Health Care Sciences, Department of Family and Preventive Medicine, University of California, San Diego, La Jolla, California 92093-0622.

Social Support and Cardiovascular Disease, edited by Sally A. Shumaker and Susan M. Czajkowski. Plenum Press, New York, 1994.

the conceptualization and measurement of health outcomes, and problems in relating health status measures to social support measures will be simulated. Finally, directions for future research are suggested.

The Conceptualization and Measurement of Social Support

Although definitions vary, most measures of social support include tangible components (e.g., financial assistance or physical aid) and intangible components (e.g., encouragement and guidance). As noted above, social support has been implicated in the mediation of stressful life events, recovery from illness, and increased program adherence. Some measures emphasize the instrumental function of social support, whereas others focus on its stress-buffering function.

Heitzmann and Kaplan (1988) reviewed the literature on the assessment of social support and identified at least 23 different measurement techniques. Most of the measures had suitable reliability; however, only about half of the measures had any evidence of validity, defined as the correlation between the measures of social support and well-defined criterion measures. This was particularly problematic for studies concerning the relationship of social support to health, because there are few well-validated measures of health status.

Chapters 2 and 3 in this volume consider the conceptualization and measurement of social support. In concert with Heitzmann and Kaplan (1988), these writings suggest that problems in the conceptualization and measurement of social support still remain. Few studies, however, have seriously considered problems in the conceptualization and measurement of the other side of the equation—health status. Some would question why health measures should be used as validity criteria for measures of social support. The rationale is that social support interventions are justified on the basis of their presumed relationships to health outcomes. Authors repeatedly evoke the social support–health outcome connection in discussions of either direct effects or buffering models. It is the evidence for these support–health relationships that I examine here.

Table 1 provides a summary of scales used as validity criteria for social support measures. The left-hand column of the table lists the social support scale, the next column gives the measure the scale was validated against, and the remaining columns describe the nature of the criterion measure and the association. In the Heitzmann and Kaplan (1988) review, 11 of 23 measures were validated against some external criterion. In three of the studies, measures were validated against other social support measures. In another three studies, they were validated against symptom

Table 1. Summary of Scales Used as Validity Criteria for Social Support Measures

Scale	Validity criterion	Nature of criterion measure	Correlation
Norbeck Social Support Questionnaire Norbeck (1981)	SSQ Schaefer et al., (1981)	Social support scale	-.03 to .56
Personal Resource Questionnaire (PRQ; Brandt & Weinert, 1981)	Family integration measure	Social support scale	.21 to .44
Arizona Social Support Interview Schedule (ASSIS; Berrera 1981a)	Inventory of Socially Supportive Behaviors (ISSB; Berrera, 1981b)	Social support measure	.42 (network size)
Interpersonal Support Evaluation Schedule (ISES; Cohen et al., 1985)	Psychiatric and physical symptoms	Symptom checklists	-.60 with measures of psychiatric symptoms, -.39 with measures of physical symptomatology
Social Relationship Scale (SRS; McFarlane, et al., 1981)	Clinician reports	Clinical judgment	Specific correlations not reported
Interview Schedule for Social Interaction (ISSI; Henderson, et al., 1980)	Eysenck Personality Inventory (EPI)	Personality test	Modest correlation
Social Support Questionnaire (SSQ; Sarason et al., 1983)	Multiple Affect Adjective Checklist (MAACL) and EPI	Adjective checklist and personality test	-.43 between SSQ and MAACL, -.37 between SSQ and ERI (for women)
Social Support Scale (SSS; Lin et al., 1979)	Psychiatric symptoms	Symptom checklist	.36
Perceived Social Support from Friends (PSS-Fr; Procidano & Heller, 1983)	Psychiatric symptomatology	Symptom checklist	Modest negative correlation with psychiatric symptoms
Work Relationship Index (WRI; Billings & Moos, 1982)	Personal functioning	Personality measure	-.33 for men -.15 for women
Diabetes Family Behavior Checklist (DFBC; Schafer et al., 1984)	Adherence with diabetes regimen	Adherence behavior	Significant negative correlations with changes in 3 categories of adherence to diabetic regimen

checklists. In three further studies, the measures were validated against personality tests. One study validated the social support scales against clinical judgments, and in one case social support was validated against self-reported measures of behaviors.

Inspection of Table 1 suggests that social support measures have rarely been validated against widely accepted measures of health status. Most often, when validity data are presented, mental health measures are used as the outcome. For example, McFarlane, Neale, Norman, Rox, and Streiner (1981) validated their social relationship scale against clinical judgments (the specific correlations were not reported). Henderson, Duncan-Jones, Byrne, and Scott (1980) found modest correlations between their interview schedule for social interaction and the Eysenck Personality Inventory. Sarason, Levine, Bashom, and Sarason (1983) found substantial correlations between their social support questionnaire and the Multiple Affect Adjective Check List. Some of the studies used psychiatric symptoms as validity criteria (Cohen, Mermelstein, Kamarck, & Hoberman, 1985; Lin, Simeone, Ensel, & Kuo, 1979; Procidano & Heller, 1983). A few studies used adherence behaviors as an outcome (Schafer, McCaul, and Glasgow, 1984).

As Table 1 suggests, the "health" variables have been inconsistent across studies of social support and health. In order to understand clearly the relationship between social support and health, we need a definition of health status. The next section of this chapter considers health status in more detail.

Measurement of Health Status

The conceptualization and measurement of health status has been of interest to scholars for many decades. Following the Eisenhower administration, a President's Commission on National Goals identified health status measurement as an important objective. Shortly after, John Kenneth Galbraith, in his noted book *The Affluent Society*, described the need to measure the effect of the health care system upon quality of life. In recent years, there have been many attempts to define and measure health status (see Walker & Rosser, 1988; Wenger, Mattson, Furberg, & Elinson, 1984; Bergner, 1985).

The terms *health status, quality of life,* and *health-related quality of life* are often used interchangeably. The term *health status* is often used to describe indicators of health outcome, including mortality rates, disability days, and years of potential life lost. I reserve the term *quality of life* here for indicators that assume some valuation of states of being (see below). I use the term *health-related quality of life* to refer to the impact of health conditions upon the values associated with function, excluding those quality dimensions associated with work, housing, air pollution, and so forth. Before considering any specific approach, it is worth noting that traditional indicators of "health" have well-identified problems.

Mortality

Mortality remains the major outcome measure in most epidemiological studies and clinical trials. Typically, mortality is expressed in the form of a rate, that is the proportion of deaths from a particular cause occurring in some defined time interval (usually per year). Usually, mortality rates are age adjusted. Case fatality rates express the proportion of persons who died of a particular disease divided by the total number with the disease (including those who die and those who live). There are many advantages to reporting mortality rates: They are "hard" data (despite some misclassification bias) and the meaning of the outcome is not difficult to comprehend. But despite these advantages, there are also some obvious limitations. Mortality rates consider only the dead and ignore the living; many important health variables, including social support, might have little or no impact on mortality rates. Some very important illnesses, such as arthritis, are clearly major public health concerns, yet these conditions have relatively little impact upon mortality. Nevertheless, we would not want to conclude that they are unimportant.

Two chapters in this volume consider the relationship between social support and mortality; Chapter 5 reviews the international evidence, whereas Chapter 6 reviews the U.S. evidence. To date, the epidemiological investigations provide the best evidence of the relationship between social support and health outcomes. There is little disagreement that mortality is an important health indicator.

Morbidity

The most common approach to health status assessment is to measure morbidity in terms of function or role performance (e.g., workdays missed or bed disability days). Most approaches to health status assessment are essentially morbidity indicators. The RAND health status measures (Stewart, Ware, Brook, & Davies-Avery, 1978) include separate categories for the effects of disease or health states upon physical function, social function, and mental function. These measures do not integrate morbidity and mortality, although as each birth cohort ages, there is accrual of mortality cases.

Death is a health outcome, and it is important that this outcome not be excluded from any expression of health status. For example, suppose we were evaluating the effect of a program of integrated support and treatment, as opposed to no support or treatment, for randomly assigned groups of very ill, elderly nursing home residents. Let us suppose that the program maintained them all at a very low level of function throughout the year, while in the comparison group, the sickest 10% died. Looking just at the living in the follow-up, one finds the comparison group to be healthier, because the sickest have been removed by mortality. By this standard, the program of no supportive treatment might appear to be the better alternative. With a measure that combined morbidity and mortality, however, the story would be very different, with mortality effects dragging the overall health of the comparison group to a very low level.

Some authors believe that the idea of integrating morbidity and mortality into a single measure is problematic because death can be viewed not as a health outcome, but rather as the absence of life and of health. According to this line of reasoning, death is not a level of health but a qualitatively different outcome altogether. We assert that mortality is a very important end point; in fact, many health services are directed toward preventing premature mortality. Also, it has been suggested that mortality and morbidity should be separated because many treatments cause side effects, and those refusing treatment may die earlier but experience fewer side effects and a better quality of life before their deaths. According to this argument, if health status includes mortality, these latter individuals would be seen as having a lower quality of life despite its improvement during the period that they avoided the toxic medications. A comprehensive system that includes morbidity and mortality avoids this sort of problem. If the system includes duration of stay at different states, it may or may not suggest that the treatment is worthwhile. For example, a treatment that extends life by only one month but makes people very disabled prior to their deaths would accumulate a loss of well years of life (discussed later in this chapter) that may exceed the benefit in well years. Separating morbidity from mortality confuses rather than clarifies this issue.

I do not mean to imply that mortality should never be analyzed separately. In fact, in many studies there are separate comprehensive analyses for morbidity and mortality. Yet separating morbidity and mortality essentially forbids an analysis that compares treatment with different objectives. For example, it is sometimes of interest to compare programs that prevent early mortality for a few people versus those that reduce morbidity for a large number of people. A comprehensive system allows for these types of trade-offs.

The Value Dimension

Scholars have debated about components of "health" for many centuries. Sullivan (1966), synthesizing literature from a variety of different fields, notes that most concepts of morbidity involve three types of evidence: clinical, subjective, and behavioral. Most studies in social support focus on either clinical or subjective outcomes. Clinical outcomes might include clinical judgment as well as the results of tests obtained during physical examination or invasive procedures; subjective evidence might include symptoms and complaints. Clinical evidence is valuable only if it is clearly related to well-defined behavioral health outcomes. For example, significant abnormalities in certain blood proteins are only of concern if these deviations correlate with dysfunction and early mortality. The burden of proof is on the scientist to demonstrate these associations.

Subjective symptoms are also very important in health care, because symptoms are a major correlate of health care utilization. Not all symptoms, however, should be given equal weight. It is not obvious that the number of symptoms depicts the severity of health status. For example, an adult with an acute 24-hour flu may have an enormous number of symptoms, including nausea, headache, aches and pains, vomiting and diarrhea. Yet it is not clear that this condition is more severe than the single symptom of a very severe headache. Several factors need to be taken into consideration. First, we must determine the degree to which the symptoms limit function. One individual may have five symptoms—an itchy eye, a runny nose, coughing, fatigue, and headache. Yet he or she may still feel well enough to work and to perform all usual activities. Another person with the single symptom of a severe headache may be limited to bed and unable to move around. Would we want to call the person with five symptoms less well? Another dimension is the duration of the symptoms; a year in pain is certainly worse than a day in pain. Finally, and perhaps the most often neglected, is the value or preference associated with different types of dysfunction.

Biomedical investigators often avoid reference to values or preferences because these constructs are not considered scientific; however, the value dimension in health status is inescapable. Fishburn (1964) defined value as the quantification of the concept of worth, importance, or desirability. Ultimately, our judgment of the value of health states depend upon subjective evaluations. The judgment that one level of functioning is better than another level of functioning is ultimately tied to this appraisal. If we advise individuals to change their diet in order to avoid heart disease, we inherently assume that the reduced probability of heart disease later in life is valued more than the immediate but enduring mild displeasure of dietary change. The term *quality of life* presumes a qualitative judgment.

Behavioral Dysfunction

When Sullivan (1966) reviewed the literature on health measurement, he emphasized the importance of behavioral outcomes. Bolstered by the proud accomplishments of behavioral scientists, a convincing argument was developed suggesting that such behavioral indicators as absenteeism, bed disability days, and institutional confinement would be the most important consequences of disease and disability. Ability to perform activities at different ages could be compared to societal standards for these behaviors; restrictions in usual activity were seen as prima facie evidence of deviation from well-being. Many other investigators focus on point-in-time measures of dysfunction as measures of health (Bergner, 1985; Katz, Ford, Moskowitz, Jackson, & Jaffe, 1963; Stewart et al., 1978). Clearly point-in-time dysfunction is crucial in our quantification of health, but it is important not to neglect what will happen in the future. The spectrum of medical care ranges from public health, preventive medicine, and environmental control, through diagnosis and medical care, to convalescence and rehabilitation. Many programs affect the probability of occurrence of dysfunction in the future, rather than altering present functional status. For example, a socially supportive family that instills proper health habits in its children may also promote better health in the future, yet it may be years until this benefit is realized. A positive future orientation might lead to the exercise of better health habits or better planning for future health care.

The concept of health must consider not only the ability to function now, but also the probability of future changes in function. A person who is very functional and asymptomatic today may harbor a disease with a poor prognosis. Thus, many individuals are at high risk for mortality attributable to heart disease even though they are perfectly functional today. The term *severity of illness* should take into consideration both dysfunction and prognosis, as many medical treatments may cause near-term dysfunction in order to prevent future dysfunction. For example, coronary artery bypass surgery causes severe dysfunction for a short period of time, but it is presumed that the surgery will enhance function or decrease mortality at a later point in time. Patients may be incapacitated following myocardial infarction and restricted to coronary care units, yet the treatment is designed to help them achieve better future outcomes. Pap smears are performed and hysterectomies are executed in order to decrease the probability of future deaths caused by cancer. Much of health care involves looking into the future in order to enhance outcomes over the life span, and therefore it is essential to separate out the current and future components of health. I prefer the term *prognosis* to describe the probability of transition among health states over the course of time (Fanshel & Bush, 1970).

Health-Related Quality of Life

There is a growing sentiment that the objectives of health care are twofold. First, health care and health policy should be designed to increase the life expectancy. Second, the health care system should improve the quality of life during the years that people are alive. It is instructive to consider various measures in health care in light of these two objectives. Traditional biomedical indicators and diagnoses are important to us because they may be related to mortality or to quality of life. I prefer the term *health-related quality of life* to refer to the impact of health conditions upon function. Thus, health-related quality of life may be independent of quality of life relevant to work setting, housing, air pollution, and so forth (Rice, 1984).

Numerous new quality-of-life measurement systems have evolved since 1965, representing various traditions in measurement. In the late 1960s and early 1970s, the National Center for Health Services Research funded several major projects to develop general measures of health status. Those projects resulted in the Sickness Impact Profile (Bergner, Bobbitt, Carter, & Gilson, 1981), the Quality of Well-Being Scale (Kaplan & Bush, 1982), and the RAND health status measures (Stewart, et al., 1978). A variety of other measures resulted from this work. Most of these efforts involved extensive multidisciplinary collaboration between behavioral scientists and physicians and focused on the impact of disease and disability upon function and observable behaviors. For example, many of these measures examined the role of disease or disability upon performance of social roles, ability to get around the community, and physical functioning. Some of the systems include separate components for the measurement of social and mental health. All of the systems were guided by the World Health Organization definition of health status: "Health is a complete state of physical, mental, and social well-being and not merely absence of disease" (WHO, 1948). Three of the more commonly used methods include the Sickness Impact Profile (SIP), the Index of Activities of Daily Living scales, and the RAND measures.

Sickness Impact Profile (SIP)

The Sickness Impact Profile (SIP) is one of the best-known and widely used quality-of-life measures. It is a general measure applicable to any disease or disability group, and it has been successfully used with a variety of different cultural subgroups. The SIP includes 136 items describing the effect of sickness upon behavioral function. These items are divided into 12 categories, which are further clustered into three groups: independent, physical, and psychosocial. The independent categories include sleep and rest, eating, work, home management, and recreation/pastimes. Physical categories include ambulation, mobility, and body care and movement. The psychosocial categories are social interaction, alertness behavior, emotional behavior, and communication. Examples of SIP items include "I sleep or nap during the day" (sleep and rest), "I am not doing heavy work around the house" (home management), and "I have difficulty reasoning and solving problems—for example, making plans, making decisions, learning new things" (alertness behavior).

Each SIP item has been evaluated by an independent group of judges on a 15-point scale of dysfunction. Using these independent weights, a respondent taking the SIP endorses or does not endorse each of the 136 items. The overall SIP percentage score is obtained by separating the items endorsed by the respondent, summing their scale values, and dividing by the sum of all values for all items on the SIP. This proportion is then multiplied by 100; scores are obtained similarly for each category. Percentage scores for each category can be plotted on a graphic display that looks similar to an MMPI profile. A variety of studies attest to the substantial reliability and validity of the SIP (see Bergner et al., 1981).

Two minor issues are relevant to general use of the SIP. First, it does not integrate morbidity and mortality, and thus it is less appropriate than some other measures for policy analysis. The second problem is that the SIP is sometimes cumbersome to administer. With 136 items, it can be time-consuming, and it requires alertness and attention by the respondent. The SIP, however, is an example of a measurement system that has undergone systematic methodological refinements over many years. It has been widely used, widely tested, and well evaluated.

Index of Activities of Daily Living

Perhaps the oldest general quality-of-life measure is the Index of Activities of Daily Living (ADL) most commonly used in studies of the elderly. Katz was very early to argue that the major importance of disease and disability was upon function and ability to perform role activities (Katz et al., 1963).

The system includes six subscales: bathing, dressing, toileting, transfer, continence, and feeding. For each category, a judgment is made as to whether the person is independent or dependent. For the category of bathing, people are judged to be independent if they need assistance only in bathing a single part of the body or can bathe themselves; they are judged to be dependent if they need assistance in bathing more than one part of the body. Once a judgement of dependence or independence is obtained for each of the six categories, an overall grade is assigned. To receive the top grade of A, the person must be independent in all six categories. A grade of B is assigned to those who are independent in all but one of these functions. The bottom grade, G, is assigned to those who are dependent in all six functions. Several reliability and validity studies for the ADL have been reported (Katz, Downs, Cash, & Grotz, 1970).

Despite its many important applications in studies of aging, the ADL has been criticized because it does not make distinctions toward the well end of the quality-of-life continuum. Stewart and colleagues (1978) suggest that nearly 80% of the noninstitutionalized population have no functional limitations and would obtain the top score in the ADL system. Other population surveys, however, demonstrate that more than 50% of the population experience one or more symptoms on a given day (Kaplan, Bush, & Berry, 1976). Given the wide array of challenges for a quality-of-life measure, the ADL has some significant limitations. Other measures are required in order to distinguish between those individuals who are toward the healthy end of the functioning continuum.

RAND Health Status Measures

Perhaps the most thorough review in the conceptualization of health-related quality-of-life measures yet available has been accumulated by the RAND Corporation. The RAND group adapted questionnaires developed by Bush, Kaplan, and others to describe physical activity, social activity, and mobility. The social activity category was subdivided to include social activity, role activity, household activity, and leisure activity. The RAND group also adapted Dupey's (1969) General Well-Being Index. In addition, they have added a General Health Perceptions Questionnaire (Ware & Karmos, 1976) and a variety of other measures. Finally, the RAND group uses self-report questionnaires to assess the clinical status associated with a wide variety of medical conditions (Brook et al., 1979). Through considerable testing and evaluation the RAND group revised the measure for the

Medical Outcomes Study (MOS) and eventually shortened it to 36 items. The measure is now known as the 36 item short form, or SF-36.

The RAND approach has the advantage of being very comprehensive. Perhaps the major disadvantage is that it is sometimes difficult to aggregate the measures in order to provide a comprehensive expression of quality of life. For example, the approach may demonstrate that patients with cardiovascular disease have shown minor improvements in certain aspects of mobility and role performance, but are experiencing side effects such as mental confusion and headaches. Unlike some other systems, the RAND approach does not allow a comprehensive statement about whether the patients are getting better or worse on a composite index.

In addition to these approaches that focus on health status, other authors refer to quality of life as something that is independent of health status. Although many investigators believe that symptoms and mortality represent quality of life (see Bush, 1984), Croog et al. (1986) used a wide variety of outcome measures to define the term. Some investigators now use traditional psychological measures and call them quality-of-life outcomes; for instance, Follick et al. (1988) include the patient's subjective evaluation of well-being, physical symptoms, sexual function, work performance and satisfaction, emotional status, cognitive function, social participation, and life satisfaction. Other investigators, including Hunt and McEwen (1983) regard quality of life as subjective appraisals of life satisfaction. In summary, there is no agreement on which dimensions should be considered the standard for assessing quality of life in research studies, yet consideration of recurrent themes in the methodological literature can assist in the evaluation of existent instruments.

Measurement Issues

Unidimensional versus Multidimensional

There is essentially no disagreement that quality of life is a multidimensional construct, yet there is considerable debate about whether outcome measures must necessarily represent this multidimensional structure. There are essentially two major approaches to quality of life assessment: a psychometric approach, and a decision theory approach. The psychometric approach attempts to provide separate measures for the many different dimensions of quality of life. Perhaps the best-known example of the psychometric tradition is the Sickness Impact Profile (above).

The alternative is the decision theory approach, which attempts to weight the different dimensions of health in order to provide a single unitary expression of health status. Supporters of this approach argue that psychometric approaches fail to consider that different health problems are not of equal concern; 100 runny noses are not the same as 100 severe abdominal pains (Bush, 1984). In an experimental trial using the psychometric approach, it is not uncommon to find that some aspects of quality of life improve while others get worse. For example, a medication might reduce high blood pressure but also be associated with headaches and impotence. The decision theory approach attempts to place an overall value on health status by weighting the different dimensions and combining them into an aggregate quality score. It is argued that "quality" is the subjective evaluation of observable or objective health states. The decision theory approach attempts to provide an overall summary of quality of life that integrates subjective function states, preferences for these states, morbidity, and mortality.

Ware et al. (1981) argue that the psychometric approach has greater validity for studies in quality of life. Citing studies on factor analysis, they suggest that different components of health (including mental, physical, and social aspects) might be statistically independent dimensions, and thus any aggregate measure of health status might be considered the same as adding apples to oranges. In rebuttal, Bush (1984) argued that different components of quality-of-life measures indeed are different from one another and might be considered analogous to different pieces of fruit; however, it is the overall evaluation of the basket of fruit that is important. A fruit peddler who regularly delivers a full basket of fruit is preferred over one who delivers a half-empty basket. A basket of fruit in which all pieces are fresh and none are rotten is preferred over one in which some pieces are either missing or decayed. Baskets of fruit thus are associated with preferences or levels of desirability. Even though the contents of baskets may differ, some baskets are preferred over others, and there is a differential willingness to pay for different baskets. Bush argued that the psychometric approach was analogous to comparing one full bowl of fruit to a second bowl of fruit with a banana rotted and a pear missing. Both are bowls of fruit, but they may have different values. Health status often represents combinations of function, symptoms, and disabilities in different systems. Ultimately, our concern is with the overall desirability of the aggregate.

Many investigators prefer the profile approach for assessing side effects of medications. For example, measures such as the SIP allow the investigators to determine if some dimensions of health are getting better while others are getting worse. In other cases, focus on the aggregate may be more desirable. The aggregate approach allows the investigator to state comprehensibly whether the treatment makes people better or worse. There may be instances in which individual preferences rather than societal preferences are used for these decision processes. Knowing the aggregate may be important for some purposes, but the ability to disaggregate may be important for other purposes. Some investigators may want to know whether or not lowering blood pressure makes people dizzy; here a profile approach would be preferable. Others want to know if, considering all of the benefits and all the side effects, blood pressure treatment improves health status; in this case, the aggregate approach may be more desirable.

Disease-Specific versus General Approaches

Most health-related quality-of-life measures are designed for use with any population. Some investigators, however, feel it is necessary to develop quality-of-life measures for specific diseases. For example, the RAND Corporation has produced a series of booklets describing the conceptualization and measurement of "physiologic health." Each booklet describes the problems in conceptualization and measurement of a specific condition, such as coronary heart disease. The rationale underlying these measures is largely clinical, based on the idea that medical conditions have very specific outcomes: Heart patients are evaluated according to ejection fractions, blood gases, etc. Clearly there are advantages to the clinician in considering outcomes relative to specific diseases. In addition to general physiological indicators, there are also quality-of-life measures designed specifically for particular disease groups, best represented in the arthritis literature (Liang, Cullen, & Larson, 1982).

In contrast to those using disease-specific approaches, many investigators believe that all diseases and disabilities have a general effect upon quality of life. In fact, the purpose of quality-of-life measurement is not to identify clinical information relevant to the disease; instead, it seeks to determine the impact of the disease on general function. For example, a lower ejection fraction may be associated with shortness of breath, weakness, and increased risk of mortality, and medications used to control cardiovascular diseases might cause headaches, irritability, and general confusion. By focusing too specifically on clinical correlates of disease, it is argued that the general impact is overlooked. It has also been argued that the general quality-of-life measures adequately capture a wide variety of dysfunctions associated with cardiovascular diseases. These dysfunctions might be in many different systems and recognized in symptoms such as confusion, tiredness, sexual impotence, and depression. These outcomes may not be specific to disease condition.

There is considerable debate over generalized versus disease-specific measures. Although my colleagues and I have argued for the more generalized approach, we recognize the value of disease-specific measures in some clinical studies (R. Kaplan & Anderson, 1988). We urge investigators who choose disease-specific approaches, however, not to limit their measures to symptoms or clinical indicators of a specific disease.

Risk Factors and Outcomes

Epidemiological studies identify a variety of risk factors for coronary heart disease. (N. Kaplan & Stamler, 1983). Among the most important of these is blood pressure. Studies consistently show that elevated blood pressure is a predictor of mortality, nonfatal heart attack, and stroke; thus, important interventions have been developed to lower blood pressure. Many studies use blood pressure reduction as the outcome, and interventions that lower blood pressure are deemed successful. Yet blood pressure is a risk factor for bad health outcomes, but not an outcome itself.

One example that might illustrate this point concerns cigarette smoking. The evidence that cigarette smoking is detrimental to health is overwhelming (Holbrook, 1986; Surgeon General of the United States, 1979). In addition, cigarette smoking interacts with other risk factors such as hypercholesterolemia and hypertension to enhance the risk of coronary heart disease (Gotto, 1986). Nevertheless, the effect of cigarette smoking upon blood pressure is difficult to evaluate. Cigarette smoking may cause an acute rise in blood pressure (Benowitz, Kuyt, & Jacobs, 1984). Epidemiological studies, however, consistently find that smokers have lower blood pressure than nonsmokers. In addition, ex-smokers have blood pressures similar to nonsmokers, even after adjustments for the confounding effects of age and weight. Toshima (1987) recently reviewed this literature and found that across a remarkably diverse set of studies, the effects of cigarette smoking on blood pressure are consistent. Yet they go in the unexpected direction: Cigarette smoking may reduce rather than increase blood pressure.

Toshima also evaluated prospective changes in blood pressure across a variety of epidemiologic studies. Again, in several prospective studies, relationships between cigarette smoking and blood pressure were in the unexpected direction. For example, the Normative Aging Study (Seltzer, 1974) found that systolic blood pressure increases when smokers discontinue cigarette use. The Framingham Heart Study (Gordon et al., 1975) also observed slight increases in systolic blood pressure in ex-smokers in comparison to continuing smokers. Dietary changes were not capable of explaining these changes. Other studies have not observed these relationships, Greene, Aavedel, Tyroler, Davis, & Hames, 1977; Paffenbarger, Thorne, & Wing, 1968); however, most studies simply do not demonstrate that quitting smoking reduces blood pressure.

What can we make of these results? If our outcome measure is blood pressure, we might come to the conclusion that cigarette smoking is good. After all, it appears that habitual cigarette use lowers blood pressure. In addition, we might advise cigarette smokers to continue to smoke; again, the studies consistently demonstrate that smoking cessation is associated with increased blood pressure. But advising smokers to continue would clearly be the wrong conclusion, because the evidence that cigarette smoking has detrimental effects upon health status is overwhelming (Holbrook, 1986). Blood pressure is a risk factor, but not an outcome. Focus of attention on a risk factor may misdirect the purpose of a health care intervention.

Finally, consider the case of insulin-dependent diabetes mellitus. Several studies, including the Diabetes Control and Complications Trial (DCCT, 1993), have suggested that degree of hyperglycemia is associated with the long-term risk of diabetic complications (Tchobroutsky, 1978). A general quality-of-life scale may have substantial advantages for estimating the treatment benefits in diabetes care. In addition to mortality, diabetes may be associated with poor outcomes in a variety of organ systems; for example, poor control may lead to differential rates of retinopathy, kidney failure, and foot infection. The difficulty is in finding one common expression of these outcomes, when some patients may have foot infections that result in amputations while others have eye problems that result in blindness. One purpose of a general quality-of-life measurement system is that it can aggregate these outcomes with death to provide a single expression of the impact of poor control.

In addition to the benefits of the tight management of diabetes, we must also consider the consequences or side effects. Some data suggest that as many as one third of patients who are aggressively managed experience nausea and weakness associated with hypoglycemia on as many as half of the days. A comprehensive view of the benefits of tight control in diabetes must trade the expected benefits against the consequences of tight control. If poor outcomes can be established, they must be represented as probabilities. Retinopathy, for example, may occur in about 50% of insulin-dependent diabetic cases; tight control may reduce this rate to 30%. The real question in diabetes care is how to exchange minor symptoms that occur over an extended period of time with major symptoms that occur later in the life cycle.

Decision Theory Approaches

Within the last few years there has been growing interest in using quality-of-life data to help evaluate the cost/utility or cost-effectiveness of health care programs. Cost-effectiveness analysis typically quantifies the benefits of health care intervention in terms of years of life or *quality-adjusted life years* (QALYs). Cost/utility is a special use of cost-effectiveness that takes expressed preference for health status into consideration (Kaplan & Bush, 1982). In cost/utility analysis, the benefits of medical care, behavioral interventions, or social support are expressed in terms of *well years*; others have chosen to describe the same outcome as QALYs (Weinstein & Stason, 1976) or healthy years of life (Russell, 1986). Because the term *quality-adjusted life years* has become most popular, I will use it in this presentation. QALYs integrate mortality and morbidity to express health status in terms of equivalents of well years of life. If a man dies of heart disease at age 50 and we would have expected him to live to age 75, it might be concluded that the disease was associated with 25 lost life years. If 100 such men died at age 50, we might conclude that 2,500 (100 men times 25 years) life years had been lost.

Yet death is not the only outcome of concern in heart disease. Many adults suffer myocardial infarctions that leave them somewhat disabled over longer periods of time; although they are still alive, the quality of their lives has diminished. QALYs take into consideration the quality-of-life consequences of these illnesses. For example, a disease that reduces quality of life by half will take away 0.5 QALYs over the course of 1 year. If it affects two people, it will take away a total of 1.0 years over the same period. A medical treatment that improves quality of life by 0.2 for each of five individuals will result in the equivalent of 1.0 QALY if the benefit is maintained over a 1-year period. This system has the advantage of considering both benefits and side effects of programs in terms of the common QALY units.

The need to integrate mortality and quality-of-life information is clearly apparent in studies of heart disease. Consider the case of hypertension. People with high blood pressure may live shorter lives if they are untreated; thus, one benefit of treatment is to add years to life. For most patients, however, high blood pressure is not associated with symptoms for many years. Conversely, the treatment for high blood pressure may cause a variety of symptoms. In other words, in the short run, patients taking medication may experience more symptoms than those who avoid it. If a treatment is evaluated in terms of changes in life expectancy, the benefits of the program will be overestimated, because side effects are not taken into consideration. In contrast, considering only current quality of life will underestimate the treatment benefits, because information on mortality is excluded. A comprehensive measurement may take into consideration side effects and benefits and provide an overall estimate of the net effectiveness of treatment (Russell, 1986).

Although there are several different approaches for obtaining quality-adjusted life years, most of them are similar (R. Kaplan, 1985b). The approach that I prefer involves several steps. First, patients are classified according to objective levels of functioning represented by scales of mobility, physical activity, and social activity. The dimensions and steps for these levels of functioning are shown in Table 2. (The reader is cautioned that these steps are not actually the scale, only listings of labels representing the scale steps.) Standardized questionnaires have been developed to classify individuals into one of each of these scale steps (Anderson, Bush, & Berry, 1986). In addition to classification into these observable levels of function, individuals are also classified by the symptom or problem that bothered them most (see Table 3).

Many measures include separate dimensions for emotional and sexual functioning. In this system, these problems are captured in the list of symptoms and problems (i.e., problems in sexual interest or performance, spells of feeling upset, depressed, or crying, etc.). Systems vary in the attention they give to these symptoms, although most agree on the importance of the problems. Depression is a symptom, though, just as is a cough. It has a duration, and its severity might be judged by the degree to which it inhibits role performance. Although it could be regarded as its own dimension, depression disrupts function just as other symptoms do. There are also advantages in keeping the number of dimensions to a minimum. On any particular day, nearly 80% of the general population is optimally functional; however, fewer than 15% of the population experience no symptoms. Symptoms may be severe (e.g., serious chest pain) or minor (e.g., taking medication or a prescribed diet for health reasons). The functional classification and the accompanying list of symptoms or problems was created after extensive reviews of the medical and public health literature (Kaplan et al., 1976).

Once levels of functioning for observable behavior have been classified, the observable health states are weighted by ratings for the desirability of these conditions on a preference continuum with an anchor of 0 for death and 1.0 for completely well. In several studies, random samples of citizens from a metropolitan community evaluated the desirability of more than 400 case descriptions. Using these ratings, a preference structure that assigned the weights to each combination of an observable state and a symptom or problem was developed (R. Kaplan et al., 1976). Cross-validation studies show that the model can be used to assign weights to all

Table 2. Quality of Well-being/General Health Policy Model: Elements and Calculating Formulas (Function Scales, with Step Definitions and Calculating Weights

Step number	Step definition	Weight
	Mobility Scale (MOB)	
5	No limitations for health reasons	−.000
4	Did not drive a car, health related; did not ride in a car as usual for age (younger than 15 yr), health related, *and/or* did not use public transportation, health related; *or* had or would have used more help than usual for age to use public transportation, health related	−.062
2	In hospital, health related	−.090
	Physical Activity Scale (PAC)	
4	No limitations for health reasons	−.000
3	In wheelchair, moved or controlled movement of wheelchair without help from someone else; *or* had trouble or did not try to lift, stoop, bend over, or use stairs or inclines, health related; *and/or* limped, used a cane, crutches, or walker, health related; *and/or* had any other physical limitation in walking, or did not try to walk as far as or as fast as other the same age are able, health related	−.060
1	In wheelchair, did not move or control the movement of wheelchair without help from someone else, *or* in bed, chair, or couch for most or all of the day, health related	−.077
	Social Activity Scale (SAC)	
5	No limitations for health reasons	−.000
4	Limited in other (e.g., recreational) role activity, health related	−.061
3	Limited in major (primary) role activity, health related	−.061
2	Performed no major role activity, health related, but did perform self-care activities	−.061
1	Performed no major role activity, health related, *and* did not perform or had more help than usual in performance of one or more self-care activities, health related	−.106
	Calculating formulas	
	Formula 1. Point-in-time well-being score for an individual (W): W = 1 + (CPXwt) + (MOBwt) + (PACwt) + (SACwt) where "wt" is the preference-weighted measure for each factor and CPX is Symptom/Problem complex. For example, the W score for a person with the following description profile may be calculated for one day as:	
CPX-11	Cough, wheezing or shortness of breath, with or without fever, chills, or aching all over	−.257
MOB-5	No limitations	−.000
PAC-1	In bed, chair, or couch for most or all of the day, health related	−.077
SAC-2	Performed no major role activity, health related, but did perform self-care	
	W = 1 + (−.257) + (−.000) + (−.077) + (−.061) = .605	
	Formula 2. Well-years (WY) as an output measure: WY = [No. of persons × (CPXwt + MOBwt + PACwt + SACwt) × Time]	

Table 3.   Quality of Well-being/General Health Policy Model:
Symptom/Problem Complexes (CPX) with Calculating Weights

CPX number	CPX description	Weight
1	Death (not on respondent's card)	−.727
2	Loss of consciousness such as seizure (fits), fainting, or coma (out cold or knocked out)	−.407
3	Burn over large areas of face, body, arms, or legs	−.387
4	Pain, bleeding, itching, or discharge (drainage) from sexual organs—does not include normal menstrual (monthly) bleeding	−.349
5	Trouble learning, remembering, or thinking clearly	−.340
6	Any combination of one or more hands, feet, arms, or legs either missing, deformed (crooked), paralyzed (unable to move), or broken—includes wearing artificial limbs or braces	−.333
7	Pain, stiffness, weakness, numbness, or other discomfort in chest, stomach (including hernia or rupture), side, neck, back, hips, or any joints or hands, feet, arms, or legs	−.299
8	Pain, burning, bleeding, itching, or other difficulty with rectum, bowel movements, or urination (passing water)	−.292
9	Sick or upset stomach, vomiting or loose bowel movement, with or without chills, or aching all over	−.290
10	General tiredness, weakness, or weight loss	−.259
11	Cough, wheezing, or shortness of breath, *with* or *without* fever, chills, or aching all over	−.257
12	Spells of feeling upset, being depressed, or of crying	−.257
13	Headache, or dizziness, or ringing in ears, or spells of feeling hot, nervous or shaky	−.244
14	Burning or itching rash on large areas of face, body, arms, or legs	−.240
15	Trouble talking, such as lisp, stuttering, hoarseness, or being unable to speak	−.237
16	Pain or discomfort in one or both eyes (such as burning or itching) or any trouble seeing after correction	−.230
17	Overweight for age and height or skin defect of face, body, arms, or legs, such as scars, pimples, warts, bruises or changes in color	−.188
18	Pain in ear, tooth, jaw throat, lips, tongue; several missing or crooked permanent teeth—includes wearing bridges or false teeth; stuffy, runny nose; or any trouble hearing—includes wearing a hearing aid	−.170
19	Taking medication or staying on a prescribed diet for health reasons	−.144
20	Wore eyeglasses or contact lenses	−.101
21	Breathing smog or unpleasant air	−.101
22	No symptoms or problems (not on respondent's card)	−.000
23	Standard symptom/problem	−.257
X24	Trouble sleeping	−.257
X25	Intoxication	−.257
X26	Problems with sexual interest or performance	−.257
X27	Excessive worry or anxiety	−.257

X—Specific weight not available.

possible states of functioning with a high degree of accuracy ($R^2 = .96$); the regression weights obtained in these studies are given in Tables 2 and 3. Finally, it is necessary to consider the duration of stay in various health states. For example, 1 year in a state that has been assigned the weight of .5 is equivalent to 0.5 QALYs. Table 2 provides an illustrative example of such a calculation.

The *well life expectancy* is the current life expectancy adjusted for diminished quality of life associated with dysfunctional states and duration of stay in each state. Using the system, it is possible to consider simultaneously mortality, morbidity, and the preference weights for these behavioral states of function. When the proper steps are followed, the model quantifies the health activity or treatment program in terms of the quality-adjusted life years that it produces or saves. A quality-adjusted life year is defined conceptually as the equivalent of a completely well year of life, or a year of life free of any symptoms, problems, or health-related disabilities. More detailed descriptions of this system are available in other publications (R. Kaplan, 1985a; R. Kaplan & Bush, 1982).

There are other approaches to integrating values into a quality-of-life measure. DuPuis (1989) argues for a subjective approach to quality-of-life measurement. According to this method, preferences are completely unstandardized; quality of life becomes an individual's preference for states. Many investigators favor this approach because it allows the individual to estimate how treatments affect him or her. The disadvantage is that these approaches are completely unstandardized, do not allow for comparisons between different treatment approaches, and forbid policy analysis because the outcomes are not in the same unit. These subjective approaches are valuable for learning how patients react to their treatments, may give guidance with regard to compliance decisions, and may be held as subjective reactions to treatment.

Reliability and Validity

Measures of health status are often evaluated using common psychometric methods. Despite the attractiveness of applying commonly used psychometric methods to health measures, there are several inherently difficult problems. Some of these problems concern validity, and others concern reliability.

The reliability of a health status measure is difficult to assess, particularly if we consider test-retest reliability (Kaplan & Saccuzzo, 1993). Conceptually, test-retest methods were developed to measure traits— characteristics of individuals that are stable over the course of time. Thus, variation in test scores over the course of time is attributable to measurement error. Health, in contrast, is not assumed to be constant; indeed, it is the variability in health status that is of major interest. Traditional methods of reliability assessment will overestimate measurement error for measures of health status because true changes in health status will be counted as errors. Internal consistency methods are commonly used, but they are limited to assessing error associated with item sampling.

Reliability refers to the portion of variance in a measure that is "true score," or free of measurement error. There are difference sources of unreliability in scores. For example, some methods for evaluating reliability consider the internal consistency of the measure. Using this model, it is assumed that all items in the measure tap the same construct, and that these items are independent samples of characteristic under study. Other methods for evaluating reliability assume that such characteristics as social support or health are stable over the course of time; thus, different scores obtained at different points in time are attributable to measurement error. Reliability is a problem in research because it reduces the chances of finding significant relationships between measures.

Problems in the assessment of the validity of health status measures have been outlined by R. Kaplan et al. (1976). Validity, a frequently misunderstood concept in health status measurement, describes the range of inferences that are appropriate when interpreting a measurement, a score, or the result of a test. In other words, the validity of a measure defines the meaning of a score. Validity is not absolute: It is relative to the domain about which statements are made. If we want to measure what society means by health, then an indicator or index is a valid measure of total health status only to the extent that it expresses or correlates with that construct.

Criterion validity is the correspondence of a proposed measure with some other observation that accurately measures the phenomenon of interest. By definition, the criterion must be a superior, more accurate measure of the phenomenon if it is to serve as a verifying norm. If a criterion exists, only greater practicalities or less expense justify the use of concurrent measures as proxies. If the criterion is not a superior measure, then failure of correspondence by any new measure may be a defect of the criterion itself, making it insufficient as a reference for validity.

Most exercises in validation of health status measures involve construct validity. Construct validation is a process required when "no criterion or universe of content is accepted as entirely adequate to define the quality to be measured" (Cronbach & Meehl, 1955). Construct validation involves assembling empirical evidence to support the inference at a particular level that has meaning. It is an ongoing process, akin to amassing support for a complex scientific theory for which no single set of observations provides crucial or critical evidence. It is difficult to define a point at which an investigator can declare that his or her measure is valid; instead, the meaning of the measure is established by its empirical connections to other defined measures.

Simulations

The purpose of this chapter is to identify some of the psychometric issues in research linking social support and health outcomes. Most of the focus has been on the definition and measurement of health. I will now return to the measurement issues in identifying relationships between imperfect measures of health and social support.

Some of the psychometric problems associated with establishing the relationship between social support and health can be understood through simulation. The effect of low reliability on correlations has been well documented in the psychometric literature. Observed correlations between two variables are attenuated when either or both variables are measured with error; formulas that describe this relationship are available (R. Kaplan & Saccuzzo, 1993).

In our simulations, my colleagues and I made the following assumptions. First, we assumed that the maximum true correlation between social support and various outcome measures would not exceed .5. This seems reasonable, because most health outcome variables are affected by multiple sources of variability. For example, one of the variables in our simulation is blood pressure; we would not expect the true correlations between social support and blood pressure to exceed .5, because blood pressure is affected by hereditary factors, age, weight, diet, and so forth. The outcome variables selected for the simulation were chosen because they were used in a variety of studies and may reasonably be expected to correlate with social support.

Five outcome variables were chosen somewhat arbitrarily to represent different observed levels of reliability. In a similar fashion, four social support questionnaires were chosen to represent different levels of reliability. Because the simulation is for illustrative purposes only, the outcome variables chosen may or may not actually bear significant relationships to social support. But because social support has been shown to affect physical (Cohen & Syme, 1985; DiMatteo & Hays, 1981) and psychological health (Dean, Lin, & Ensel, 1981; Sarason & Sarason, 1985) and may serve as a buffer against life stress (Cohen & Wills, 1985) it seems reasonable to select outcome variables associated with health concerns.

The first outcome variable used in the simulation was the Mental Health Questionnaire of the Older American Research and Service Center

instrument (OARS). The OARS is a multipurpose assessment questionnaire for evaluating the elderly; it was developed at Duke University and
has been used in a wide variety of studies. Although the psychometric
data for the OARS are generally good, the test-retest coefficient for the 15-
item mental health screening tool was only .32. This measure was chosen
for use in the simulation because this relatively low coefficient (Fillenbaum, 1978).

Social scientists often attempt to correlate their measures with ratings
by trained medical practitioners. Clinical ratings are known to be fallible,
however, and are often measured with considerable error. To demonstrate
this point, we chose clinical ratings of dysfunction provided by active
medical practitioners for use in the simulation. The reliability obtained in a
careful study by Bergner et al. (1981; see their Table 5) of these ratings of
dysfunction was .41.

Our next range of reliability was taken from a measure of life stress.
Although the Schedule of Recent Events (SRE) has been used successfully
in many studies, early reports suggested that it had a test-retest reliability
of only .55 (Holmes & Rahe, 1967). A measure of life change was chosen
because many investigators hope to demonstrate a relationship between
life events and social support.

Some investigators use risk factors as criteria against which to evaluate social support variables. To simulate one physical risk factor, we chose
blood pressure. A variety of different studies demonstrate that blood
pressure, even when measured under the most rigorous criteria, has a
reported reliability of approximately .65 (Hypertension Detection and
Follow-Up Program Cooperative Group, 1979). Finally, we used the Sickness Impact Profile (SIP), a widely used general health outcome measure
that has a reported reliability for an interviewer-administered form of .97
(Bergner et al., 1981).

The first social support measure was the Dean et al. (1981) Social
Support Scale (SSS), which was chosen for its low reliability level of .28.
Various studies show a range of reliability coefficients for this measure; the
.28 value was chosen because it was the lowest observed reliability coefficient. The second social support measure used for the simulation was the
support need measure from Barrera's (1981a) Arizona Social Support
Interview Schedule (ASSIS). The reliability coefficient for that measure was
.52. The third social support measure, the Social Support Satisfaction Scale
(SSSS; Blaik & Genser, 1980) has an internal consistency reliability of .69
for the short form; it was also used in this simulation. Finally, a portion of
the Sarason et al. (1983) Social Support Questionnaire (SSQ), which
enumerates the number of people in one's social network, was chosen
because of its very high (.97) level of reliability.

The expected observed correlations between each social support measure and each outcome measure was estimated using the formula $R = .5\sqrt{r_{11}r_{22}}$, in which R is the expected observed correlations, r_{11} is the reliability of the social support questionnaire, r_{22} is the reliability of the outcome measure, and .5 is the expected true correlation. The simulation is summarized in Table 4. The entries in the table represent the expected observed correlation between each social support and outcome measure pair if the true correlation is .50. Asterisks are also used to identify those that would be statistically significant at the 0.5 level in a study with 50 respondents.

As the table demonstrates, the expected observed correlations between measures is affected by their reliability. If the true correlations between variables were .5, the SSQ would still find a statistically significant correlation when used with all outcome measures except the OARS Mental Health Questionnaire. Conversely, the SSS, with a reliability of .28, would not be able to detect a .5 correlation with any of the chosen outcome measures. In other words, it would be a frustrating effort to employ the SSS and to expect to obtain any significant correlations under our assumptions. The other social support questionnaires represent intermediate capabilities to detect correlations; for example, the ASSIS might be expected to detect a correlation with blood pressure or the SIP, but not with the SRE, the OARS measure, or clinical judgments. Again, this simulation assumes that the true correlations would be .5. Many of the relationships

Table 4. *Correlations between Selected Social Support and Criterion Measures*

Scale	OARS Mental Health (.32)	Clinical ratings (.41)	SRE (.55)	Blood pressure (.65)	SIP (.97)
Social Support Questionnaire (SSQ; .97) (Sarason et al., 1983)	.278	.32*	.37*	.40*	.48*
Social Support Satisfaction Scale (short form; .69) (Blaik & Genser, 1980)	.24	.27	.31*	.33*	.41*
Arizona Social Support Interview Schedule (ASSIS; support need measure; .52) (Barrera, 1981a)	.20	.23	.27	.29*	.36*
Social Support Scales (Lowenthal & Haven items; .28) (Dean et al., 1981)	.15	.17	.20	.21	.26

*p < .05 (.2818)

between social support and health outcomes involve measures with less than optimal reliability.

Despite this, a researcher may select a measure with moderate or even low reliability because of the instrument's ease of administration, simplicity in scoring, or appropriateness to the variable being examined. Although determining the reliability of scales is a well-established standard in terms of assessment, it may be legitimate to use a less reliable tool if the dependent measure has high enough reliability on its own to make the inquiry worthwhile. In any case, the researcher should be cognizant of the approximate reliability of measures and the potential impact of low reliability on observed correlations. Other outcome measures used in social support research (e.g., mortality) are considerably more reliable; however, they may also occur with a relatively low probability. In a prospective study, only a small proportion of the participants will die in any defined time period. As a result, sample sizes for observational studies that use mortality as an outcome often need to be in the thousands or even tens of thousands.

Summary

Several chapters in this volume describe problems in the conceptualization and measurement of social support. Lack of a consensual definition of social support has made it difficult, if not impossible, to compare studies linking social support to stress, health outcomes, and general psychological and physical well-being. Many authors attribute the problems in this field to the inadequate definitions of social support (Heitzmann & Kaplan, 1988); however, there are equally serious problems in the conceptualization and measurement of health status. The definition of health has been ambiguous for several centuries. Within the last 25 years, several groups have attempted to define health status using quantitative measures. Although progress is being made, large conceptual problems still remain.

Perhaps the best consensus on a measure of health status is for mortality. Indeed, there is some convincing evidence that social support is associated with a lower rate of mortality from cardiovascular disease. Beyond mortality, studies linking social support to health become very problematic. The number of reported symptoms is not a strong outcome measure, because symptom reporting is highly subjective, unreliable, and subject to various biases.

Another problem in research on social support and health concerns the ratio of the number of subjects to variables. It is not uncommon for investigators to capture health status by measuring or tabulating an enormous number of indicators; some studies, for example, use as many as 100 indicators of life quality. Such approaches greatly inflate the probability of spurious findings. Studies focusing on one well-defined outcome, such as mortality, may also encounter problems in sample size if only a small number of cases actually die.

In summary, the problems in the conceptualization and measurement of social support are well recognized. As noted above, though, there are equally, if not more serious, problems in the conceptualization and measurement of health status. The literature on health status is well documented (Patrick & Erickson, 1988; Walker & Rosser, 1988). Future studies should embrace state-of-the-art technologies for both health status and social support measurements.

References

Anderson, J. P., Bush, J. W., & Berry, C. C. (1986). Classifying function for health outcome and quality of life evaluation: Self-versus-interviewer modes. *Medical Care, 24,* 454–469.

Barrera, M. (1981a). Preliminary development of a scale of social support. *American Journal of Community Psychology, 9,* 435–447.

Barrera, M. (1981b). Preliminary development of a scale of social support. *American Journal of Community Psychology, 9,* 435–447.

Benowitz, N. L., Kuyt, T., & Jacobs, P. (1984). Influence of nicotine on cardiovascular and hormonal effects of smoking. *Clinical Pharmacological Therapeutics, 36,* 74.

Bergner, M. (1985). Measurement of health status. *Medical Care, 23,* 696–704.

Bergner, M., Bobbitt, R. A., Carter, W. B., & Gilson, B. S. (1981). The Sickness Impact Profile: Development and final revision of a health status measure. *Medical Care, 19,* 787–786.

Berkman, L. F. (1982). Social networks and analysis and coronary heart disease. *Advances in Cardiology, 29,* 37–49.

Billings, A. F., & Moos, R. H. (1982). Social support and functioning among community and clinical groups: A panel model. *Journal of Behavioral Medicine, 5,* 295–311.

Blaik, R., & Genser, S. G. (1980). Perception of Social Support Satisfaction: Scale development. *Personality and Social Psychology Bulletin, 6,* 172.

Brandt, P. A., & Weinert, C. (1981). The PRQ—a social support measure. *Nursing Research, 30,* 277–280.

Broadhead, W. E., Kaplan, B. H., James, S. A., Wenger, E. H., Schoenbach, V. J., Grimson, R., Heyden, S., Tibblin, G., & Gehlback, S. H. (1983). The epidemiologic evidence for a relationship between social support and health. *American Journal of Epidemiology, 117,* 521–537.

Brook, R. H., Goldberg, G. A., Harris, L. J., Applegate, K., Rosenthal, M., & Lohr, K. N. (1979). *Conceptualization in measurement of physiologic health in the health insurance study.* Santa Monica, CA: RAND Corporation.

Bush, J. W. (1984). Relative preferences versus relative frequencies in health-related quality of life evaluations. In N. K. Wenger, M. E. Mattson, C. D. Furberg, & J. Elinson (Eds.), *Assessment of quality of life in clinical trials of cardiovascular therapies* (pp. 118–139). New York: LaJacq.

Cohen, S., Mermelstein, R., Kamarck, T., & Hoberman, H. N. (1985). Measuring the functional components of social support. In I. Sarason & B. Sarason (Eds.), *Social support: Theory, research, and applications* (pp. 73–94). Dordrecht, Netherlands: Martinus Nijhoff.

Cohen, S., & Syme, S. L. (1985). *Social support and health*. New York: Academic Press.

Cohen, S., & Wills, T. A. (1985). Stress, social support, and the buffering hypothesis. *Psychological Bulletin, 98*(2), 310–357.

Cronbach, L. J., & Meehl, P. E. (1955). Construct validity in psychological tests. *Psychological Bulletin, 52*, 281.

Croog, S. H., Levine, S., Testa, M. A., Brown, D., Bulpitt, C. J., Jenkins, C. D., Klerman, G. L., & Williams, G. H. (1986). The effects of anti-hypertensive therapy on quality of life. *New England Journal of Medicine, 314*, 1657–1664.

Davidson, T. N., Bowden, L., & Tholen, D. (1979). Social support as a moderator of burn rehabilitation. *Archives of Physical Medicine and Rehabilitation, 60*, 556.

Dean, A., Lin, N., & Ensel, W. M. (1981). The epidemiological significance of social support systems in depression. *Research in Community Mental Health, 2*, 77–109.

Diabetes Control and Complications Group (1993). The effect of intensive treatment of diabetes on the development and progression of long term complications in Insulin Dependent Diabetes Mellitus. Results of the Diabetes Control and Complications Trial. *New England Journal of Medicine, 329* (14), 977–986.

DiMatteo, M. R., & Hays, R. (1981). Social support and serious illness. In B. H. Gottlieb (Ed.), *Social networks and social support* (pp. 117–148). Beverly Hills, CA: Sage.

Dupey, H. J. (1969). *The psychological examination: Cycle IV*. Washington, DC: National Center for Health Statistics.

Fanshel, S., & Bush, J. W. (1970). A health-status index and its applications to health-services outcomes. *Operations Research, 18*, 1021–1066.

Fillenbaum, G. C. (1978). Validity and reliability of the multidimensional functional assessment questionnaire. In *Multidimensional functional assessment: The OARS methodology* (pp. 25–35). Durham, NC: Duke University, Center of the Study of Aging and Human Development.

Fishburn, P. (1964). *Decision and value theory*. New York: Wiley.

Follick, M. J., Gorkin, L., Smith, T., Capone, R. J., Visco, J., & Stabein, D. (1988). Quality of life post-myocardial infarction: The effects of a transtelephonic coronary intervention system. *Health Psychology, 7*, 169–182.

Gordon, T., Kannel, W. B., & McGee, D. (1974). Death and coronary attacks in men after giving up cigarette smoking. *Lancet, 2*, 1345–1348.

Gotto, A. M. (1986). Interaction of the multiple risk factors of coronary heart disease. *American Journal of Medicine, 80*, 48–55.

Greene, S. B., Aavedel, M. J., Tyroler, H. A., Davis, C. E., & Hames, C. G. (1977). Smoking habits and blood pressure change: A seven year follow-up. *Journal of Chronic Diseases, 30*, 410.

Heitzmann, C. A., & Kaplan, R. M. (1988). Assessment of the methods for measuring social support. *Health Psychology, 7*, 75–109.

Henderson, S., Duncan-Jones, P., Byrne, D. G., & Scott, R. (1980). Measuring social relationships: The Interview Schedule for Social Interaction. *Psychological Medicine, 10*, 723–734.

Holbrook, J. H. (1986). *Cigarette smoking*. Washington, DC: The Brookings Institution.

Holmes, T. H., & Rahe, R. H. (1967). The Social Readjustment Rating Scale. *Journal of Psychosomatic Research, 11*, 213–218.

Hunt, S. M., & McEwen, J. (1983). The development of a subjective health indicator. *Sociology of Health and Illness, 2*, 231–245.

Hypertension Detection and Follow-Up Program Cooperative Group. (1979). Five years findings of the Hypertension Detection and Follow-up Program: I. Reduction in mortality of persons with high blood pressure, including mild hypertension. *Journal of the American Medical Association, 242,* 2562–2571.

Kaplan, N. M., & Stamler, J. (1983). *Prevention of coronary heart disease.* Philadelphia: Saunders.

Kaplan, R. M. (1985a). Quality of life measurement. In P. Karoly (Ed.), *Measurement strategies in health psychology* (pp. 115–146). New York: Wiley-Interscience.

Kaplan, R. M. (1985b). Quantification of health outcomes for policy studies in behavioral epidemiology In R. M. Kaplan & M. H. Criqui (Eds.), *Behavioral epidemiology and disease prevention.* New York: Plenum.

Kaplan, R. M., & Anderson, J. P. (1988). A general health policy model: Update and applications. *Health Services Research, 23*(2), 203–235.

Kaplan, R. M., & Bush, J. W. (1982). Health-related quality of life measurement for evaluation research and policy analysis. *Health Psychology, 1,* 61–80.

Kaplan, R. M., Bush, J. W., & Berry, C. C. (1976). Health status: Types of validity for an index of well-being. *Health Services Research, 11,* 478–507.

Kaplan, R. M., & Saccuzzo, D. S. (1993). *Psychological testing: Principles, applications, and issues* (3rd ed.). Pacific Grove, CA: Brooks-Cole.

Katz, S. T., Downs, H., Cash, H., & Grotz, R. (1970). Progress and development of an index of ADL. *Gerontologist, 10,* 20–30.

Katz, S. T., Ford, A. D., Moskowitz, R. W., Jackson, B. A., & Jaffe, M. W. (1963). Studies of illness in the aged: The index of ADL. *Journal of the American Medical Association, 185,* 914–919.

Liang, N. H., Cullen, K., & Larson, M. (1982). In search of a more perfect mouse trap (health status or a quality of life instrument). *Journal of Rheumatology, 9,* 775–779.

Lin, N., Simeone, R., Ensel, W., & Kuo, W. (1979). Social support, stressful life events and illness: A model and an empirical test. *Journal of Health and Social Behavior, 20,* 108–119.

McDowell, I., & Newell, C. (1987). *Measuring health: A guide to rating scales and questionnaires.* New York: Oxford.

McFarlane, A. H., Neale, K. A., Norman, G. R., Roy, R. G., & Streiner, D. L. (1981). Methodological issues in developing a scale to measure social support. *Schizophrenia Bulletin, 7,* 90–100.

Norbeck, J. S., Lindsey, A. M., & Carrieri, V. L. (1981). The development of an instrument to measure social support. *Nursing Research, 30,* 264–269.

Paffenbarger, R. S., Thorne, M. C., & Wing, A. L. (1968). Chronic disease in former college students: Characteristics in youth predisposing to hypertension in later years. *American Journal of Epidemiology, 88,* 25.

Patrick, D. L., & Erickson, P. (1988). Assessing health-related quality of life in clinical decision making. In S. R. Walker & R. M. Rosser (Eds.), *Quality of life: Assessment and applications* (pp. 9–19). London: MTP Press.

Porrit, D. (1979). Social support in crisis: Quantity or quality. *Social Science and Medicine, 13,* 715–721.

Procidano, M. E., & Heller, K. (1983). Measures of perceived social support from friends and from family: Three validation studies. *American Journal of Community Psychology, 11*(1), 1–24.

Rice, R. M. (1984). Organizational work and the overall quality of life. In S. Oscamp (Ed.), *Applied social psychology annual: Applications in organizational settings, vol. 5* (pp. 155–178). Beverly Hills, CA: Sage.

Russell, L. B. (1986). *Is prevention better than cure?* Washington, DC: Brookings Institution.

Sarason, I. G., & Sarason, B. R. (1985). *Social support: Theory, research, and applications.* Boston: Martinus Nijhoff International.

Sarason, I. G., Levine, H. M., Basham, R. B., & Sarason, B. R. (1983). Assessing social support: The Social Support Questionnaire. *Journal of Personality and Social Psychology*, 44(1), 127–139.

Schaefer, C., Coyne, J. C., & Lazarus, R. S. (1981). Health related functions of social support. *Journal of Behavioral Medicine*, 4, 381–406.

Schafer, L. C., McCaul, K. D., & Glasgow, R. E. (1984). *Supportive and nonsupportive family behaviors: Relationships to adherence and metabolic control in persons with Type I diabetes*. Unpublished manuscript, North Dakota State University, Fargo.

Seltzer, C. C. (1974). Effect of smoking on blood pressure. *American Heart Journal*, 87, 558.

Stewart, A. L., Ware, J. E., Brook, R. H., & Davies-Avery, A. (1978). *Conceptualization and measurement of health for adults: vol. II: Physical health in terms of functioning*. Santa Monica, CA: RAND Corporation.

Sullivan, D. F. (1966). Conceptual problems in developing an index of health. Office of Health Statistics, National Center for Health Statistics, Monograph Series II, No. 17.

Surgeon General of the United States. (1979). *Smoking and health*. (Publication No. 79–50066). Washington, DC: Department of Health, Education, and Welfare.

Tchobroutsky, G. (1978). Relation of diabetic control to development of microvascular complications. *Diabetologia,*, 15, 143–152.

Toshima, M. T. (1987). *Cigarette smoking cessation*. Unpublished manuscript, San Diego State University, San Diego, CA.

Walker, S., & R. M. Rosser (Eds.). (1988). *Quality of life: Assessment and applications*. London: MTP Press.

Wallston, B. S., Alagna, S. W., DeVellis, B. M., & DeVellis, R. F. (1983). Social support and physical health. *Health Psychology*, 2, 367–391.

Ware, J. E., Brook, R. H., Davies-Avery, A. R., et al. (1981). Choosing measures of health status for individuals in general populations. *American Journal of Public Health*, 71, 620–625.

Ware, J. E., & Karmos, A. H. (1976). *Development and validation of scales to measure perceived health and patient role propensity, Vol. 2*. Carbondale: Southern Illinois School of Medicine.

Weinstein, M. C., & Stason, W. B. (1976). *Hypertension: A policy perspective*. Cambridge, MA: Harvard University Press.

Wenger, N. K., Mattson, M. E., Furberg, C. D., & Elinson, J. (1984). *Assessment of quality of life in clinical trials of cardiovascular therapies*. New York: LaJacq.

World Health Organization. (1948). *Constitution of the World Health Organization*. Geneva: Author.

PART II

Establishing a Relationship between Social Support and Cardiovascular Disease

International Epidemiological Evidence for a Relationship between Social Support and Cardiovascular Disease

Kristina Orth-Gomér

The concept of social support is almost as old as the Old World. Aristoteles argued around 350 B.C. that friendship was a basic human need along with food, shelter, and clothing. "We naturally desire to love other human beings and to be loved by them. A totally loveless life—a life without friends of any sort—is a life deprived of much needed good" (Alcalay, 1983). Several centuries later, Paracelcus (1599), a physician, alchemist, and natural scientist, prescribed "love as the best possible cure for several diseases." The first scientific evidence of a link between social support and health was offered by Durkheim (1897/1951) in his extensive sociological studies on the origins of suicide and self-destructive behavior, in which he found that marriage and religion were the best protectors against such deviant behavior. Kropotkin (1908), a Russian ethologist and psychobiologist, stated that "mutual help and support is a factor of great significance for the maintenance of life and health in animals and in humans."

Most of the modern epidemiological studies from the Old World concerning the relationship of social support and cardiovascular disease (CVD) have been inspired by studies from the United States, such as the Alameda County study (Berkman & Syme, 1979). Because Chapter 6 discusses U.S. epidemiological evidence, this chapter focuses on internal studies only.

KRISTINA ORTH-GOMÉR • National Institute for Psychosocial Factors and Health, 171 77 Stockholm, Sweden.

Social Support and Cardiovascular Disease, edited by Sally A. Shumaker and Susan M. Czajkowski. Plenum Press, New York, 1994.

Before reviewing the international evidence, though, a few basic characteristics of epidemiological studies should be noted. As with any study based on statistical associations, results from epidemiological studies cannot be interpreted as providing conclusive evidence about causal relationships. Unlike experimental studies, in which virtually all external influences are kept under control, in observational studies one cannot control for all possible confounding factors or processes that may be underlying causes of the relationships found. One can minimize the possible bias, however, by adhering to some established standards for causal interpretation, such as the eight criteria suggested by Hill (1965):

1. *Temporality of events.* With reference to prospective studies, does the exposure precede the disease outcome?
2. *Strength of the association.* How much of the variance in the outcome variable is explained by the exposure variable? How great is the relative risk associated with the exposure?
3. *Consistency of associations.* Do several studies demonstrate similar results?
4. *Biological gradient.* Is there an increased risk of adverse outcome with increased exposure?
5. *Biological plausibility.* Is there evidence of a plausible pathogenic mechanism linking the exposure to the outcome variable?
6. *Coherence.* Do the conclusions from several kinds of studies (e.g., using animals, human populations, and human patient studies) point in the same direction?
7. *Experimental/intervention evidence.* Is there evidence from such studies that supports the associations found?
8. *Specificity of outcome.* Are several different effects of the exposure variable observed, or are the findings specific to one outcome?

In this chapter several of these criteria, such as temporality, strength, and consistency of the associations, are applied. For example, if it is found that different studies come to similar conclusions about an effect over time, about the strength of an effect and about the kind of pathogenic outcome involved, then the probability of a causal relationship is increased. Another criterion to be addressed is the role of intervention studies. Not only are these studies a test of preventive or therapeutic effects, but they can also be interpreted as experimental support for a causal relationship. For example, if it can be shown that increasing social support leads to a decrease in systolic blood pressure, the inference of a causal relationship between social support and blood pressure is strengthened.

The epidemiological studies reviewed in this chapter are mainly of two kinds. First I discuss longitudinal studies, which analyze the impact of social support on cardiovascular end points over a period of time. A methodological strength of this type of study is the measurement of social support before clinical signs of disease are present. With this design, we can conclude that the presence or absence of support influences the disease process, rather than the reverse (i.e., that the disease causes lack of support). A problem with many of these studies, however, is the measurement of social support at only one point in time. This assumes that social support is relatively stable over time. Characteristics of the longitudinal studies are reviewed and their results are summarized in Table 1.

The second type of study reviewed in this chapter addresses possible mechanisms of the social support–cardiovascular disease (CVD) relationship. These studies have documented associations between various social support measures and standard risk factors for cardiovascular diseases. They are cross-sectional in nature, involving the measurement of social support and the risk factor at the same point in time. Consequently it is impossible to draw inferences about the temporal nature of the social support–CVD relationship. Therefore, these studies do not provide conclusive evidence concerning the role of social support in the development of standard risk factors for CVD. Table 2 summarizes characteristics and results of these cross-sectional studies.

In discussing the evidence for a social support–CVD relationship based on population studies, measurement problems require special attention. The difficulties involving identifying social support measures suitable for population surveys are widely recognized by epidemiological investigators. In response to this problem, an international workshop on the measurement of social support was sponsored by the World Health Organization (1986) and held in Stockholm in September, 1985. One outcome of the workshop was a review of available social support measures (Orth-Gomér & Undén, 1987) that identifies instruments suitable for population surveys and reviews the instruments in terms of the conceptual framework used, ability to predict chronic disease outcome, and psychometric properties. Although no social support measure was found to satisfy all the proposed requirements, some were found to be acceptable based on their previous use in population surveys and prior evaluation of their psychometric properties.

Finally, this review focuses on the following questions, which are of particular interest for studies on social support and health:

1. Is there evidence for a main effect of the social support measure? In addition, has the "buffer effect" hypothesis been tested (i.e., does social support buffer against the harmful effects of stressful life events)? Is there evidence for both effects?

Table 1. Longitudinal Population Studies of Social Support and Cardiovascular Disease

Study	Population characteristics	Follow-up time	Social support measure	Outcome variable	Findings (RR)	Control variables
Israeli Ischemic Heart Study	10,000 Israeli male employees	5 years	Qualitative emotional support	Angina pectoris	1.8	Age, blood pressure, cholesterol, diabetes, ECG abnormalities
Gothenburg Study	937 men aged 50 or 60	20 and 10 years	Quantitative social activity index	All-cause mortality	3.4	Age, blood pressure, cholesterol, smoking,
Swedish Survey of Living Conditions	17,433 men and women aged 29 to 74	6 years	Quantitative social network interaction index	All-cause mortality, CVD mort	1.4 (men) 1.6 (women)	Age, education, employment, initial health status, smoking, exercise, ethnic origin
Swedish Survey of Living Conditions	13,779 employed men and women aged 16 to 65		Quantitative workers' social support index	All-cause mortality		
North Karelia Study	13,300 men and women aged 39–59 years	5 years	Quantitative social network index	All-cause mortality, CVD mortality, CHD mortality	2.0, 1.8, and 1.7, respectively (men only)	Age, education, urban/ rural residence, initial health status, blood pressure, body mass index, family history

Table 2. Cross-Sectional Studies of Social Support and Cardiovascular Risk Factors

Study and site	Population characteristics	Social support measure	Risk factors examined	Findings
Gothenburg Study	850 men aged 50 years	Qualitative measure of social interaction and attachment	Exercise Smoking Body mass index Cholesterol Blood pressure	Low social interaction associated with poor exercise, smoking habits
Malmö Study	500 men aged 68 years	Qualitative measure of social anchorage, social participation, social influence, material support, information support, and emotional support	Nutrition habits Smoking habits Blood pressure Cholesterol Exercise	Low social anchorage associated with inadequate nutrition, little physical exercise, and high diastolic blood pressure
Marburg Study of Factory Workers	416 men aged 25–65 years	Qualitative/quantitative social integration, emotional support, workers support, strain from family, work problems, and social mobility	Blood pressure Body mass index Smoking Cholesterol	High strain from family problems and social mobility associated with excessive smoking
Whitehall Study of Civil Servants	17,500 men aged 20–64 years	Quantitative measure of worker contacts, friend contacts, neighbor contacts, and relative and family contacts	Social class	Worker and friend contacts less frequent in lower social class

2. Is there evidence of a graded relationship (i.e., the more support, the less the risk of adverse health outcome)? Or is there evidence of a threshold effect (i.e., is there a critical amount of social support which is conducive to health, with no further beneficial effect above that level)?
3. Have both men and women been studied, and has the question of gender differences been addressed?
4. Are there specific cultural patterns in the populations studied? Can comparisons be made between populations in terms of the influence of cultural characteristics on the social support–CVD relationship?
5. Has the question of specificity been addressed? Are the results specific to cardiovascular disease, or can the effects be generalized to overall health outcomes?
6. Do the results suggest ways in which social support can be used to prevent disease? In other words, are the components of social support studied amenable to improvement through advice, recommendations, or other intervention strategies directed toward individuals or health professionals?
7. How was the social support measure operationalized? Was a qualitative perceptual support measure or a quantitative network measured used? In other words, was the issue of the function of support (quality) or of its structure (quantity) addressed?

Longitudinal Studies of General Population Samples

One of the first studies of social support outside the United States, the Israeli Ischemic Heart Study, was designed to investigate psychosocial as well as standard risk factors for the development of angina pectoris and myocardial infarction. Ten thousand adult, male Israeli civil service and municipal employees were examined and followed for 5 years. A number of psychosocial risk factors for angina pectoris were identified; among the strongest predictors were reported family problems. Furthermore, self-reported love and support from the spouse was found to be protective against angina pectoris. This, however, was only true for men who also reported symptoms of anxiety, so that love and support from the wife appears to buffer or ameliorate the effects of anxiety. The risk of contracting angina pectoris for anxious men without support from their wives was 1.8 ($p < .05$), relative to men with support from their wives. This result was obtained even after controlling for age, high blood pressure, high serum cholesterol, diabetes, and ECG abnormalities (Medalie, Kahn, et al., 1973;

Medalie, Snyder, et al., 1973). No support was found for the main effect hypothesis (i.e., that social support affects angina independently of anxiety or stress).

The association reflected a graded or dose-response relationship, with a consistent increase in risk across five social support strata ranging from high to low support. Women were not studied, thus gender differences could not be addressed. It is interesting to note that this association held across a variety of cultural backgrounds. The study sample was selected as representing both subjects born in Israel and those who were immigrants from eastern Europe, central Europe, southeastern Europe, the Middle East, and North Africa. In spite of considerable differences in CVD incidence among these cultural groups, results concerning social support could be generalized to the entire study population. In summary, the Israeli study showed an effect of a qualitative, perceptual social support measure (emotional support) that was specific to angina pectoris and buffered the effects of anxiety.

The subsequent longitudinal studies to be reviewed are all based on quantitative measures of social networks or social activity levels. A Swedish study of men born in 1913 and in 1923 in Gothenburg utilized a concept that is related to but not entirely synonymous with social support (Welin et al., 1985). This index of social influences was based on the social activities reported by these men, aged 50 and 60 at examination. Such social activities were both informal (e.g., entertaining, dancing) and more formal (e.g., organized sports, trade union meetings). The probability sample consisted of almost 1,000 men, who were followed for 20 years (men aged 50) or 10 years (men aged 60). Only the findings for total mortality have been reported, but preliminary results indicate that the findings for cardiovascular mortality are similar (World Health Organization, 1986).

Results show an inverse, graded relationship between social activity levels and mortality. After controlling the results for age, systolic blood pressure, serum cholesterol, and smoking, a mortality risk of 3.4 for the lowest quintile of the social activity index (relative to the highest quintile) was found. The same quintile comparison using numbers of persons living in the household yielded a mortality risk of 2.5 for those living with few others relative to those living with many persons. Women were not examined, and the buffer-effect hypothesis was not addressed in this study. Few cultural differences existed within the population studied, because the population of Gothenburg is primarily of European descent. Thus the study supports the hypothesis of a nonspecific main effect of social support on total mortality, with the suggestion of a similar effect on cardiovascular mortality.

A similar conclusion can be drawn from a study using the Swedish nationwide Survey of Living Conditions. Starting in 1974, these annual surveys of representative samples of the entire adult Swedish population were originally intended to describe welfare and well-being in non-economic terms (Vogel, 1982). In 1976 and 1977, the survey included a structured interview on the availability and frequency of social contacts and social ties, which was used to create a comprehensive, quantitative description of all relevant social contacts. Seven distinct sources of social contacts were identified using factor analysis: parents, siblings, nuclear family (i.e., spouse and children), neighbors, coworkers, youth friends, and more distant friends and relatives. A social network interaction index was obtained by summing across items. 17,433 men and women between the ages of 29 and 74 were interviewed, and their cause-specific mortality was followed for 6 years. The age-adjusted relative risk of dying from cardiovascular disease in the lower as compared to the upper social network index tertile was 1.4 for men and 1.6 for women ($p < .001$). Controlling for presence of cardiovascular disease at entry, smoking and exercise habits, educational level, employment status, and ethnic origin did not alter the size of the relative risk (Orth-Gomér & Johnson, 1987).

Further examination of the nature of the association revealed evidence of a threshold effect for the social network index. The highest mortality risk was found in the lower third of the distribution, the lowest mortality risk was found for the middle tertile, and the highest tertile had a similar or even slightly higher mortality than the middle tertile. Further analyses of relative risks using quintiles or even deciles of the distribution of social network scores were not helpful in identifying the most vulnerable group. Thus the lower 33% of the population seemed to be at increased risk; the magnitude of the risk was similar for total and cardiovascular mortality and similar in men and women. The results support the hypothesis of a nonspecific main effect of social support on cardiovascular mortality.

In a more detailed analysis of the working members of this population (13,779 men and women), the buffer-effect hypothesis was tested. All employed men and women were examined for work strain using the Karasek model, which postulates that work strain is increased under conditions that combine high work demand, low work control, and low levels of support at work (Karasek, Baker, Marxer, Ahlbom, & Theorell, 1981). More specifically, support at work has been found to buffer against work strain with respect to prevalence of cardiovascular disease (Johnson, 1986) and subsequent mortality from cardiovascular diseases (see Chapter 8).

Concomitantly with the Swedish studies, a similar study of social connections was conducted in North Karelia, Finland. This study of social ties was part of a large community intervention trial against standard risk factors for cardiovascular diseases. As North Karelia (a rural area bordering Russia) had been found to have the highest known incidence rate of coronary heart disease (CHD) in the industrialized world, this trial was initiated in 1972 in order to modify CHD risk factors and thus reduce its incidence (Puska et al., 1981). A total of 13,300 men and women aged 39 to 59 years participated in the study of social connections. The study group was followed for 5 years, mortality from all causes, as well as specifically from cardiovascular and coronary heart diseases, was recorded. The social connections index was based on five items: marital status, frequency of visiting friends and relatives (two items), number of people encountered every day, and participation in formal and informal groups and organizations. For men, there was an increased relative risk of CHD mortality of 1.7 in the two lower quintiles of the social connections index as compared to the upper quintile; this difference remained significant after controlling for age, education, urban/rural residence, cardiovascular disease at entry, and standard risk factors.

For women there was also an increased mortality risk in the lower social connections strata, but it was not as consistent as for men and not statistically significant. Furthermore, in multivariate analyses, after controlling for other predictors of cardiovascular mortality, the social connections index was not found to be a significant predictor (Kaplan et al., 1986). Thus the North Karelia results support the hypothesis of a nonspecific main effect of social support on CHD mortality in men, but not in women. The effect in men was of a threshold nature, identifying a vulnerable group of 40% of the study population.

These three studies have several features in common. In terms of methodology, the measures of social support represent quantitative descriptions of social connections or social activity patterns. Thus they describe potential supportive resources, although no information is given about the actual provision or quality of support. The study populations are representative of a city, county, or an entire nation, which permits considerable generalization of the results. In addition, attrition rates were within acceptable limits. This is important, because nonrespondents often have higher mortality and morbidity rates, as well as a greater prevalence of unmarried (single, widowed, and divorced) individuals (Lindström, 1981). Consequently, the magnitudes of the relative risks obtained probably represent underestimations of the true risk. In terms of the results of these studies, the magnitude of the risk found in any given study is dependent on the type of social support measures used, their variability and distribution in the population, and to some extent the type of data analysis performed. In terms of the latter consideration, if extremes like the lowest and highest deciles are compared, risk ratios will be greater than in a more conservative comparison (e.g., using tertiles).

In spite of differences both in measures and methods of analyses, some general conclusions can be drawn about the magnitude of the risks in these population studies. In general, the risk ratios are modest; they vary from 1.4 to somewhat more than 3, with most of them falling between 1.5 and 2. Thus the effects of social support on cardiovascular health seem moderate. Furthermore, in general, the risk ratios are higher before adjusting for standard risk factors for cardiovascular disease. This suggests that part of the effects of lack of social support may be mediated by the standard risk factors, indicating a possible biological pathway of the effect. It is possible that the traditional method of analysis in epidemiological studies (adjusting for possible confounders) is not necessarily the most meaningful in this context.

Outcome measures in these studies are "hard" end points that, at least in the case of total mortality, are 100% reliable. Similar effects are found for cardiovascular and for all-cause mortality. This finding would support the hypothesis of an increased vulnerability for any kind of disease agent, rather than an effect specific to cardiovascular diseases. This fact has important consequences for the effects of social support as an intervention, given that it may affect not only cardiovascular disease but several different conditions. Both the Swedish and the Finnish studies have found such an increased general vulnerability in 30% to 40% of the population.

The studies are not consistent in regard to gender. In North Karelia, after controlling for confounders, no effects were found in women for either total or cardiovascular mortality. In the two Swedish studies, the effects were similar for men and women, both with regard to the entire nationwide population sample and the one representing only the working population. These apparently contradictory findings can be compared to North American studies, where an effect in women was found in the Alameda County study (Berkman & Syme, 1979) and in the Durham study of the elderly (Blazer, 1982), but not in Tecumseh (House, Robbins, & Metzner, 1982) or in Evans County (Schoenbach, Kaplan, Fredman, & Kleinbaum, 1986).

One possible explanation for the inconsistent findings regarding gender is that there may be differences in the effects of social supports for women who work outside the home compared to homemakers. In the Swedish survey of living conditions, a majority of women were working outside their homes, whereas in North Karelia, a mainly agricultural and forestral area, the primary occupation of many of the women was home-making (Puska et al., 1981). Perhaps the dual-work situation for the Swedish women made them more vulnerable, and hence in greater need of social supports of various kinds, than their Finnish sisters. Consequently, one would examine this hypothesis concerning gender differences by applying the buffer hypothesis; this has only been done in a few of the population studies examining social supports and health. One is the analysis of the Swedish working force, in which support at work was found to buffer against psychological strain in men as well as in women (Johnson, 1986). To confirm this hypothesis, however, further analyses of gender differences are needed in both U.S. and international studies.

A further extension of this line of reasoning concerns women and the coronary-prone behavior pattern. In the Framingham study, women employed outside the home were found to exhibit coronary-prone behavior to a greater extent than homemakers (Haynes & Feinleib, 1980). Given the differences in employment rates between the North Karelian and Swedish women, one might assume that coronary-prone behavior was less prevalent among the North Karelian women. An interactive effect of coronary-prone behavior and social support has been demonstrated on an outcome measure related to cardiovascular mortality, the extent of coronary atherosclerosis as visualized on coronary angiography (Cohen & Matthews, 1987). The protective effect of social support was found only in those who exhibited coronary-prone or a related behavior pattern. Thus, a possible explanation for the gender differences found in the North Karelia study may be that men more often exhibit coronary-prone behavior and thus are in greater need of social support as a buffer. It could also be argued that because women constitute almost half of the work force in Sweden, gender differences in the prevalence of coronary-prone behavior would be small. If social support serves as a buffer, then differences between men and women in the presence and strength of the association between social support and ill health would also be expected to be small.

Cross-Sectional Studies of General Population Samples

As a consequence of the results from longitudinal studies of social ties and mortality, a number of investigators are now asking how the beneficial effects of social support are mediated, and what behavioral and biological mechanisms are involved. Two major and theoretically different pathways have been suggested: first, social support may help the individual to avoid or give up unhealthy behaviors (e.g., excessive smoking or drinking) or help to enforce healthy behaviors (e.g., physical exercise); second, the effects of social support may be mediated by emotional reactions and their neuroendocrine responses (see Chapter 9). It is probable that both of these mechanisms are relevant.

In ongoing population studies, the emphasis has been on the role of social support in inducing behavioral change, and this interest has involved moving beyond the structural measures of social support used in the longitudinal studies to measures of the functional aspects of social support as well. As mentioned above, longitudinal studies have used primarily quantitative measures of social contacts, social activities, and social network structure. These measures do not explicitly address the function of the social network, which is believed to be most relevant for cardiovascular health. More recently, qualitative measures of social support functions are used in longitudinal population studies.

The most widely used functional measure in ongoing Scandinavian studies is an abbreviated version of the social support measure created by Henderson, Duncan-Jones, and Byrne (1980). This measure, the Interview Schedule for Social Interaction (ISSI), has been adapted for use in population surveys and found to be valid, reliable, and applicable in cross-cultural comparisons (Undén & Orth-Gomér, 1984). In this measure, a distinction is made among attachment or emotional support, social interaction (which is related to belongingness), and material and informational support.

The instrument was used in a study of psychosocial influences on cardiovascular risk factors in men born in 1933 in Gothenburg. Risk factors assessed were smoking, physical exercise and dietary habits, serum lipids, body mass index, and systolic and diastolic blood pressure. Preliminary results from the study of 850 randomly obtained 50-year-old men indicate that the scale that measures social interaction is the one most closely related to standard cardiovascular risk factors (Orth-Gomér, Rosengren, Undén, & Wilhelmsen, 1987). The items that describe belongingness, comradeship, and having the sense of sharing interests and values with a stable group of people are most strongly related to healthy behavior; specifically, the number of men smoking was lower, and the number of men engaging in regular physical exercise was higher, among those who reported a high sense of belongingness.

Another Swedish group from Malmö, an industrial city in the south of Sweden, has developed several interconnected measures of social networks and social supports including: social anchorage, social participation, social influence, material and informational support, and emotional support. Of these subscales, social anchorage has been shown to be the one most strongly related to standard cardiovascular risk factors. Social anchorage describes the extent to which one is rooted in the neighborhood, belongs to a stable group of friends or associates, and belongs to organizations and clubs. It differs from the structural measures of social networks in that it is a perceptual qualitative assessment.

In a probability sample of 500 randomly selected 68-year-old men born in 1914 in Malmö, low social anchorage was independently and significantly related to inadequate nutritional habits (Hanson, Mattisson, & Steen, 1987). Men with inadequate nutrition were defined as those who had a low intake of protein, calcium, iron, or vitamins according to recommendations by the Food and Nutrition Board. These men (about 20% of the sample) were also more obese, less physically active, and more often engaged in heavy alcohol drinking.

Furthermore, a significant association was found between low social anchorage and elevated diastolic blood pressure (DBP). Men who reported low anchorage had an average DBP of 94 mm Hg, whereas men with high anchorage had a DBP of 90 mm Hg. This association was independent of smoking habits, physical activity and body mass index. In this study a thorough analysis of nonrespondents by means of telephone interviews was also performed; there were 19.5% nonrespondents among these elderly men. In comparison with respondents, nonrespondents were more often living alone, which was particularly true of those from lower social classes. They had more signs of alcohol dependency, but were not more often found to be smokers. The prevalence of hypertension, myocardial infarction, and stroke was not higher in nonrespondents than in respondents (Janzon, Steen, Hanson, Isacsson, & Lindell, 1986).

Little work outside Scandinavia has systematically addressed the relationship between social support and risk factors for CVD. One study from Germany found an association between low social support and smoking. This longitudinal study of 416 factory workers (skilled and semiskilled workers and factory group leaders) between 25 and 55 years of age found a remarkable degree of social stability among the men studied. Most of the men were born in the area in which they lived and worked, the provinces of Hessen and North Rhine–Westphalia. Lack of social support was not related to cardiovascular risk factors; however, chronic familial difficulties associated with excessive smoking did relate to CVD. These few men who had experienced occupational and residential instability, as well as those whose wives were working full-time outside the home, were heavier smokers (Siegrist, 1986). In summary, among German blue-collar workers, daily stress from family problems and social instability may be more strongly related to cardiovascular risk than lack of social support. Unfortunately, the possible buffering effect of social support on daily hassles was not examined in this study.

The issue of social class differences has been addressed in great detail in the Whitehall study of British civil servants. The study demonstrates an inverse relationship between employment grade and cardiovascular disease incidence involving a threefold increase in CVD in the lowest as compared to the highest occupational class. Furthermore, because only a fraction of the social class gradient could be accounted for by differences in traditional risk factors for cardiovascular disease, it is possible that psychosocial factors (e.g., social support) may contribute to some of this social gradient. In fact, social class differences in the availability of social support were demonstrated; the proportion of men reporting that they had no contacts with other friends was 20% in the highest and 40% in the lowest grade, and those reporting that they had no social contact with people at work were 55% of the highest as opposed to 82% of the lowest grade (Marmot, Kogevinas, & Elston, 1987). Whether this social class gradient has an impact on cardiovascular disease outcome and whether it is operating via standard risk factors or directly influencing cardiovascular diseases will be addressed in future analyses.

In conclusion, associations have been found between lack of social support and unhealthy life-style factors that are known to increase the risk of cardiovascular disease. In one study poor social integration was related to both smoking and lack of exercise, in another insufficient social anchorage was associated with poor nutrition, and in a third study social instability was associated with heavy smoking. These results suggest that individuals who are socially integrated are more prone to engage in and maintain healthy life-styles. Caution is needed, as this conclusion is based on cross-sectional analyses, in which the direction of causality cannot be determined. Further longitudinal studies are greatly needed.

Longitudinal Studies of Patient Populations

Very few investigators outside the United States have specifically addressed the impact of social support in the therapy and rehabilitation of cardiac patients. In many of the studies on secondary prevention, it is implied that interaction with and support from others (both health professionals and family and friends) are important. Only studies that explicitly deal with social support as a factor influencing health outcome in cardiac patients are reviewed below.

The issue of cardiac rehabilitation in European countries is the subject of much debate. In the countries of central Europe (e.g., Germany), cardiac rehabilitation occurs in specialized rehabilitation clinics throughout the country. In contrast, in the Scandinavian countries, most of the patients who suffer a myocardial infarction are rehabilitated as outpatients living in their homes; hence they are released as soon as possible after the acute event. In addition, it is generally assumed that return to work—at first often on a part-time basis—may even be a helpful and health-promoting measure, rather than an additional strain preventing recovery. This is true primarily for myocardial infarctions without major clinical complications, which do not require special diagnostic and therapeutic measures.

In Germany, there are several reports that specifically dealt with social support and health effects in a patient group. Perhaps the most extensive of these is the Oldenburg longitudinal study (Badura et al., 1987). The study group consisted of a probability sample of 841 male patients under the age of 60 with a first acute myocardial infarction. Patients were obtained from 213 cardiology clinics throughout the western part of the country. All men were employed before the acute event.

Patients were examined on three different occasions: immediately before discharge from the acute care unit; after 6 months, a point of time at which a majority had completed their rehabilitative clinical treatment and returned to their regular familial environment, and after 12 months, when a majority were expected to be back to a normal life with respect to family, work, and other roles. The outcome measures consisted of instruments concerning psychological adjustment and quality of life. Interestingly, biomedical factors had very little impact on global quality of life, whereas social support and subjective health perceptions were the best predictors of quality of life after myocardial infarction. The effects of social support on physical health outcomes were not analyzed, which is unfortunate because the findings may suffer from a redundancy in the measurement of "exposures" and "outcomes." Both measures were self-reported and related to subjective ratings of good health and well-being; thus, the possibility of circular evidence unrelated to hard cardiovascular disease end points cannot be ruled out.

As mentioned above, therapeutic and rehabilitative traditions in Sweden are somewhat different from those of central Europe: Patients are quickly discharged from the hospital and then treated in outpatient cardiology clinics or by general practitioners. Therefore the impact of the social context may be greater, because the patient goes home and back to work as soon as possible after a myocardial infarction. In a Swedish study (Orth-Gomér, Undén, & Edwards, 1988), the long-term effects of social support on survival in cardiac patients and controls were investigated and compared to the effects of clinical factors. One hundred and fifty middle-aged men (one third were men with clinical signs of coronary heart disease, one third had elevated standard risk factors, and one third were originally healthy) were extensively examined in terms of both clinical and psychosocial predictors of outcome. They were followed for 10 years, and their cause-specific mortality was recorded during that period. Clinical predictors of mortality included biochemical variables (serum lipids, glucose and uric acid), X rays of the heart and lungs, resting and exercise

ECG, and 24-hour Holter monitoring in ordinary work and home settings. The psychosocial predictors included basic sociodemographic factors, a semistructured interview on work and life stressors, and an assessment of social activities and social participation. Particular efforts were made to disentangle the influences of clinical from psychosocial predictors of mortality. This was done through the use of canonical correlations analysis, which evaluates both the independent effect of each of the predictors on the outcome variable and the interrelationship among factors in the model (Hotelling, 1936).

In univariate analyses, several predictors of mortality were found. The most important clinical predictors were increased ventricular irritability (classified according to Lown's criteria), elevated systolic blood pressure, cardiac enlargement, and elevated serum glucose. Among psychosocial predictors, the following were significant in univariate analyses: age, low educational level, low social class, a subjective rating of poor general health, and low social activity and social participation rates. Two kinds of results are obtained from the canonical model: the factors that have an independent effect on the outcome variable, and the strength of this effect, and the strength of associations between factors in the model, controlling for the influence of other factors. Three factors had an independent effect on ten year total mortality:

1. Increased ventricular irritability on a 24-hour electrocardiogram
2. Poor self-rating of general health
3. Social isolation as assessed by lack of social activities

When analyzing mortality from coronary heart disease, the canonical correlation coefficient of ventricular irritability increased from 0.24 ($p < 0.01$) to 0.38 ($p < 0.001$). The impact of the social support measure, however, remained the same. These results indicate that there is an effect of social support on mortality in cardiac patients independent of other prognostic factors. The effects of social support were demonstrated regardless of severity of cardiac disease, as assessed by a number of clinical investigative methods. Thus the often-used argument that social isolation in patients is merely a consequence of their disease does not appear valid.

Evidence from Intervention Studies

The clinical approach to cardiac rehabilitation often includes elements of increased social support, from both health professionals and family members. As these effects are often not scientifically evaluated, it is difficult to conclude anything about their magnitude and impact. A few studies, however, have deliberately attempted to stimulate social interactions, to form new bases for friendships and social ties among participants, and to measure the effects of these interventions on cardiovascular outcome variables.

In a study of elderly women in the greater Stockholm area, 108 women, all living alone, were selected for either intervention (68 women) or a control group (40 women) (Andersson, 1985). Their mean age was 77 years, and they were all rated as being in good physical health. The intervention consisted of organized meetings with other women in the neighborhood at which specific themes were discussed and new social ties were formed. Measurements of psychological, social, and biological outcome variables were made at baseline. Six months after beginning participation in the program, intervention subjects rated themselves as less lonely and as having more social contacts, higher self-esteem, a greater ability to trust others and lower demonstrated systolic and diastolic blood pressure than controls. Systolic blood pressure decreased an average of 8.8 mm Hg, and diastolic blood pressure decreased by 5.6 mm Hg. Although these women were not judged to be initially hypertensive, and the main aim of the study was not hypertensive treatment (Andersson, 1984), the results show that it is possible to influence a cardiovascular risk factor by altering the social environment and by increasing social supports.

Some indirect evidence of the impact of social support can be drawn from experimental animal studies. The remarkable studies by von Holst and coworkers in Bayreuth can be interpreted as being supportive of the role of social support on cardiovascular outcomes. The authors have studied three shrews (*Tupaia belangeri*) in a series of elegant experiments. These animals are diurnal mammals approximately the size of squirrels who, in the wild, live in pairs and within territories that they vigorously defend. In experiments the researchers randomly allocated a male and female animal to the same cage, in which they were observed for several weeks.

In about 20% of the cases, aggressive behavior (e.g., fighting) occurred, similar to that observed when two male animals are left together. After a stronger animal emerged, the conquered animal died within a few days. In another 60% of the cases, the animals were apparently indifferent to each other, as they tried to avoid each other as much as possible. Concomitant biological reactions were elevated heart rates and increased excretion rates of cortisol and norepinephrine. Few puppies were born, and if they were, they were severely neglected by their parents.

In about one fifth of the cases, however, a "happy marriage" occurred. The male and female immediately began affectionate behaviors, such as cuddling, that continued for at least a half hour every day. They lay beneath each other during resting periods in the day and always slept together. Their offspring was well cared for and they lived longer than average (up to 10 years). When exposed to experimental stressors, their excretion of hormones was lower, and their ambulatory heart rates were lower throughout the day than in the other groups (Von Holst, 1986).

Summary

Evidence has been presented here showing a relationship between social support and cardiovascular disease. Although systematic efforts in the field are rare, there are data from many different kinds of sources indicating that social support is protective of cardiovascular health. This conclusion is supported in cross-sectional and longitudinal population studies, in intervention studies, with humans and animal experiments.

Recently the relationship was further corroborated, as the previously mentioned population study of 50-year-old men in Gothenburg was able to demonstrate a prospective and substantial effect of lack of support on myocardial infarction risk. In a 6-year follow-up of the population the MI

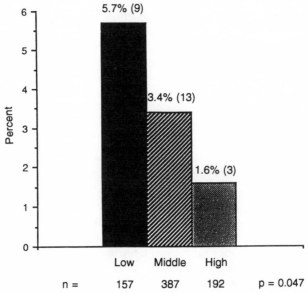

Figure 1. Six-year incidence of myocardial infarction by social integration (749 men, 50 years of age).

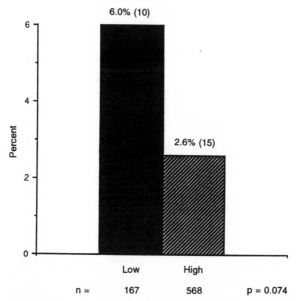

Figure 2. Six-year incidence of myocardial infarction in men with low versus high attachment (749 men, 50 years of age).

incidence was more than three times higher in poorly socially integrated (as compared to well-integrated) men. Also, the MI risk associated with poor attachment to the closest family members was of almost similar magnitude (Figures 1 and 2).

In multivariate analyses controlling for standard risk factors (blood pressure, lipids, coagulation factors, family history, sedentary life style, etc.), two factors emerged as the strongest independent risk factors for MI in these middle-aged men: smoking and lack of social support (Orth-Gomér, Rosengren, & Wilhelmsen, 1993). As far as we are aware, this is the first study to prospectively link social support to the occurrence of coronary heart disease. If these findings are repeated in further studies, a new psychosocial cardiovascular risk factor has been identified that needs to be considered in future investigative and preventive efforts.

References

World Health Organization. (1986). *Consultation on psychosocial determinants of cardiovascular diseases* (Second MONICA Psychosocial Meeting, Stockholm, September 21–22, 1985). Copenhagen: Author.

Alcalay, R. (1983). Aristoteles. In R. Alcalay (Ed.), *Ethics* (pp. 71–88). Holland: Elsevier.

Andersson, L. (1984). Intervention against loneliness in a group of elderly women: A process evaluation. *Human Relations, 37*(4), 295–310.

Andersson, L. (1985). Intervention against loneliness in a group of elderly women: An impact evaluation. *Social Science and Medicine, 4,* 355–364.

Badura, B., Kaufhold, G., Lehmann, H., Pfaff, H., Schott, T., & Waltz, M. (1987). *Leben mit dem Herzinfarkt*. Berlin: Springer-Verlag.

Berkman, L. F., & Syme, S. L. (1979). Social networks, host resistance and mortality: A nine-year follow-up study of Alameda County residents. *American Journal of Epidemiology, 109,* 186–204.

Blazer, D. G. (1982). Social support and mortality in an elderly community population. *American Journal of Epidemiology, 115,* 684–694.

Cohen, S., & Matthews, K. A. (1987). Social support, Type A behavior, and coronary artery disease. *Journal of Psychosomatic Medicine, 49,* 325–330.

Durkheim, E. (1951). *Suicide*. New York: Free Press. (Original work published in 1897)

Hanson, B. S., Mattisson, I., & Steen, B. (1987). Dietary intake and psychosocial factors in 68-year-old men. A population study. *Comprehensive Gerontol., 1*(2), 62–67.

Haynes, S., & Feinleib, M. (1980). Women, work and coronary heart disease: Prospective findings from the Framingham Heart Study. *American Journal of Public Health, 70,* 133–141.

Henderson, S., Duncan-Jones, P., & Byrne, D. (1980). Measuring social relationships. The Interview Schedule for Social Interaction. *Journal of Psychological Medicine, 10,* 723–734.

Hill, A. B. (1965). The environment and disease: Association or causation? *Proceedings of the Royal Society of Medicine, 58,* 295–300.

Hotelling, H. (1936). Relations between two sets of variables. *28,* 321–377.

House, J. D., Robbins, C., & Metzner, H. L. (1982). The association of social relationships and activities with mortality: Prospective evidence from the Tecumseh Community Health Study. *American Journal of Epidemiology, 116,* 123–140.

Janzon, L., Steen, B., Hanson, B., Isacsson, S. O., & Lindell, S. E. (1986). Factors influencing participation in health surveys: Results from prospective population study of men born in 1914 in Malmö, Sweden. *Journal of Epidemiology and Community Health, 40*(2), 174–177.

Johnson, J. V. (1986). *The impact of workplace social support, job demands and work control upon cardiovascular disease in Sweden* (Report No. 1). Department of Psychology, University of Stockholm.

Kaplan, G. A., Salonen, J. T., Cohen, R. D., Brand, R. J., Syme, S. L., & Puska, P. (1986). *Social connections and mortality from all causes and cardiovascular disease: Prospective evidence from eastern Finland*. Irvine: University of California.

Karasek, R., Baker, D., Marxer, F., Ahlbom, A., & Theorell, T. (1981). Job decision latitude, job demands, and cardiovascular disease: A prospective study of Swedish men. *American Journal of Public Health, 71,* 694–705.

Kropotkin, P. (1908). *Gegenseitige Hilfe in der Tier—und Menschenwelt*. Leipzig: Thomas.

Lindström, H. (1981). *Bortfallsfel vid uppskattning av sjukfrånvaro* [Errors in disability estimates, due to nonresponse] (Report No. 24). Stockholm: Central Bureau of Statistics.

Marmot, M. G., Kogevinas, M., & Elston, M. A. (1987). Social/economic status and disease. *Annual Review of Public Health, 8,* 111–135.

Medalie, J H., Kahn, H. A., Neufeld, H. N., Riss, E., Goldbourt, U., Perlstein, T., & Oron, D. (1973). Myocardial infarction over a five-year period: 1. Prevalence, incidence and mortality experience. *Journal of Chronic Disease, 26,* 63–84.

Medalie, J. H., Snyder, M., Groen, J. J., et al. (1973). Angina pectoris among 10,000 men: 5 year incidence and univariate analysis. *American Journal of Medicine, 55,* 583–594.

Orth-Gomér, K., & Johnson, J. V. (1987). Social network interaction and mortality. *Journal of Chronic Disease, 40,* 949–957.

Orth-Gomér, K., Rosengren, A., Undén, A. L., & Wilhelmsen, L. (1987). *Social environmental factors and cardiovascular risk in 50-year-old men in Gothenburg.* Paper presented at the 96th annual meeting of the Swedish Medical Association.

Orth-Gomér, K., & Undén, A. L. (1987). The measurement of social support in population surveys. *Social Science and Medicine, 24,* 83–94.

Orth-Gomér, K., Undén, A. L., & Edwards, M. E. (1988). Social isolation and mortality in ischemic heart disease. *Acta Medica Scandinavia, 224,* 205–215.

Orth-Gomér, K., Rosengren, A., & Wilhelmsen, L. (1993). Lack of social support and incidence of coronary heart disease in middle-aged Swedish men. *Psychosomatic Medicine, 55:* 1, 37–43.

Paracelsus. (1599). *Theophrastus, Bombastus von Hohenheim. Labyrinthus medicorum errantium.* Hanoviae:

Puska, P., et al. (1981). *The North Karelia project.* Copenhagen: World Health Organization.

Schoenbach, V., Kaplan, B. H., Fredman, L., & Kleinbaum, D. (1986). Social ties and mortality in Evans County, Georgia. *American Journal of Epidemiology, 123,* 577–691.

Siegrist, K. (1986). *Sozialer Rückhalt und kardiovaskuläres Risiko.* Munich: Minerva.

Undén, A. L., & Orth-Gomér, K. (1984). *Social support and health, report no. 2: Development of a survey method to measure social support in population studies* (Stress Research Report No. 178). Stockholm: Karolinska Institute.

Vogel, J. (1982, August). *The Swedish annual Level of Living Surveys: Social indicators and social reporting as an official statistics program.* Mexico City,

Von Holst, D. (1986). Psychosocial stress and its pathophysiological effects in tree shrews (*Tupaia belangeri*). In *Biological and psychological factors in cardiovascular disease.* Berlin: Springer-Verlag.

Welin, L., Tibblin, G., Svardsudd, K., et al. (1985). Prospective study of social influences on mortality. *Lancet, 1,* 915–918.

CHAPTER 6

A Critical Evaluation of U.S. Epidemiological Evidence and Ethnic Variation

Helen P. Hazuda

The purpose of this chapter is (a) to review critically epidemiological studies of social support and cardiovascular disease conducted in the United States, (b) to examine ethnic differences in the social support–cardiovascular disease relationship, and (c) to summarize the current status of U.S. epidemiological research on social support and cardiovascular disease. Because of page limitations, cardiovascular end points will be limited to those categorized under ischemic heart disease (IHD), including myocardial infarction (MI), angina pectoris (AP), and coronary atherosclerosis.

The review is organized around the stages of disease: studies of IHD risk factors are reviewed first, followed by studies of manifest IHD and IHD onset, and then studies of outcomes of the disease process (i.e., case fatality or recovery). Within stages of disease, studies are grouped according to research design—case-series studies, case-control studies, cross-sectional (prevalence) studies, prospective (incidence, cohort) studies, and randomized clinical trials. To facilitate ethnic comparisons, studies are further grouped by ethnicity of target population, as shown in Table 1.

A summary of reviewed studies for each stage of disease is presented in Tables 2 through 5, which describe the research design, ethnicity of target population, study name or site, sample characteristics, IHD end

HELEN P. HAZUDA • Division of Clinical Epidemiology, Department of Medicine, University of Texas Health Science Center, San Antonio, Texas 78284-7873.

Social Support and Cardiovascular Disease, edited by Sally A. Shumaker and Susan M. Czajkowski. Plenum Press, New York, 1994.

Table 1.   U.S. Evidence for the Relationship
between Social Support and Ischemic Heart Disease (IHD)
among White and Ethnic Population Subgroups

Type of data and IHD end point	Population subgroup			
	White Americans	Japanese Americans	Mexican Americans	Black Americans
Prevalence data				
Risk factors	×	×	×*	
Total IHD		×		
Morbidity	×	×		
Mortality	×*	×		×*
Incidence data				
Risk factors				
Total IHD		×		
Morbidity		×		
Mortality	×	×		
Survival after MI	×			

*Includes ethnic and white comparison groups within the same study.

points, social support/social network measures, and results and covariates for each study. Each table is accompanied by several pages of text that provide a summary of results, an assessment of strengths and limitations, and a comment on observed ethnic variation. The chapter ends with a brief summary of the current status of U.S. epidemiological research on social support and cardiovascular disease and offers several recommendations for future research.

IHD Risk Factors

Summary of Results

A preventive health practices model, which posits that members of one's social network are always willing to offer advice about prudent health habits, was not supported (see Table 2). Studies of a direct effects model, which posits that having a social network is in itself beneficial to health, uncovered no consistent pattern of statistically significant associations between social networks and IHD risk factors that would support the model. Several studies did support a stress-buffering model, which posits that the negative health consequences of stress are reduced or eliminated by social support.

Table 2. U.S. Studies of Social Support and IHD Risk Factors

Study/site and reference	Sample	Risk factor	Social support/ social network measure	Results and covariates[a]
Population-based prevalence studies				
The Health Examination Survey, 1960–1962 (Weiss, 1986)	5,372 men and women, ages 25–79, who consitituted a national probability sample of the civilian, noninstitutionalized population (whites and nonwhites pooled)	Systolic and diastolic BP, serum cholesterol, ponderal index (height/cubic root of weight)	Self-reported marital status: married and living with spouse vs. D, W, and/or NM; individuals separated/ not living with spouse were excluded from analyses	There were no consistent differences in any of the risk factor levels by marital status (married vs. nonmarried).[c]
An urban, southwestern community (Thomas, Goodwin, & Goodwin, 1985)	197 male and female healthy volunteers, ages 61–89, who were mostly middle class (whites and nonwhites pooled)	Serum cholesterol, serum uric acid	Presence of satisfying confiding relationships with trusted individuals, measured by a self-administered form of the ISSI	All associations were in the expected inverse direction and were statistically significant in the pooled sample. In men, only the association with uric acid and, in women, only the association with cholesterol were significant. Findings supported the stress-buffering hypothesis.

(Continued)

Table 2. (Continued)

Study/site and reference	Sample	Risk factor	Social support/ social network measure	Results and covariates[a]
Honolulu Heart Program, 1971–1979 (Reed et al., 1983)	4,653 Japanese American men living in Hawaii, ages 52–71, who received an initial medical exam in 1965–68 and responded to a mailed psychosocial questionnaire in 1971; 61% of eligibles returned questionnaires	Systolic BP, serum cholesterol, serum glucose, serum uric acid, forced vital capacity, BMI, physical activity, smoking, alcohol, Japanese diet, complex carbohydrate, SES	A conceptual social network score constructed post hoc from 9 existing items: 5 measuring available intimate ties (heavier weighting), and 4 measuring actual ties at work, church, and social organizations; a factor-derived score included the first 5 items.	For both measures, there was a trend for men with higher social network scores to have lower risk levels of BP, serum glucose, alcohol intake, physical activity, and diet, but the trend was statistically significant only for physical activity and Japanese diet. A preventive health practices model received little support.
San Antonio Heart Study, Phase, I & II, 1979–82 & 1984–85 (Patterson et al., 1986)	1,975 MA and 1,142 NHW men and women, ages 25–64, randomly sampled from a low, middle, and high SES neighborhood in San Antonio, TX; 64.6% response rate	Systolic and diastolic BP; total, LDL, and HDL cholesterol; HDL ratio; TG; BMI; cigarettes per day	Living alone vs. living with others, ascertained from a household enumeration form; an NIH workshop recommended this measure (Ostfeld & Eaker, 1985)	For women, there were no significant differences on any risk factor; for men, those living alone had lower risk levels of TG, total and LDL-cholesterol, but higher systolic BP.[c,d,h]
San Antonio Heart Study, Phase I, 1979–82 (Hazuda, 1986)	1,230 MA and 890 NHW men and women, ages 25–64, randomly sampled from a low, middle, and high SES neighborhood in San Antonio, TX; 64% response rate	Systolic and diastolic BP; total, LDL, and HDL cholesterol; HDL ratio; TG; BMI; cigarettes per day	Self-reported marital status (M vs. S, D, W vs. NM), organizational membership (member vs. nonmember), and church participation (active vs. occasional vs. none)	There were few statistically significant associations, and the pattern of significant results was not consistent: Some social support measures were associated with greater risk, whereas others were assoicated with lower risk.[c]

Organization-based, prospective comparison studies

3 manufacturing plants in a large city and 3 manufacturing plants in a small rural community (Cobb, 1974)	54 rural and 46 urban male blue-collar job terminees and 74 continuously employed controls, ages 35–62; all subjects were married; 10% were black (whites and blacks pooled)	Serum cholesterol, serum uric acid	A 13-item ad hoc index: 8 items tapped perception of wife, friends, and relatives as supportive or unsupportive; 3 items tapped frequency of activities outside the home with wife, friends, and relatives; and 2 items tapped the perceived opportunity to engage in satisfying social relations and discuss personal problems; men in the lowest population tertile were considered unsupported	Among job terminees who were supported, changes in levels of serum cholesterol from termination to 2 years following termination remained very similar to levels of cholesterol among controls, whereas cholesterol levels among unsupported terminees over the same time period remained significantly higher. A similar pattern was observed for uric acid up to 1 year following job termination. Findings supported the stress-buffering hypothesis.
Same as above (Gore, 1978)	Same as above *except* controls were not included in the statistical analyses because of observed self-selection bias	Serum cholesterol	Same as above	Among job terminees who remained unemployed at end of study, there was a significant drop in mean levels of serum cholesterol from the time termination was anticipated to 2 years following termination. Among unsupported terminees who remained unemployed, there was no significant drop in serum cholesterol over the same period.

Note: BP = blood pressure, LDL = low-density lipoprotein, HDL = high-density lipoprotein, HDL ratio = ratio of HDL cholesterol to total cholesterol; TG = triglycerides, BMI = body mass index (weight in kilograms/height in meters^2), SES = socioeconomic status, M = currently married, S = separated, D = divorced, W = widowed, NM = never married, ISSI = Interview Schedule for Social Interaction, MA = Mexican American, NHW = non-Hispanic white.

[a]Covariates: c = age, d = BMI, e = cigarette smoking, f = alcohol intake, g = self-reported psychological distress, h = SES.

Strengths and Limitations

Negative studies of social networks and IHD risk factors were large, population-based prevalence studies carried out in several distinct ethnic populations. All relied on post hoc social network measures with undetermined psychometric properties. Measurement error or suppression of network effects by uncontrolled confounders may account for the negative findings, but the consistency of results across studies cannot be ignored. Positive studies of social support were specifically designed to test a stress-buffering model. Serum cholesterol and uric acid were treated as indicators of physiological stress rather than IHD risk factors. All were based on small samples subject to volunteer bias (Sackett, 1979), relied on social support measures constructed on an ad hoc or post hoc basis and subject to an unknown degree of measurement error, and did not adjust for several potential confounders.

Comment on Ethnic Variation

Berkman (1985, 1986) suggests that group differences in the availability of network ties may affect the strength of observed associations between social networks and health outcomes. A group's ethnic composition may be an important determinant of available network ties. Gore (1978) notes, for example, that subjects in a largely Polish-American rural area had higher mean social support scores than those in a non-Polish-American urban area. Nonetheless, negative findings related to the social network–IHD risk factor association were similar across several ethnically varied populations. Studies of multiple IHD risk factors in a biethnic population found little evidence of ethnic-by-social-network interaction effects. Available social ties among Mexican Americans varied directly with their level of acculturation (i.e., adoption of the values, attitudes, and behaviors of mainstream, non-Hispanic white society), but the impact of acculturation on the social network–IHD risk factor association was not examined.

IHD Morbidity

Summary of Results

All five studies supported a direct effects model of social networks or support on IHD morbidity (see Table 3). Assessment of discrete network characteristics suggested that (a) instrumental support and emotional support, assessed by a measure of perceived positive appraisal from

Table 3. U.S. Studies of Social Support and IHD Morbidity

Hospital-based case-series studies (ethnic/racial composition not specified)

Study/site and reference	Sample	IHD end points	Social support/ social network measure	Results and covariates[a]
Four teaching hospital medical centers in northeastern U.S. that performed more than 150 cardiac surgical procedures per year (Jenkins et al., 1983)	204 male CABG patients, 25–69 years old, who met highly restrictive eligibility criteria, including medical, language, residential, and availability criteria, and volunteered to be in the study; 84% of eligibles participated.	AP categorized as exertional, emotional, postprandial, and resting; diagnosed using the London School of Hygiene Angina Questionnaire and questions about the circumstances triggering the AP, its intensity, response to rest and medication, and frequency of sublingual nitroglycerin use	Three types of psychosocial supports related to religion, security, and frequency of visiting preoperatively; the number and content of items in these three measures were not provided	None of the social support measures were related to emotional or resting AP. Support involving religion was significantly and inversely related to exertional and emotional AP. After adjustment for all covariates[c-l], the latter associations remained statistically significant only for exertional AP.

(*Continued*)

Table 3. (*Continued*)

Study/site and reference	Sample	IHD end points	Social support/ social network measure	Results and covariates[a]
Six hospitals in the San Francisco Bay Area, CA (Seeman, 1984)	120 men and 41 women, ages 30–70, referred by 25 participating cardiologists for angiography with a diagnosis of AP, CAD, recent MI, and/or asymptomatic CAD; exclusion criteria to eliminate patients with *known* history of IHD were MI more than 6 months prior to angiography or previous catheterization; 88% of eligibles participated.	CAD, assessed by angiography and evaluations of the four major arteries as recommended by the AHA; a summary measure of total % occlusion equal to the sum of occlusions for all four arteries was the outcome measure	Four aspects of social networks: (1) structure—closely approximated Berkman-Syme SNI (ties to spouse, close friends and relatives, church, and other groups); (2) Instrumental support—number of times subject relied on family and/or friends for help with minor household tasks, a ride, or financial assistance; (3) Emotional support—number of times subject relied on family and/or friends for information, discussing health or personal problems, and being cheered up; (4) Adequacy of social support and caring, and positive appraisal provided by the network	There was a significant inverse association between CAD and both instrumental support and perceived positive appraisal from the network independent of age, sex, and all major IHD risk factors.[c,m–u] Network structure and emotional support were not related to CAD. For men, perceived network adequacy was inversely associated with CAD, but for women it was positively associated with CAD. This sex difference was particularly salient for the item measuring loneliness.

Hospital-based, retrospective case-control studies (ethnic/racial composition not specified)

The university hospital, VA hospital, and several major community hospitals in Oklahoma City, Oklahoma (Thiel, Parker, & Bruce, 1973)	50 male cases, age 40–60, admitted consecutively to the hospital following a recent, initial MI; and 50 age-matched healthy controls selected from volunteer patients seen for routine physical examinations; eligibility criteria for cases included general good health and no prior history of diabetes	MI diagnosed on basis of typical changes of ECG, history, or enzyme elevation	Self-reported marital status at time of MI (currently married vs. divorced; handling of single, separated, and widowed men was not described)	Men suffering an initial, nonfatal MI were significantly more likely than healthy controls to be divorced.[c]

(Continued)

Table 3. (*Continued*)

Study/site and reference	Sample	IHD end points	Social support/ social network measure	Results and Covariates[a]
Population-based prevalence studies				
Japanese-American Health Research Project (Joseph, 1980)	Japanese-American men, ages 30–74: 2,974 enumerated by a special census of the SFBA, and a convenience sample of 835 from Japanese-American groups in Santa Clara County, California received medical exams and completed questionnaires; 889 more SFBA men completed questionnaires only	Definite and probable IHD, defined by Minnesota codes for major ECG abnormality and by the London School of Hygiene Cardiovacular Questionnaire; the case mix was 38% definite IHD and 62% probable IHD (total N = 394)	Two measures constructed post hoc from available data: (1) structural affiliation—relational ties to spouse, church, and formal organizations; and (2) attitudinal affiliation—importance placed on the latter ties and on the group in general	Attitudinal affiliation was not related to IHD prevalence. Structural affiliation was strongly and inversely related to IHD prevalence: after adjusting for covariates[c,f,g,n,p,v,w] and for attitudinal affiliation, the RR for men in the lowest structural affiliation category vs. the highest was 1.94. No support was found for a buffering hypothesis.
Honolulu Heart Program, 1971–1979 (Reed et al., 1983)	4,653 Japanese ancestry men living in Hawaii, ages 52–71, who received an initial medical exam in 1965–68 and responded to a mailed psychosocial questionnaire in 1971; 61% of eligibles returned questionnaires	Nonfatal MI and AP diagnosed on basis of examination findings and medical staff review of hospital discharge records; total IHD was defined as both diagnoses combined; the case mix was 49% AP and 51% nonfatal MI (total N = 267)	A conceptual social network score constructed post hoc from 9 existing items: 5 measuring available intimate ties (heavier weighting), 4 measuring actual social ties to work, church, and social organizations; a factor-derived score included only the first 5 items	After adjustments for covariates,[c,e,n,v,x] the conceptual network score was significantly and inversely related only to prevalence of total IHD; the factor-derived score was significantly related to prevalence of total IHD and AP, but not to MI.

Population-based incidence studies

Honolulu Heart Program, 1971–1979 (Reed et al., 1983)	4,389 Japanese ancestry men living in Hawaii, ages 52–71, who received an initial medical exam in 1965–68, responded to a mailed psychosocial questionnaire and were free of IHD in 1971	Same as above *except* the case mix was 33% AP and 67% nonfatal MI (total $N = 142$; fatal MI accounted for 76 additional incident cases)	Same as above	After age adjustment, the conceptual network score was not significantly related to incidence of any IHD end point, whereas the factor-derived score was related to incidence of nonfatal MI and total IHD. After adjustment for other covariates,[e,n,v,x] the association was no longer significant. A buffering hypothesis was not supported.

Note: IHD = ischemic heart disease, CABG = coronary artery bypass graft, AP = angina pectoris, CAD = coronary artery disease, AHA = American Heart Association, VA = Veterans Administration, BP = blood pressure, MI = myocardial infarction, ECG = electrocardiogram, SFBA = San Francisco Bay Area, SNI = Social Network Index, SES = socioeconomic status, BMI = body mass index (weight in kilograms/height in meters²)
[a]Covariates: c = age, d = degree of coronary occlusion and number of involved vessels, e = sleep disturbances, f = physical inactivity, g = cigarette smoking, h = distressed response to life crises, i = life dissatisfactions, j = hostility, k = propanolol use, l = duration of cardiac illness, m = hypertension, n = serum cholesterol, o = diabetes, p = family history of IHD, q = AP, r = Type A behavior pattern, s = trait anxiety, t = sex, u = income, v = systolic BP, w = social disconnections, x = BMI, serum glucose, serum uric acid, forced vital capacity, Japanese diet, complex carbohydrate, and SES.

network members, but not by a measure of aid given in specific situations of emotional need, may have a greater impact than network structure on cardiovascular health; and (b) actual social ties (i.e,. network structure) may have an impact on IHD morbidity independent of the value attached to those ties by the individual or group. A buffering model, which posited that social networks are most beneficial to persons at high risk of IHD, was not supported. Stratified analyses suggested the potential importance of examining age and gender differences in the social network and support–IHD relationship.

Strengths and Limitations

Generalizability of study results is limited by the use of specialized ethnic or high-risk populations. Two broadly focused studies, which used inadequately described "psychosocial support" scales or measured only marital status, were particularly vulnerable to established biases (Sackett, 1979) in case-series and case-control designs. The other three studies were specific attempts to expand the scope of social network or support research by assessing network characteristics other than structure or testing hypotheses generated by previous epidemiological investigations. Several different models were examined, and alternative hypotheses were carefully assessed. Potential gender differences in the meaning of social networks and support were uncovered by carrying out stratified analyses. Covariate adjustments for physical risk factors were made in all three studies, with additional adjustment for Type A behavior patterns in one of them.

Psychometric properties of the social network and support indices used in these three studies were not formally documented. The two Japanese-American studies were based on post hoc measures that may have been strongly influenced by the study population's ethnic composition. Joseph's (1980) measure of "attitudinal affiliation," in particular, appears to be closely bound to the concept of acculturation rather than to any distinctive characteristic of social networks themselves. Network indices constructed by Reed, McGee, Yano, and Feinleib (1983) were named for the methods by which they were derived rather than the type of social ties measured, with the unfortunate result that conceptual distinctions which may explain disparate results obtained with the two indices were missed.

Seeman's (1984) measures, constructed with original data specifically collected to test the effects of social networks *and* support on IHD morbidity, are the most advanced to date. Indices related to social support should be further refined, however, by positing two distinct dimensions of a single underlying construct: (a) the frequency with which network members actually provide aid in specific situations of emotional need, and (b) the individual's general feeling that his or her personal worth is affirmed by network members. The second dimension of emotional support appears to be related to CAD; the first does not.

Comment on Ethnic Variation

Japanese Americans are an ethnically distinct population subgroup known for their maintenance of traditional Japanese customs, religion, and attitudes and an emphasis on the group. It has been suggested that the meaning of bonds and social isolation in such highly cohesive groups may differ from that in groups which are less cohesive (Berkman, 1985). More specifically, differences in the extent of social isolation may have less impact on differences in disease risk in groups with high overall levels of support, or high levels of social contact may be so much a part of such groups that they go unnoticed and unreported by group members (Berkman, 1985). It is possible, then, that the social network effects observed among Japanese Americans *under*estimate the strength of the true effects.

Two alternative hypotheses should be considered: (a) The greater the cohesion of the social group, the greater the effect of isolation on health; and (b) the effect of social isolation on health is relatively constant across groups regardless of their level of cohesion. If the first hypothesis is correct, associations observed among Japanese Americans *over*estimate the true association. If the second hypothesis is correct, observed associations among Japanese Americans closely approximate the true associations. Because neither hypothesis can be ruled out on the basis of the studies reviewed here, future studies should focus on resolving this issue. The finding that race was not associated with either CAD or network characteristics in a pooled sample of whites and nonwhites (Seeman, 1984) suggests that ethnic and racial variation in the association between social network and support and CAD may be negligible.

IHD Mortality

Summary of Results

A direct effects model was supported by seven of the nine studies, including four large, population-based incidence studies (see Table 4). The relative risk (*RR*) associated with low social network scores ranged from 2.0 to 3.0; some gender differences and variation in the predictive capacity of specific social ties were observed within and across studies. The two

Table 4. U.S. Studies of Social Support and IHD Mortality

Study/site and reference	Sample	IHD end points	Social support/ social network measure	Results and covariates[a]
Case-control study within a population-based, prospective investigation				
Washington County, MD (Comstock, 1971)	A private county census in 1963 identified all white males, ages 45–64. Cases were 185 men who died of ASDHD during the subsequent 3-year period. 2 controls per case were randomly selected from the census list and matched on race, sex, and age.	ASDHD death, ascertained from death certificates matched to the 1963 census listing	Three measures: (1) marital history (categories not defined), (2) affiliation with a particular religious sect (yes-no), (3) frequency of church attendance (less than once per week vs. more frequently)	Marital history and religious affiliation were not associated with fatal ASDHD. After covariate adjustments, [c,d] the RR for men attending church less than once per week versus those attending more frequently was 1.7.
Population-based prevalence studies, whites and nonwhites stratified				
NCHS national vital statistics data, 1959–61 (Carter & Glick, 1970)	Men and women 15–64 years old	Age-standardized deaths from coronary disease and other myocardial degeneration	Marital status (currently married vs. nonmarried)	Nonmarried persons had an excess of IHD deaths relative to married persons. The excess was greater among men than women and among nonwhites than whites.[c]
Same as above (Ortmeyer, 1974)	Men and women 15 years and older	Ratio of expected to standard deaths from ASHD, including coronary disease	Same as above	Same as above.

Tecumseh Community Health Study (House et al., 1982)	1,322 white men and 1,432 white women, ages 35–69, who participated in the third round of study (1967–69). The baseline response rate was 71%. Follow-up ascertainment was 100%.	Primary endpoint: all-cause mortality, verified by death certificate. Endpoint for exploratory analyses: IHD, ascertained by underlying cause on death certificates. 5.1% of male and 1.7% of female deaths were attributed to IHD.	Four types of social relationships/activities and perceived satisfaction from them: (1) intimate social relationships, (2) formal organizational involvements outside of work, (3) active and relatively social leisure, and (4) passive and relatively solitary leisure. A "count index" consisted of the number of variables in activities 1–3 on which the respondent scored above the lowest level; a "mean index" was the average of actual responses on the same variables.	After covariate adjustments,[c,f,g,l,o] the two social support indices were significantly and inversely associated with all-cause mortality only in men. Perceived satisfaction had no significant independent effect. No clear dose-response relationship was observed for any social support variable. Exploratory analyses of IHD mortality showed that social relationships/activities were generally strong and significant predictors among women, but less strong and predictive among men. Details about the associations and supporting data were not provided.
Rancho Bernardo, an upper-middle-class Caucasian community in Southern California (Wingard et al., 1983)	1,535 men and 1,981 women, ages 30–69, followed since 1972 for a minimum of 7 years. Follow-up ascertainment was 99%.	All-cause and IHD-mortality, ascertained by underlying cause of death on death certificates as coded by a certified nosologist (ICDA-8)	Marital status (married vs. unmarried)	Marital status was a significant predictor of all-cause mortality in men, but not in women.[c,f,m,j,n,k] The number of IHD deaths in women was too small to permit sex-specific analyses; however, in multivariate analyses adjusted for sex, marital status was not a significant predictor of IHD mortality.

(Continued)

Table 4. (*Continued*)

Study/site and reference	Sample	IHD end points	Social support/ social network measure	Results and covariates[a]
Alameda County, CA, 9-year follow-up, 1965–1974 (Berkman & Syme, 1979)	2,229 men and 2,469 women, ages 30–69, included in the 1965 Human Population Laboratory (HPL) survey of a random sample of noninstitutionalized adults residing in the county. Respondents were judged to be a representative sample of adults in the county. Baseline response was 86%. Follow-up ascertainment was 96%.	Primary endpoint: all-cause mortality, ascertained through death certificates. Secondary endpoint: four specific causes of death, including IHD, probably ascertained from underlying cause on death certificates.	Four sources of social contact available in HPL data base: (1) marriage, (2) close friends and relatives, (3) church, and (4) informal and formal group associations. A Social Network Index (SNI) was developed to summarize type and extent of social contacts (intimate contacts weighted more heavily). Response categories were ordered from least to most social connections.	Each contact source predicted all-cause mortality independently of the other 3; but intimate ties were stronger predictors (*RR* range: 1.3–2.9). Age-adjusted *RRs* for persons in the lowest SNI category compared to the highest were 2.3 for men and 2.8 for women. Associations persisted after covariate adjustments.[c,d,f,p] *RRs* were reportedly similar for IHD mortality, but no data were provided.
Alameda County, CA, 9-year follow-up, 1965–1974 (Kaplan, 1985)	2,352 male and female respondents to the HPL 1965 survey, who were 50 years old or over at that time	IHD mortality (ICD-8: 410–414); ascertainment method not described, but probably coded form underlying cause on death certificates	The Berkman-Syme SNI	After adjustment for age, sex, and physical health status, the *RR* of IHD mortality associated with few versus many social ties was 3.55. After additional covariate adjustments,[f,q] the *RR* was still 2.86.

| Alameda County, CA, 9-year follow-up, 1965–1974 (Wingard & Cohn, 1987) | 1,699 men and 2,052 women, who were 40 years old and over when they responded to the 1965 HPL survey | IHD mortality, ascertained from underlying cause on death certificates (ICD-8: 410.0–414.9) | The four separate components of the Berkman-Syme SNI: marital status, index of contacts with close friends and relatives, church membership, and formal and informal group affiliation | In sex-specific analyses adjusting for covariates,[c,d,f,g,j-l,r-v] only group affiliation was associated with 9-year IHD mortality *and* only in women (*RR* for nonaffiliation = 2.1.) In a combined model with sex as an added covariate, no SNI component was significantly related to IHD mortality. |
| Honolulu Heart Program, 1971–1979 (Reed et al., 1983) | 4,653 Japanese ancestry men living in Hawaii, ages 52–71, who received an initial medical exam in 1965–68 and responded to a mailed psychosocial questionnaire in 1971 | Fatal MI diagnosed on basis of medical staff review of mortality records (*N* = 76; nonfatal MI and AP accounted for 142 additional incident cases) | A conceptual social network score constructed post hoc from 9 existing items: 5 measuring available intimate ties (heavier weighting); and 4 measuring actual social ties to work, church, and social organizations; a factor-derived score included only the first 5 items | After age adjustment, neither social network score was significantly related to incidence of fatal MI. A buffering hypothesis was not supported. |

Note: ASHD = arteriosclerotic heart disease, ASDHD = arteriosclerotic and degenerative heart disease, NCHS = National Center for Health Statistics, *RR* = relative risk, SES = socioeconomic status, IHD = ischemic heart disease, BP = blood pressure, BMI = body mass index (weight in kilograms/height in meters[2]), ICD = International Classification of Diseases, HPL = Human Population Laboratory, SNI = Social Network Index.

[a]Covariates: c = age; d = sex; e = race; f = SES; g = cigarette smoking; h = cigar smoking; i = water hardness; j = high BP; k = BMI; l = alcohol intake; m = serum cholesterol; n = serum glucose; o = baseline morbidity (diagnosis of suspect or probable IHD, chronic bronchitis or persistent cough or phlegm), probable hypertension, systolic/diastolic BP, serum cholesterol, blood glucose, forced expiratory volume, BMI); p = indices of health practices, preventive utilization of health services, and baseline health status; q = measures of perceived health, health practices, life satisfaction, depression, and helplessness; r = chest pain; s = diabetes; t = physical activity; u = sleeping patterns; v = life satisfaction.

incidence studies that failed to support the direct effects model included an investigation of fatal MI in Japanese-American men and an investigation of marital status and total IHD deaths among middle-class whites. Examination of direct and indirect effects models indicated that social network ties not only have a direct effect on IHD mortality ($RR = 2.86$ after covariate adjustments) but account for some of the associations of health practices, life satisfaction, and depression with IHD death. Testing of a multivariate model showed that perceived network satisfaction has no effect on IHD mortality once frequency of relationships and activities is controlled.

Strengths and Limitations

This group of studies includes Berkman and Syme's (1979) seminal work on network ties and mortality, and several studies (House, Metzner, & Robbins, 1982; Kaplan, 1985; Reed et al., 1983) that attempted to confirm and expand this work by examining a broader range of ties and activities, measuring structural characteristics other than size (i.e., intensity), and assessing models that included nonstructural network characteristics, buffering effects, and interrelationships between network structure and psychosocial and behavioral variables. Other studies (Wingard & Cohn, 1987; Wingard, Suarez, & Barrett-Connor, 1983) expanded the field by examining social ties as one of a larger set of IHD risk factors. All of the incidence studies were large, population-based investigations that reported negligible bias from baseline nonresponse and loss to follow-up. Most included covariate adjustments for baseline health status, although some used self-report rather than clinical measures.

All nine studies were carried out as secondary analyses. Social network measures were created post hoc, primarily on the basis of face validity, and had otherwise undocumented psychometric properties. Two of the most influential studies examined all-cause rather than IHD mortality as the primary outcome; analyses related specifically to IHD were summarized briefly and presented as "exploratory and suggestive." Three of six incidence studies were conducted on overlapping age groups of the Alameda County Human Population Laboratory data base. Among this group were the only studies that found a clear dose-response relationship between network ties and IHD mortality. Two of three incidence studies conducted on other data bases failed to support the social network–IHD mortality association.

Comment on Ethnic Variation

Several hypotheses were formulated to explain differences in the sex-specific associations observed in Tecumseh and Alameda counties (House et al., 1982). Their underlying premise is that the meaning of social ties for particular individuals or subgroups varies according to the social context in which people carry out their day-to-day activities. Ethnic variation may be a special case of social context effects; thus, the meaning of ties and strength of their association with IHD mortality may vary across population subgroups as a function of their ethnic makeup. Finding that excess IHD mortality among the nonmarried is greater for nonwhites than whites (Carter & Glick, 1970; Ortmeyer, 1974) is consistent with this premise.

Survival Following Acute IHD Episodes

Summary of Results

A direct effects model was supported in all three studies (see Table 5). Severity of manifest disease at time of hospitalization partially explained the positive findings in one of these (Hrubec & Zukel, 1971). Social networks were protective against in-hospital and longer-term fatalities in both men and women. Examination of the joint effects of social networks and life stress indicated that isolated men with high life stress had four to five times greater risk of death from all causes and six times greater risk of sudden cardiac death than men with adequate social ties and low life stress.

Strengths and Limitations

These studies broke new ground by focusing on the potentially protective effect of social networks against fatal outcomes following an acute IHD event. Several testable hypotheses were formulated to account for observed network benefits: (a) Presence of a spouse at the time of MI may be lifesaving because the spouse will seek and/or render first aid (Chandra et al., 1983); (b) persons who live alone may have lower survival chances because they cannot physically care for themselves (Chandra, Szklo, Goldberg, & Tonascia, 1983); and (c) married men may find it easier than nonmarried men to follow prescribed medical programs (Hrubec & Zukel, 1971). Studies were limited by the use of relatively specialized hospital-based samples subject to varying degrees of admission and selection bias (Sackett, 1979), and by the social network measures utilized.

Comment on Ethnic Variation

Race was treated as a covariate. Information about racial or ethnic variation was not provided.

Table 5.   U.S. Studies of Social Support and Survival Following an Acute IHD Episode

Study/site and reference	Sample	IHD end points	Social support/ social network measure	Results and covariates[a]
Hospital-based incidence studies				
Veterans Administration (Hrubec & Zukel, 1971)	1,495 white males admitted to VA hospitals for first acute episodes of IHD (MI, CO, CT, AP, CI, & other) between June, 1943 and December, 1944, and who were still alive 6 months after admission	18-year survival status ascertained by VA Master Index records verified as 98% complete	Marital status at entry into military service, ascertained by review of induction or enlistment records (married vs. S, D, or W)	Married men in both major IHD categories had a better survival prognosis than nonmarried men. This relationship was at least partially influenced by differences in severity of disease manifestation at time of hospital admission.[c,h]
20 hospitals in the Baltimore, MD, SMSA (Chandra et al., 1983)	1,401 men and women, who constituted a 1-in-3 systematic sample of patients discharged with a diagnosis of acute MI between the periods July 1, 1966–June 30, 1967 and January 1–December 31, 1971	Survival status in-hospital and 3, 5, and 10 years following hospital discharge, ascertained by review of hospital records, contacts with attending physicians, patients, or next-of-kin and a search of death records in the Baltimore SMSA. Survival status was ascertained on 95%, 90%, and 46% of patients, respectively, at the three follow-up periods.	Marital status at time of diagnosis, ascertained from medical records. 4.4% of patients whose marital status could not be determined were excluded from the study. An interview with 32% of patients or their next-of-kin showed 91% agreement between medical records and interview-reported marital status. Type of disagreements not reported.	After adjustment for covariates,[c,d,e,g,i] the in-hospital and 3-year survival rate of married persons were significantly higher than those of unmarried persons. The crude 10-year survival rate was also significantly better for married persons, but had been ascertained on only 46% of the original sample.

Incidence studies within multicenter, randomized clinical trials

Health Insurance Plan ancillary study of the Beta-Blocker Heart Attack Trial (BHAT; Ruberman et al., 1984)	2,320 men hospitalized for acute MI, ages 30–69, randomly assigned to treatment in 25 of 31 BHAT centers. The sample included 90% of men in the 25 cooperating centers and 79% of men in all 31 BHAT centers. BHAT eligibility included medical exclusion criteria.	3-year cumulative probability of death (all causes and sudden ASHD considered separately) after acute MI, among men surviving the acute event by at least 2.6 months. Ascertainment method not specified.	Two measures: (1) social isolation (dichotomized as high vs. low), and (2) a combined index of social isolation and life stress (subjects categorized as high on both, high on only one, or low on both).	Men who scored high on isolation had roughly 2 times the mortality risk of those who scored low. After covariate adjustments,[c,f,j] men high on both social isolation and life stress were at 4–5 times greater risk of death from all causes and 6 times greater risk of sudden cardiac death than men who scored low on social isolation and stress.

Note: IHD = ischemic heart disease, VA = Veterans Administration, MI = myocardial infarction, CO = coronary occlusion, CT = coronary thrombosis, AP = angina pectoris, CI = coronary insufficiency, S = separated, D = divorced, W = widowed, SMSA = Standard Metropolitan Statistical Area, CCU = coronary care unit, ECG = electrocardiogram, CHF = congestive heart failure, ASHD = arteriosclerotic heart disease.

[a]Covariates: c = age; d = sex; e = race; f = SES; g = cigarette smoking; h = severity of disease; i = admission to a CCU; type of hospital (teaching vs. nonteaching); history of AP, clinical complications during admission, initial or recurrent MI, location and depth of MI, administration of anticoagulant therapy in hospital; j = myocardial function, ventricular arrhythmia, AP, treatment group, cigarette smoking.

Summary and Recommendations

U.S. epidemiological studies have investigated the association between social networks or support and several stages of cardiovascular disease, including risk factor development, morbidity, mortality, and survival following an acute IHD episode. The theoretical model most frequently guiding these studies has been a direct effects model, which posits that social ties in themselves are beneficial for IHD. Several studies have been guided by either a stress-buffering model, which posits that negative consequences of stress on IHD are reduced or eliminated by social support, or a buffering model, which posits that social networks are protective against IHD only for persons at high physiological risk of disease. The relative contribution of structural and nonstructural network characteristics (e.g., instrumental support, perceived satisfaction from network relationships and activities) to IHD has also been assessed. A direct effects model has been supported for IHD morbidity (including AP, CAD, MI, and total IHD), IHD mortality, and survival prognosis following acute IHD, but it has received little or no support for IHD risk factors. A stress-buffering model has been supported only for IHD risk factors, whereas a buffering model has received no support. Assessments of the relative importance of structural and nonstructural network characteristics in IHD have suggested that structural characteristics may be more important than the value placed on network ties or the perceived satisfaction they provide, but less important than instrumental support or a dimension of emotional support reflecting an individual's general feeling that network members affirm his or her personal worth.

Notable strides thus have been made in the relatively new area of U.S. epidemiological research on social support and CVD, and there is reason to be encouraged that certain social network characteristics potentially amenable to therapeutic intervention play a role in several stages of the IHD disease process. Supporting evidence is primarily suggestive, however, rather than conclusive. With only a single exception, even the most reliable studies available have been secondary analyses, based on unvalidated, post hoc network measures of unknown reliability. Several promising hypotheses have been generated about the importance of structural versus nonstructural network characteristics, the role of social context (including ethnic composition) in modifying network effects, and the mechanisms through which network effects operate, but these have not yet been systematically tested in other epidemiological investigations.

If cardiovascular epidemiological research on social support is to provide a solid foundation for designing public health interventions, future investigations must address several issues. First, standardized instruments with well-documented validity and reliability (and suitable for large- and small-scale epidemiological investigations) must be developed to measure discrete dimensions of structural and nonstructural network characteristics. As a starting point the validity and reliability of previously used measures, particularly the composite indices used in large-scale incidence studies and in Seeman's (1984) study, should be formally documented. Second, validated and reliable measures of social networks and support should be included in original studies designed to test and refine promising hypotheses, including those generated by the existing body of research and those derived from current theory linking social networks and support to health. These original studies should be informed by theoretical models with the potential for identifying specific mechanisms through which social networks and support are linked to discrete stages of the IHD process. Finally, attention should be given to identifying possible variations in the association between social networks and support and IHD among men and women, among persons of varying ages or at different stages in the life cycle, and among persons in varying social contexts (e.g., rural vs. urban settings, and population subgroups that vary in ethnic composition or, within ethnic groups, in their level of acculturation).

References

Berkman, L. F. (1985, March). Measures of social networks and social support: evidence and measurement. In A. M. Ostfeld & E. D. Eaker (Eds.), *Measuring psychosocial variables in epidemiological studies of cardiovascular disease: Proceedings of a workshop* (NIH Publication No. 85–2270). Washington, DC: Department of Health and Human Services.

Berkman, L. F. (1986). Social networks, support, and health: Taking the next step forward. *American Journal of Epidemiology, 123*, 559–562.

Berkman, L. F., & Syme, S. L. (1979). Social networks, host resistance, and mortality: A nine-year follow-up study of Alameda County residents. *American Journal of Epidemiology, 109*, 186–204.

Carter, H., & Glick, P. C. (1970). *Marriage and divorce: A social and economic study* (American Public Health Association, Vital and Health Statistics Monograph). Cambridge, MA: Harvard University Press.

Chandra, V., Szklo, M., Goldberg, R., & Tonascia, J. (1983). The impact of marital status on survival after acute myocardial infarction: A population based study. *American Journal of Epidemiology, 117*, 320–325.

Cobb, S. (1974). Physiologic changes in men whose jobs were abolished. *Journal of Psychosomatic Research, 18*, 245–258.

Comstock, G. (1971). Fatal arteriosclerotic heart disease, water hardness at home, and socioeconomic characteristics. *American Journal of Epidemiology, 94*, 1–10.

Gore, S. (1978). The effect of social support in moderating the health consequences of unemployment. *Journal of Health and Social Behavior, 19*, 157–165.

Hazuda, H. P. (1986). *Social support and cardiovascular risk factors in Mexican Americans and non-Hispanic whites: Findings from the San Antonio Heart Study.* Presented at the Workshop on Social Support and Cardiovascular Disease, sponsored by the Behavioral Medicine Branch, National Heart, Lung, and Blood Institute (NHLBI), and the University of California, Irvine, April 2–4.

House, J. S., Robbins, C., & Metzner, H. D. (1982). The association of social relationships and activities with mortality: Prospective evidence from the Tecumseh Community Health Study. *American Journal of Epidemiology, 116,* 123–140.

Hrubec, Z., & Zukel, W. J. (1971). Socioeconomic differential in prognosis following episodes of coronary heart disease. *Journal of Chronic Diseases, 23,* 881–889.

Jenkins, C. D., Stanton, B. A., Klein, M. D., Savageau, J. A., & Harkin, D. E. (1983). Correlates of angina pectoris among men awaiting coronary bypass surgery. *Psychosomatic Medicine, 45,* 141–153.

Joseph, J. (1980). *Social affiliation, risk factor status, a, d coronary heart disease: A cross-sectional study of Japanese-American men.* Unpublished Ph.D. thesis, University of California, Berkeley.

Kaplan, G. A. (1985). Psychosocial aspects of chronic illness: Direct and indirect associations with ischemic heart disease mortality. In R. M. Kaplan & M. H. Criqui (Eds.), *Behavioral epidemiology and disease prevention* (pp. 237–269). New York: Plenum.

Ortmeyer, C. F. (1974). Variations in mortality, morbidity, and health care by marital status. In L. L. Erhardt & V. E. Berlin (Eds.), *Mortality and morbidity in the United States* (pp. 159–188). Cambridge, MA: Harvard University Press.

Ostfeld, A. M., & Eaker, E. D. (Eds.). (1985, March). *Measuring psychosocial variables in epidemiological studies of cardiovascular disease. Proceedings of a workshop.* (NIH Publication No. 85–2270). Washington, DC: Department of Health and Human Services.

Patterson, J. K., Haffner, S. M., Stern, M. P., & Hazuda, H. P. (1986, March). *Social support and cardiovascular risk factors in Mexican Americans and non-Hispanic whites.* Presented at the 7th Annual Scientific Sessions, Society of Behavioral Medicine, San Francisco, CA. March.

Reed, D., McGee, D., Yano, K., & Feinleib, M. (1983). Social networks and coronary heart disease among Japanese men in Hawaii. *American Journal of Epidemiology, 117,* 384–396.

Ruberman, W., Weinblatt, E., Goldberg, J. D., & Chaudhary, B. S. (1984). Psychosocial influences on mortality after myocardial infarction. *New England Journal of Medicine, 311,* 552.

Sackett, D. L. (1979). Bias in analytic research. *Journal of Chronic Diseases, 32,* 51–63.

Seeman, T. (1984). *Social networks and coronary artery disease.* Ph.D. thesis, University of California, Berkeley.

Thiel, H. G., Parker, D., & Bruce, T. A. (1973). Stress factors and the risk of myocardial infarction. *Journal of Psychosomatic Research, 17,* 43–57.

Weiss, N. S. (1973). Marital status and risk factors for coronary heart disease: The United States Health Examination Survey of Adults. *British Journal of Preventive & Social Medicine, 27,* 41–43.

Thomas, P. D., Goodwin, J. M., & Goodwin, J. S. (1985). Effect of social support on stress-related changes in cholesterol level, uric acid level, and immune function in an elderly sample. *American Journal of Psychiatry, 142,* 735–737.

Wingard, D. L., & Cohn, B. A. (1987). Coronary heart disease mortality among women in Alameda County, 1965 to 1973. In E. D. Eaker, B. Packard, N. K. Wenger, T. B. Clarkson, & H. A. Tyroler (Eds.), *Coronary heart disease in women: Proceedings of an NIH workshop* (pp. 99–105). New York: Haymarket Doyma.

Wingard, D. L., Suarez, L., & Barrett-Connor, E. (1983). The sex differential in mortality from all causes and ischemic heart disease. *American Journal of Epidemiology, 117,* 165–172.

PART III

Individual, Environmental, and Cultural Factors in Social Support and Cardiovascular Disease

CHAPTER 7

Social Support in the Work Environment and Cardiovascular Disease

Jeffrey V. Johnson and Ellen M. Hall

Since the early 1980s considerable scientific attention has been focused on how psychosocial work organization influences physical and mental health. These issues are currently of particular concern because of the rapid changes occurring in the nature of work, including the large-scale introduction of new technological systems, the decline in manufacturing and farming, and the rise in service industries. Work environment researchers are confronted with a central question: How can we delineate what constitutes a healthy (as opposed to harmful) workplace? In responding to this question, we first examine epidemiological and other nontheoretical studies of the general relationship between work, social relations, and cardiovascular health status. We then examine theoretical formulations and related findings from two research traditions: sociomedical research and the sociology of work. Because of the relatively sparse evidence concerning the specific relationship between workplace social support and cardiovascular disease, we broaden our discussion to include other stress-related outcomes. Although we refer to empirical research (both our own and that of others), we also develop theoretical linkages between the study of work relations, social support, behavior, and cardiovascular disease.

JEFFREY V. JOHNSON AND ELLEN M. HALL • Division of Behavioral Sciences and Health Education, Department of Health Policy and Management, Johns Hopkins School of Hygiene and Public Health, Baltimore, Maryland 21205.

Social Support and Cardiovascular Disease, edited by Sally A. Shumaker and Susan M. Czajkowski. Plenum Press, New York, 1994.

Work Support and Cardiovascular Disease

We begin with a review of some of the relevant epidemiological studies, many of which do not fit neatly into the theoretical categories of social support research that we will examine in the next section. Rather, such studies have addressed the most basic question: Is there *any* evidence that we should consider social support in the workplace to be of importance in the development of cardiovascular disease risk?

A number of prospective studies have been performed. Medalie et al. (1973) have shown that there is a higher incidence of angina pectoris among men who report lack of appreciation by coworkers and supervisors. In an analysis of the Framingham data, female clerks with an unsupportive supervisor were shown to have a greater incidence of coronary heart disease than other working women and housewives (Haynes & Feinleib, 1980). The strongest prospective study to date utilized a natural experiment involving changes in two cohorts of male bank clerks (Kittel, Kornitzer, & Dramaix, 1980). The work processes and social climates of the two banks were initially quite similar, but one bank (a commercial bank) undertook a reorganization that both increased the responsibility of the clerks for investing funds and created a highly competitive and unsupportive work setting. The other bank, which was semipublic, did not undergo any organizational change and had a much less demanding and competitive work setting. At the end of the 10-year follow-up period, employees at the commercial bank had a significantly higher incidence of coronary heart disease than those at the semipublic bank. In a case-control study of Swedish men below the age of 65 in the greater Stockholm area, Alfredsson, Karasek, and Theorell (1982) reported that those with no social contact at work had a 24% excess risk of myocardial infarction compared to men with work-related social contact, though the effect was of borderline statistical significance.

A number of studies have examined the relationship between social support and hypertension. An investigation of air traffic controllers (Rose, Hurst, & Herd, 1979) found that those seeking contact during times of stress had less severe blood pressure elevation than "loners." Van Dijkhuizen and Reiche (1980) reported that poor relations with management were related to blood pressure elevation among individuals employed in 17 companies in the Netherlands. Knox, Theorell, Svensson, and Waller (1985) used causal modeling techniques (Lisrel) to identify a pathway that links poor social stimulation, measured by lack of learning opportunities and lack of social networks, to elevated plasma adrenaline at rest and to high systolic resting blood pressure. This same research group (Theorell, Knox, Svensson, & Waller, 1985) found that subjects who had high blood pressure at age 18 were more likely to develop elevated systolic blood pressure at work if they were in an occupation characterized by low discretion latitude and high psychological job demands. Many of the occupations considered as high-strain jobs in this study (cook, truck driver, taxi driver, ticket clerk, tax collector, assembler, head waiter) also represent work processes performed in relative social isolation.

One of the stronger cross-sectional studies linking workplace social support with elevated diastolic blood pressure was reported by Matthews, Cottington, Talbot, Kuller, and Siegel (1987). In a study of 288 male hourly workers, aged 40 to 63 and employed for at least 10 years at one of two plants, lack of support from coworkers and supervisors and difficulties communicating with others were found to be associated with elevated diastolic blood pressure after controlling for age, body mass index, alcohol consumption, cigarette smoking habits, family history of hypertension, and severe noise-induced hearing loss. Ideally, in such studies it would be useful to analyze data according to family history of hypertension and for those with a history of negative health behaviors.

A number of negative findings concerning blood pressure have also been reported. Caplan, Cobb, French, Harrison, and Pinneau (1980) found few significant associations between blood pressure and a number of psychosocial work characteristics (including social support) in a cross-sectional study of 23 different occupations. In a cross-sectional analysis of the Framingham Heart Study (Haynes et al., 1978), nonsupportive supervision was not found to be associated with elevated blood pressure.

Several earlier studies examined physiological correlates of cardiovascular disease risk. Cassel (1963) found that shift workers who had a constant set of coworkers had considerably lower cholesterol values than those whose workmates were constantly changing. R. Caplan (1972), in a study of NASA scientists, administrators, and engineers, found that positive work relationships modified the impact of occupational stress on physiological strain, and that role ambiguity was significantly correlated with elevations in serum cortisol only for those who had poor relationships with their subordinates.

Recent findings from the Whitehall study also suggest a potential link between social support and differentials in fibrinogen (Markowe et al., 1985; Marmot, 1986): Men in lower grades of the British civil service reported fewer social supports than those in the higher grades. The investigators also reported that the lower the occupational grade, the higher the fibrinogen level, meaning that the lower-grade men had an increased potential to form blood clots.

In summary, there is evidence of a relationship between occupational social support and cardiovascular health status. No study, however, has demonstrated a biologically plausible causal pathway between human connections in the workplace and an elevated or decreased risk of cardio-vascular disease. Social support research still lacks a consensus about both the definitions of basic terms and physiological mechanisms.

Traditionally biomedical researchers have concentrated on finding a significant association between social support and health and have not been concerned with theoretical formulations or findings drawn from more qualitative research. But much of what is known about social support and its function in adult life has been generated by sociologists, work relations researchers, and others whose research combines scientific considerations with a more humanistic or theoretical orientation.

Theoretical Frameworks Linking Work, Social Support, and Health

There is a convergence of disciplines and orientations that have contributed to the understanding of social connections and their importance in mental and physical health. A number of theories have been presented in the literature that distinguish the various functions social support may serve in the workplace, ranging from the individual (internally perceived) to the collective (externally functional).

1. Social Support in the Workplace Meets Basic Human Needs for Companionship

Group Affiliation Can Generally Reduce the Impact of Life Stresses

Much of the earlier work on the need for social affiliation was psycho-analytically oriented. Bowlby's (1969) theories of attachment, based on his studies of infants separated from their mothers, suggested that the human need for attachment is as powerful and instinctual as the need for food. Psychiatric epidemiological studies have indicated that particular events that involve the loss or disruption of human contact (e.g., divorce, death of a spouse, or job loss) may have negative mental health consequences (Dohrenwend & Dohrenwend, 1974; Paykel, 1973, 1975). Others (e.g., Theorell, 1974) have reported that the risk for premature myocardial infarction increased following stressful life events involving loss. Prospec-tive epidemiological investigations of mortality, discussed elsewhere in this volume, provide additional evidence of the importance of human ties to health and longevity (Berkman, 1985; Berkman & Syme, 1979; Blazer,

1982; House, Robbins, & Metzner, 1982; Orth-Gomér & Johnson, 1987; Schoenbach, Kaplan, Fredman, & Kleinbaum, 1986).

Why should workplace relationships be of socioaffiliative importance? One answer involves the increasing fragmentation and decline of older forms of social cohesion, such as the village, the neighborhood, and the church. Workplace interactions may be one of the few remaining sources of stable, ongoing personal contact; it is possible that work relationships are a major source of human companionship in the modern era. The effect of the loss of this workplace community was investigated by Gore (1978), who investigated the unemployment experience in a rural and in an urban setting. Although the rural group objectively had more unemployment experience, there were less pronounced changes in health status (e.g., depression, disturbances in cholesterol values) relative to the urban group. She attributes this to the sustaining mutual aid system present in the ethnically cohesive, small-town community where fellow workers were also neighbors; the urban workers, however, lost a major part of their social support resources because of the unemployment experience. Similar findings have been reported by Cobb and Kasl (1977) and Hall and Johnson (1988).

The importance of the workplace and its particular relevance for cardiovascular disease has been articulated by Matsumoto (1971) in his classic article on stress and coronary heart disease in Japan. He hypothesizes that the work community in modern Japan is an institutionalized stress-reducing mechanism that, together with diet, may help to explain the much lower rates of coronary heart disease in Japan compared to the United States. The immediate work group is of such primary and lasting importance that the Japanese develop an identification not with a particular occupation but with the workplace collectivity. This social community is characterized by continuous group membership over many years, providing emotional support and release and a haven where individuals can express both positive and negative feelings without fear of censure.

We note that there are few large-scale health studies on the relationship between personality and occupational social support. But there is a rather extensive literature offering psychological frameworks for understanding how to achieve a better match between personality type and work task characteristics. Certainly personality plays an important role in matters such as introversion or extroversion, as evidenced by the desire to work in solitude and quiet as opposed to thriving on an interactive and noisy environment. Nested within the general issue of personality, social structure, and illness is a larger question concerning the primacy of the individual versus that of the environment. Are certain personality types drawn to isolated and stressful work, or do particular environments produce isolated and stressed workers? In fact, it may be in the interactions and transactions among the individual, the group, and the environment that we find the most interesting and useful data on social support.

Social Relations Influence the Development and Maintenance of Attitudes and Behaviors

Involvement in the world of work, as in any other major social institution (e.g., marriage, family, school, the military), initiates a socialization and acculturation process by which individuals gain an occupational component to their adult identity (see Frese, 1982; and Jahoda, 1981, 1982, for excellent discussions of this topic). Occupational socialization has a variety of influences; it may be a source of injurious feelings, and it may be a way of initiating good or bad health behaviors.

Through social relationships at work, individuals and groups develop an identity, such as "I am a police officer," "I am a scientist," or "I am a farmer." Each of these examples involves both an internal and an external component, as well as a psychological and a physical aspect. For example, a police officer is socialized *within the group* concerning how to dress, how to behave, and how to think "like a cop." Eventually even his or her leisure-time identity will become that typical of other police officers. Furthermore, the long-term experience of being a police officer will mold an individual's psychological state and attitudes, in addition to affecting friendships, marriage, and family. At a physical level, police officers accept that danger is involved in their work, and that inconvenient hours and stress are to be considered part of the job. Thus the process by which 18- to 20-year-olds enter the labor force and are transformed into adults is often greatly influenced by occupational socialization. The middle-aged farmer will have a wealth of experiences in common with another middle-aged farmer, but not with a middle-aged scientist.

Paradoxically, the need for human contact also involves a susceptibility to the negative forces. Shame, disapproval, and disapprobation are used within collectivities to mold behavior. To date there has been little empirical research on this topic, and it is not possible to evaluate whether such experiences are stressful. Nevertheless, individual case studies and literature, philosophy, and psychoanalytic texts (see Wurmser, 1981, for an excellent synthesis) indicate that shame is a major force at the individual level; it may be that emotions such as shame and disapproval have physical as well as psychological consequences in human affairs. A related concern is that through socialization, workers are influenced with respect to the development of either negative or positive health behaviors. There is preliminary evidence, for example, that both smoking and smoking cessation can be influenced by social relations at work (Elden, 1981; Johansson & Gardell, 1988; Johansson, Johnson, & Hall, 1991; Taliacozzo & Vaughn, 1982). The mechanisms whereby social support could influence behavioral change have been suggested by Mermelstein, Cohen, Lichtenstein, Baer, and Kamarck (1986): (a) Support could directly influence the behavior by helping to sustain motivation or, conversely, by making a change more difficult; (b) social network members can serve as models of behavior influencing either the desired or undesired behavior; or (c) social support could modify other factors that could influence smoking (e.g., stress) and thereby exert an indirect effect.

2. Work Social Support Serves to Moderate the Impact of Job Demands

At the Individual Level, It May Buffer the Impact of Stress

How does occupational social support modify or buffer the impact of stress on health? Most, but not all of the research on this topic has been conducted within the person-environment fit theory of stress at the University of Michigan's Institute for Social Research. Kahn and Antonucci (1980), Pinneau (1975) and G. Caplan (1981) generally agree that there are three key elements: affect, affirmation, and aid. House (1981) summarizes these various formulations in a single question: "Who gives what to whom regarding which problems?" (p. 22).

Empirical tests of the stress-modifying effects of social support include an investigation of 1,809 male petrochemical-products workers by House and his colleagues (House, 1980, 1981; House & Wells, 1978). They examined the effects of social support on the impact of physical hazards and psychosocial stress and found that support, particularly from supervisors, reduced the impact of perceived stress on physical health status. Job stress had an impact on physical health symptoms (angina, ulcers, skin rashes) only for those workers with low levels of social support. When social support was high, perceived stress appeared to have little or no impact on physical health.

Although spouse and supervisor support were found to be important, House reported that coworker support had only a small effect in reducing perceived stress. But company policies, high noise levels, and the pressures of machine production militated against coworker interaction. This points to the importance of the organization of work in determining whether and in what forms social support can exist, and whether it will serve to modify or reduce stress. Research conducted within this tradition (LaRocco, House, & French, 1980; LaRocco & Jones, 1978; Pinneau, 1975) has generally found that work-related social support from coworkers and supervisors, as compared to family and nonwork friends, is most effective in reducing occupational stress and in modifying the impact of work stressors on health.

Collective Coping with Stress

The term *collectivity* and its underlying theory are based upon the work of Lysgaard (1961), a Norwegian researcher who was interested in the structurally available resources in the work environment. If one conceives of occupational social support as having a larger, structural aspect that helps groups of people to cope with stress, the closest conceptualization is found in Lysgaard's work.

It is important to distinguish between the resources available to the individual and those inherent within groups. Collective coping is not just the sum of individual coping resources; social groups can provide a more general type of protection, whereas specific persons may protect themselves through individually oriented attempts to change, cope with, or adjust their attitude. Individuals may apply talent, will, or intellect to various workplace problems, and if the environment permits, they may be able to alter certain conditions. For instance, most professional jobs permit the employee some latitude to negotiate about the conditions of employment. Many individuals have developed themselves via work so that their lives are improved intellectually, socially, and financially. For the process of development to occur, the working person must be able to maneuver within and to make use of the environment; in white-collar jobs there are usually possibilities for growth, as well as support staff and resources that are available. Professionals often provide and extract support within a system of reciprocal exchange of information and favors that functions as a sort of currency in many occupations. The "old-boy network" is a widely observed phenomenon that involves just this mixture of favors, information, and social support.

But not all occupational environments provide the same type or level of resources. In most factory and basic service work, the ability to negotiate individual wages, work space, and support services is unheard of, and often even talking on the job is forbidden. For this reason, we propose that social support emerges and is of importance in such occupations at an extraindividual (i.e., group) level. Many blue-collar jobs provide informal systems by which the most arduous work is allocated fairly, sparing elderly and inexperienced workers such work. The informal consensus of the group, not the desires of an individual worker, is the basis for such decisions. Such collective social formations may not be produced consciously. A worker is initiated into his or her job by observing and working within the group, and he or she learns that certain behaviors are expected as a means of protecting the group as a whole. Thus workers usually take all of the coffee, lunch, and vacation breaks that are provided, even if, for example, they do not particularly feel like having coffee from 2:15 to 2:30 p.m. In part this is because it would be odd not to do what is expected, but it is also because to continue working during free time would undermine the rights of the group.

In short, *this ability to control the work experience collectively is of importance in relation to those institutional structures that are relatively impervious to individual activity.* A limitation of much social support research, both conceptually and methodologically, is the emphasis on time-limited, individually based emotional transactions. This approach reduces the object of research to an atomized individual who receives supports or protection from other nodes in a network. The missing link between social support and health may be the fact that the environment permits or discourages the development of networks, and further that the transactions that connect the individual to the collective may take years to develop and may not even be consciously experienced by those involved. The importance of such collective resources at work is suggested by Pearlin and Schooler's (1978) study of general coping resources and strategies available to individuals. They found that no form of individual coping seemed to be effective in ameliorating job-related sources of stress and strain, and they concluded that in areas of life (e.g., work) that are impersonally organized, the forces affecting people are not amenable to coping either by weight of personality or individual coping responses.

When the amount of individual control over the task or career structure is relatively limited, where individual efforts are either discouraged or incapable of making any difference, social and collective forms may become even more important. Support can be understood in the words of McQueen and Celentano (1982, p. 9) as a "social mechanism of defense which can either retard or halt a pathological process." Work support then would be expected to operate in conjunction with other defense mechanisms or load controllers, such as work control.

We tested explicitly whether work support is linked to other resources, such as work control, to ameliorate the impact of job demands on cardiovascular disease (Johnson, 1985, 1986; Johnson & Hall, 1988). Using the job demand/control model (see Alfredsson et al., 1982; Baker, 1985; Karasek, 1979; Karasek, Baker, Marxer, Ahlbom, & Theorell, 1981; Karasek, Russell, & Theorell, 1982; Karasek, Theorell, Schwartz, Pieper, & Alfredsson, 1982; Theorell et al., 1984) as our starting point, we introduced a workplace social support dimension (see Figure 1). A particular concern

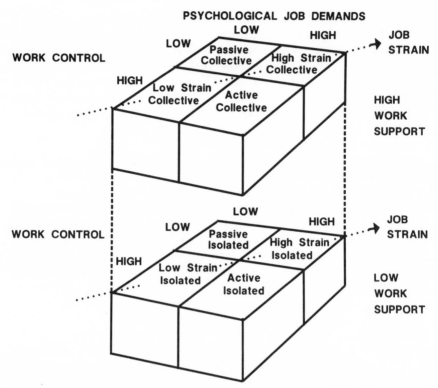

Figure 1. The demand-control-support model of work stress examines the joint effects of psychological job demands, work control, and social support on health. The model predicts that cardiovascular disease rates will be lowest in the low-strain collective group and highest in the high-strain isolated group.

was whether this addition altered or improved the already demonstrated predictive power of the model (Baker, 1985). For example, under the demand/control model, theoretically there should be no difference between a job that is performed in isolation and one that is performed collectively, so long as the levels of demand and control are similar. Thus the addition of social support expands the demand/control model into the domain of personal and collective relationships between people, as opposed to relationships between individuals and the job alone.

In a representative random sample of approximately 14,000 Swedish workers, we analyzed for the main and interactive effects of combined exposure to the three work characteristics on cardiovascular disease prevalence, and found evidence for a synergistic interaction. Combined exposure to all of the theoretically adverse conditions results in a risk 9% greater than what would be predicted in a strict multiplicative model.

Using the demand/control/support model (see Figure 2), two previously unidentified risk groups emerged: passive and active *isolated* groups were found to have significantly greater cardiovascular disease prevalence. The finding of excess prevalence risk in the passive isolated condition supports the earlier theory that "underload" can be a risk factor (Frankenhaeuser & Gardell, 1976). When examined without respect to support, the passive cell did *not* have a significant elevation in risk, suggesting that passivity becomes a risk factor when it occurs in combination with isolation. Social support interacts with control in a particular manner: The

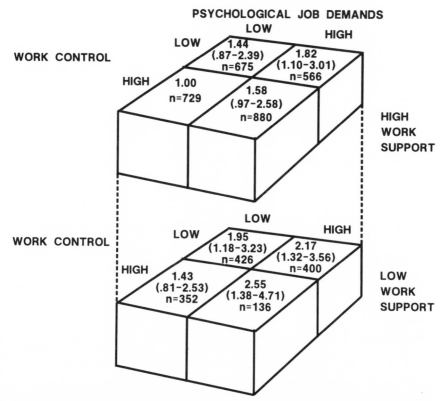

Figure 2. The demand-control-support model and cardiovascular disease prevalence:odds ratios and 95% confidence intervals in a representative random sample of Swedish male and female workers. Each cell of the model is contrasted with the reference category (the low psychological job demand, high work control, and high social support group).

combined lack of availability of both resources, is a high-risk condition for cardiovascular prevalence, even when there are low psychological job demands.

We found that social support has an effect on cardiovascular prevalence at all levels of job strain. In addition, neither control nor support alone was sufficient to modify the impact of job demands. The findings suggested that *the presence or absence of work control determines whether social support operates to reduce strain and cardiovascular disease risk*. When control is present, high support is an effective modifier; when control is absent, support no longer functions to reduce the impact of job demands. Support has an analogous impact on the effects of control: The combined presence of both resources is important both in a main and in a moderating capacity.

In summary, as noted by House, Landis, and Umberson (1988), both theoretical work and empirical evidence leads us to suspect that there is a causal impact of social relationships on health status. Despite the many questions and qualifications that may be applied to this statement, the social support literature as a whole has profound implications with respect to the organizational structure of large social institutions such as the workplace.

Substantive and Methodological Questions

Of the many challenges to etiological inference in existing research, an important problem is the lack of reliable exposure data (social support is usually evaluated on the basis of measures administered at only one point in time, rather than throughout the life course). Such an approach does not take into account various changes that might occur in an individual's working life. The intensity and sources of exposures vary over time with tasks required in a given work setting and with changes in the work process, in occupations, and in the members of a particular social network. Even in a prospective design, where the work environment variables are measured at one point and later followed up with morbidity and mortality data, we do not know the duration of individual exposure to certain work situations. Aside from making it impossible to examine dose-response relationships, we cannot determine an optimal or minimal amount of support in terms of either the frequency or the duration of social contact. It is also difficult to determine the direction of the support–illness relationship: Do people become ill and then become isolated, or is this sequence reversed?

An additional methodological difficulty is that most studies suffer from lack of generalizability resulting from restrictions of samples. Most often subjects consist of relatively healthy employed males; we know comparatively little about the experience and physical health of women with respect to their work history and family life. Life stage, age, and gender may have impacts on the need for and availability of different forms of support, but thus far we do not know how these factors interact within the workplace. The availability of family and intimate support may color the need for and the usefulness of work relationships, but there has been little research on whether support from one source may serve to compensate or replace that from another.

There is prodigious debate concerning the assessment of social support in all contexts. How do we define, operationalize, and measure both negative and positive aspects of support? Should researchers rely on subjective as opposed to objective measures? Should we evaluate total networks or only single-stranded connections? Unfortunately there is little consensus about such matters; however, the tendency has been to sum both the number of contacts and the type of functions that such contacts serve (e.g., information, self-esteem, emotional contact, instrumental aid). Though this represents both a theoretical and a methodological advance in the refinement of support research, the context of the supportive transaction is also important when linking support to occupational strain.

Determinants of Collectivity and Social Support

Thus far we have discussed investigations that attempt to elucidate linkages between social connections and health status. As in stress research more generally, these studies suffer from a black-box phenomenon: Although we have some understanding of inputs and outputs, we know relatively little about the actual functioning of human relationships within the ecology of the workplace.

Gryzb (1981) points out that informal work groups are a major source of control and personal satisfaction on the job, and that through such groups, workers devise ways of living on the job. In this subculture, norms, beliefs, traditions, and rituals are created. By discussing and interpreting the experience of work, employees defined their common situation, make sense of it, and often struggle to minimize or eliminate threats to the well-being of the group. Within the context of working life, decisions, attitudes, and activities are developed and tested for their effectiveness in solving common problems. In short, people's involvement with work promotes interaction with one another. Gryzb's insights echo the observations of Pearlin, Lieberman, Menaghan, and Mullan (1981, p. 340):

Support comes when people's engagement with one another extends to a level
of involvement and concern, not when they merely touch at the surface of each
other's lives. It appears, therefore, that being embedded in a network is only the
first step toward having access to support; the final step depends on the quality of the relations one is able to find within the network. The qualities that
seem to be especially critical involve the exchange of intimate communications
and the presence of solidarity and trust.

As we discussed earlier, Lysgaard (1961) investigated the topic of
workers' collectivity. He identified three conditions conducive to the formation of collectivity: (a) Spatial proximity is a precondition for social
interaction; (b) jointly experienced problems contribute to a common
frame of reference; and (c) having equal positions contributes to the
formation of a collective identity. We refine these observations in the
theoretical direction outlined below.

Proximity. There are different forms of structurally produced disconnections that can occur at work, involving separations both in time and
space. It is difficult to form relationships when one is physically or
temporally isolated. Time-based separations are experienced by shift
workers, whose companions are always changing. Spatial separations may
be physically determined (e.g., one person working alone in a room or at a
computer terminal), or the job itself may require privacy (e.g., writing or
precise technical work). Certain categories of workers are isolated both in
time and in space: for example, much night work involves a low level of
attendance to machines, patients, or paperwork in a relatively isolated
context. There is a similarity of experience between the accountant who
labors to get out tax forms all night long, the night janitor, the nurse on
evening duty, and the factory worker on a graveyard shift.

Ergonomic factors concerning job or machine design may also create
separations. For example, someone who must constantly be involved with
a machine (whether an instrument panel, a sewing machine, a micro-
scope, or a tractor) may be discouraged from entering into relations with
others *if* pay systems or performance evaluations are based exclusively on a
high level of individual productivity. Thus a traditional tailor may be
able to interact in an entirely different fashion with workers and customers
than an industrial garment stitcher.

The need for proximity has important implications in terms of the
design of machinery and instruments in the workplace, the scheduling of
time, and the physical layout of the work site. In settings ranging from
factories to hospitals, there is often no physical location for people to
interact comfortably. For "settingless" workers such as bus drivers, interaction on the radio or at a central terminal can function supportively, but
this is often insufficient to produce a sense of collectivity.

Shared Job Experiences. Most people are aware that a rather special bond exists between those who undergo a common experience of adversity. The emotional ties formed by soldiers in combat is a well-known example of the powerful influence of comradeship in reducing terrible strain (Grinker & Spiegel, 1963). In less dramatic situations, opportunities to talk about problems and to resolve them collectively are among the major attributes of a healthy workplace. Shared job content can also include shared knowledge and the pooling of resources to cope with high demands. Homans (1950), in his review of the Hawthorne study, argues that common experiences contribute to the development of group sentiments that form the basis of a collective approach to problem solving.

Equality. The fragmentation of production processes into many separate tasks can produce a multitude of job categories, which in turn can prevent the formation of a sense of equality among workers as a result of differences in pay and work content. Piece-rate payment systems are also antithetical to cooperation (Gardell, 1977; House, 1981). Under these systems there is no incentive to cooperate and every reason to compete with one's fellow workers, an environment that almost invariably introduces discontent into the work force. In many white-collar settings, the work is structured so that employees are in a win-lose relationship with each other. Competition, suspicion, and isolation are fostered in environments where only a select few will receive pay raises or other benefits based on their "superior" performance.

Hierarchical divisions in organizations are also expressed in the prohibition of friendships across lines of authority (e.g., between the boss and employees, or between an officer and enlisted personnel). This may present certain problems for those in positions of authority, who can become isolated if they lack a suitable group of equals with whom to form social links. Hierarchical divisions may also involve issues of race and gender.

In some jobs, all three of the above attributes of collectivity are missing. In machine-paced assembly-line jobs, for instance, high noise levels, a lack of physical proximity, rotating shifts, and piece-rate payment systems—combined with company policies that discourage socializing—can together militate against the social interaction that provides the essential basis for the development of collectivity. (See Holmila, 1986, for a recent discussion of this issue within the Finnish trade union movement.)

What enhances collectivity? We believe that social support works well when it serves the interests of the group as well as those of the individual. If social support is grounded in opportunities for reciprocity ("I'll pitch in this time, and you pitch in the next"), it is likely to have a more enduring and meaningful basis. As many managers are aware, a good team takes care of problems early and on its own, often by sharing or pooling the resources of the group. Conversely, morale problems are frequently centered on the issue of withholding of assistance and the related feelings of lack of fairness and reciprocity among members of a work group.

One of the structural preconditions for reciprocity is the extent to which there is a level of shared access to resources. It is possible to distinguish a number of different forms of resources:

- *Intellectual resources*: Knowledge and skills shared or withheld among groups of people
- *Social resources*: Formal or informal participation in the life of the group and the organization
- *Physical and material resources*: Space and access to goods and services
- *Status and/or power resources*: Political support for valued goals exchanged for the expectation of later services

In some cases the cycles involved in balancing reciprocity can be long and convoluted. There are also psychological components to conflicts about such matters, but in theory workers who are equal should have equivalent access to such resources, or there should be a reciprocity in the sharing of those resources. Social conflicts can arise in the tendency of some to accrue more than to reciprocate, especially when such acquisitiveness is a structurally determined component of advancement and is even an expectation. This occurs often in professional work, where it is necessary to put one's own interests over that of the group in order to fulfill larger expectations for career advancement. The relationship between the individual and the group theoretically will be unstable and insubstantial to the extent it is based on acquisitiveness; conversely, in those situations where members of a working group have equal positions and can anticipate working together in the same job for a relatively long period of time, there is probably a greater practical motivation for the formation of collectivity.

Traditional craft workers are a good example of employees who, for reasons of preference, tradition, or lack of other options, will remain in the same job until retirement. In such occupations, individuals and groups are embedded in a social network with relatively stable and continuous sets of expectations for reciprocity and with relative equality of access to resources. Of course, such individual factors as seniority, temperament, or proficiency may have some influence on the distribution of resources, but it is in the overall interest of the groups to achieve a state of social equity and homeostasis as a means of coping with the job and with each other.

To summarize, we would expand the Lysgaard formulation by suggesting that in those workplaces where workers are temporally and spatially proximate, and where there is shared job content and balanced reciprocity with respect to resources, we are most likely to observe a high degree of collectivity and hence social support.

Intervention in the Workplace: Formation of Autonomous Work Groups

One major job redesign strategy, originating in Scandinavia, involves the reconstruction of fragmented and isolated work through the development of autonomous work groups (T. Sandberg, 1982). More than 20 years of experimentation points to a number of significant properties of these groups (Gardell, 1982a, b):

- Work should be based on groups rather than individuals.
- The group should be given responsibility for planning and performing work within a specific area.
- Supervisors and technical experts should serve primarily as resources for these groups, rather than exerting authority or control.

This type of job design enables production groups to counteract the problems of work fragmentation and coercion that are so common in the blue-collar and lower-level white-collar sectors. Within the context of the group, individuals can enlarge their capacity for developing competence; not only are they able to increase their opportunities for learning through performing a variety of tasks, but the group is able to gain greater control over the work process. According to Gardell (1982a, b) and others (e.g., Elden, 1981; Cooper, 1981), this is attributable to the increase in social support and solidarity among group members brought about by this new type of work organization.

Unfortunately, most of the evaluations of the effects of these work experiments have concentrated on such matters as job satisfaction, turnover, and productivity rather than on cardiovascular or other health-related outcomes. One exception is a health care team at the Volvo plant in Gothenburg, Sweden (Wallin & Wright, 1986) who reports on the effects of introducing a group-oriented approach in their factory. A group of white-collar workers was examined before the introduction of a new work organization and after a 2-year follow-up period. During this time a number of major changes were introduced: Along with a smoking cessation campaign, these included key revisions in supervision and management style, combined with the introduction of a teamwork system and new work methods which involved greater personal contact between employees and customers. The authors report that after the 2-year period there was a dramatic drop in the incidence of psychosomatic symptoms such as depression and headache, a reduction in gastrointestinal symptoms, a decrease in incidence of psychological problems, the virtual cessation of smoking, and an overall reduction in work stress, monotony, and turnover. These results suggest the importance of additional intervention studies that also monitor changes in physiological functioning relevant to the cardiovascular system. Although this study does not prove that changes in social support will produce changes in health status, it suggests that we need greater understanding of how and what to change if we are concerned about health.

The Changing Nature of Work and the Labor Force

Although autonomous work groups offer a potential strategy for successful supportive interventions, larger labor market trends are a cause for genuine concern. The introduction of new technology is rapidly changing the nature of the modern working environment (P. Sandberg, 1979). It is estimated that in the 1990s more than 7 million factory jobs and 39 million office jobs will be affected by computerization and the introduction of robots (Bezold, Carlson, & Peck, 1986). This is of major concern because lower social support has been reported more frequently by workers using new-technology office equipment such as VDTs (Sauter, Gottlieb, Jones, Dondson, & Rohreer, 1983). Moreover, 9 out of 10 new jobs will be in the service sector (Bureau of Labor Statistics, 1985), which in comparison to industrial work is often characterized by greater marginality (i.e., lower pay, a less stable work force, more part-time employment, less unionization, and smaller, more scattered work sites). In short, we will see fewer opportunities for the sustained cooperative social interaction that forms the basis of collectivity in the workplace.

If these trends continue, it is likely that we will observe an increase in social disconnections in one of the few remaining sources of stable human community in our society. One must ask if requirements for short-term organizational efficiency outweigh the potential social, psychological, and physical damage that may result. The disruption of the workplace social community is neither a necessary nor inevitable consequence of technological change (Herbst, 1974). The examples of Japan and Scandinavia demonstrate that it is possible to preserve and even expand collectivity in the workplace while maintaining high levels of organizational effectiveness.

References

Alfredsson, L., Karasek, R., & Theorell, T. (1982). Myocardial infarction risk and psychosocial work environment characteristics: An analysis of the male Swedish work force. *Social Science and Medicine, 16,* 463–467.

Baker, D. (1985). The study of stress at work. *Annual Review of Public Health, 6,* 367–381.

Berkman, L. (1985). The relationship of social networks and social support to morbidity and mortality. In S. Cohen & S. L. Syme (Eds.), *Social support and health* (pp. 240–259). New York: Academic Press.

Berkman, L., & Syme, S. L. (1979). Social networks, host resistance and mortality: A nine year study of Alameda County residents. *American Journal of Epidemiology, 109,* 186–204.

Bezold, C., Carlson, R. J., & Peck, J. C. (1986). *The future of work and health.* Dover, MA: Auburn House.

Blazer, D. (1982). Social support and mortality in an elderly community population. *American Journal of Epidemiology, 115,* 684–694.

Bowlby, J. (1969). *Attachment and loss* (2 vols.). London: Hogarth.

Bureau of Labor Statistics. (1985, November). *Bureau of Labor Statistics news.* Washington, DC: Department of Labor.

Caplan, G. (1981). Mastery of stress: Psychosocial aspects. *American Journal of Psychiatry, 138,* 413–419.

Caplan, R. D. (1972). *Organizational stress and individual strain: A sociopsychological study of risk factors in coronary heart disease among administrators, engineers and scientists.* Doctoral dissertation, University of Michigan.

Caplan, R., Cobb, S., French, J., Harrison, R., & Pinneau, S. (1975). *Job demands and worker health* (NIOSH Publication No. 75-160). Cincinnati, OH: National Institute for Occupational Safety and Health.

Caplan, R. D., Cobb, S., & French, J. R. P. (1975). Relationships of cessation of smoking with job stress, personality, and social support. *Journal of Applied Psychology, 60,* 211–219.

Caplan, R. D., Cobb, S., French, J., Harrison, R., & Pinneau, S. (1980). *Job demands and worker health: Main effects and occupational differences.* Ann Arbor, MI: Institute for Social Research.

Cassel, J. (1963). The use of medical records: Opportunities for epidemiological studies. *Journal of Occupational Medicine, 5,* 185–190.

Cobb, S., & Kasl, S. (1977). *Termination: The consequences of job loss* (NIOSH Publication No. 77-224). Cincinnati, OH: National Institute for Occupational Safety and Health.

Cooper, C. L. (1981). Social support at work and stress management. *Small Group Behavior, 12,* 285–297.

Dohrenwend, B. S., & Dohrenwend, B. P. (1974). *Stressful life events: Their nature and effects.* New York: Wiley.

Elden, M. (1981). Political efficacy at work: The connection between more autonomous forms of workplace organization and a more participatory politics. *American Political Science Review, 75,* 43–58.

Frankenhaeuser, M., & Gardell, B. (1976). Overload and underload in working life: Outline of a multidisciplinary approach. *Journal of Human Stress, 2,* 35–46.

Frese, M. (1982). Occupational socialization and psychological development: An under-emphasized research perspective in industrial psychology. *Journal of Occupational Psychology, 55,* 209–224.

Gardell, B. (1977). Autonomy and participation of work. *Human Relations, 30*(6), 515–533.

Gardell, B. (1982a). Scandinavian research in stress in working life. *International Journal of Health Services, 12*(1), 31–41.

Gardell, B. (1982b). Work participation and autonomy: A multilevel approach to democracy at the workplace. *International Journal of Health Services, 12*, 527–558.

Gore, S. (1978). The effect of social support in moderating the health consequences of unemployment. *Journal of Health and Social Behavior, 19*, 157–165.

Grinker, R., & Spiegel, J. (1963). *Men under stress*. New York: McGraw-Hill.

Gryzb, G. J. (1981). Decollectivization and recollectivization in the workplace: The impact on informal work groups and work culture. *Economic and Industrial Democracy, 2*, 455–482.

Hall, E., & Johnson, J. (1988). Depression in unemployed Swedish women. *Social Science and Medicine, 27*, 1349–1355.

Haw, M. (1982). Women, work and stress: A review and agenda for the future. *Journal of Health and Social Behavior, 23*, 132–144.

Haynes, S. G., Levine, S., Scotch, N., et al. (1978). The relationship of psychosocial factors to coronary heart disease in the Framingham study: I. Methods and risk factors. *American Journal of Epidemiology, 107*, 362–383.

Haynes, S., & Feinleib, M. (1980). Women, work and coronary heart disease: Prospective findings from the Framingham Heart Study. *American Journal of Public Health, 70*, 133–141.

Henry, J. P. (1986). Mechanisms by which stress can lead to coronary heart disease. *Postgraduate Medical Journal, 62*, 687–693.

Herbst, P. (1974). *Sociotechnical design*. London: Tavistock.

Holmila, M. (1986). Life style issues—debate between men and women in the Finnish trade union movement. *Acta Sociologica, 29*, 3–12.

Homans, G. (1950). *The human group*. New York: Harcourt, Brace and World.

House, J. (1980). *Occupational stress and the mental and physical health of factory workers*. Research Report Series, Institute for Social Research, University of Michigan, Ann Arbor.

House, J. (1981). *Work stress and social support*. Reading, MA: Addison-Wesley.

House, J., & Wells, J. (1978). Occupational stress, social support and health. In A. A. McLean & M. Colligan (Eds.), *Reducing occupational stress: Proceedings of a conference*. (NIOSH Publication No. 78-140). Cincinnati, OH: National Institute for Occupational Safety and Health.

House, J., Robbins, C., & Metzner, H. (1982). The association of social relationships and activities with mortality: Prospective evidence from the Tecumseh Community Health Study. *American Journal of Epidemiology, 116*, 123–140.

House, J., Landis, K., & Umberson, D. (1988). Social relationships and health. *Science, 241*, 540–545.

Jahoda, M. (1981). Work, employment and unemployment: Values, theories and approaches to social research. *American Psychologist, 36*, 184–191.

Jahoda, M. (1982). *Employment and unemployment: A socio-psychological analysis*. Cambridge, England: Cambridge University Press.

Johansson, G., & Gardell, B. (1988). Work–health relations as mediated through stress reactions and job socialization. In S. Maes, C. Spielberger, P. Defares, & I. Sarason (Eds.), *Topics in health psychology*. New York: Wiley.

Johansson, G., Johnson, J. V., & Hall, E. M. (1991). Smoking and sedentary behavior as related to work organizations. *Social Science and Medicine, 32*, 837–846.

Johnson, J. V. (1985). *The effects of control and social support on work related strain and adverse health outcomes* (Department of Psychology Research Report No. 39). Stockholm: University of Stockholm.

Johnson, J. V. (1986). *The impact of workplace social support and work control upon cardiovascular disease in Sweden*. (Division of Environmental and Organizational Psychology Research Report No. 1). Stockholm: University of Stockholm.

Johnson, J. V., & Hall, E. M. (1988). Job strain, workplace social support and cardiovascular disease: A cross sectional study of a random sample of the Swedish working population. *American Journal of Public Health, 78,* 1336–1342.

Kahn, R. L., & Antonucci, T. (1980). Convoys over the life course: attachment, roles and social support. In P. B. Baltes & O. Brim (Eds.), *Life span development and behavior, (vol. 3).* Boston: Lexington.

Karasek, R. (1979). Job demands, job decision latitude, and mental strain: Implications for job redesign. *Administrative Science Quarterly, 24,* 285–308.

Karasek, R., Baker, D., Marxer, F., Ahlbom, A., & Theorell, T. (1981). Job decision latitude, job demands, and cardiovascular disease: A prospective study of Swedish men. *American Journal of Public Health, 71,* 694–705.

Karasek, R., Russell, R., & Theorell, T. (1982). Physiology of stress and regeneration in job related cardiovascular illness. *Journal of Human Stress, 3,* 29–42.

Karasek, R., Theorell, T., Schwartz, J., Pieper, C., & Alfredsson, A. (1982). Job, psychological factors and coronary heart disease. *Advances Cardiology, 29,* 62–76.

Kasl, S., & Wells, J. (1985). Social support and health in the middle years. In S. Cohen & S. L. Syme (Eds.), *Social support and health* (pp. 143–165). New York: Academic Press.

Kittel, F. L., Kornitzer, M., & Dramaiz, M. (1980). Coronary heart disease and job stress in two cohorts of bank clerks. *Psychotherapy and Psychosomatics, 34,* 110–123.

Knox, S., Theorell, T., Svensson, J., & Waller, D. (1985). The relation of social support and working environment to medical variables associated with elevated blood pressure in young males: A structural model. *Social Science and Medicine, 21,* 525–531.

Kohn, M. L. (1990). Unsolved issues in the relationship between work and personality. In K. Erikson & S. P. Vallas (Eds.), *The nature of work: Sociological perspectives* (pp. 36–68). New Haven, CT: Yale University Press.

LaRocco, J., House, J., & French, J. (1980). Social support, occupational stress and health. *Journal of Health and Social Behavior, 21,* 202–218.

LaRocco, J., & Jones, A. (1978). Co-worker and leader support as moderators of stress-strain relationships in work situations. *Journal of Applied Psychology, 63,* 619–634.

Lysgaard, S. (1961). *Arbeiderkollectivet* [Worker's collectivity]. Oslo: Universitets forlaget.

Markowe, H. L. J., Marmot, M. G., Shipley, M. J., Bulpitt, C. J., Meade, T. M., Stirling, T., Vickers, M. V., & Semmence, A. (1985). Fibrinogen: A possible link between social class and coronary heart disease. *British Medical Journal, 291,* 1312.

Marmot, M. G. (1986). Does stress cause heart attacks? *Postgraduate Medical Journal, 62,* 683–686.

Matsumoto, Y. S. (1971). Social stress and coronary heart disease in Japan. In H. Dreitzel (Ed.), *The social organization of health.* New York: Macmillan.

Matthews, K. A., Cottington, E. M., Talbot, E., Kuller, L. H., & Siegel, J. M. (1987). Stressful work conditions and diastolic blood pressure among blue collar factory workers. *American Journal of Epidemiology, 126,* 280–291.

McQueen, D., & Celentano, D. (1982). Social factors in the etiology of multiple outcomes. *Social Science and Medicine, 16,* 397–418.

Medalie, J. H., Snyder, M., Groen, J., Neufeld, H., Goldbourt, U., & Riss, E. (1973). Angina pectoris among 10,000 men: 5 year incidence and univariate analysis. *American Journal of Medicine, 55,* 583–594.

Mermelstein, R., Cohen, S., Lichtenstein, E., Baer, J. S., & Kamarck, T. (1986). Social support and smoking cessation and maintenance. *Journal of Consulting and Clinical Psychology, 54,* 447–453.

Orth-Gomér, K., & Johnson, J. V. (1987). Social network interaction and mortality: A six year follow-up of a random sample of the Swedish population. *Journal of Chronic Diseases, 40,* 949–957.

Paykel, E. (1973). Life events and acute depression. In J. Scott & E. Senay (Eds.), *Separation and depression* (pp. 215–237). Washington, DC: American Association for the Advancement of Science.

Paykel, E. (1975). Environmental variables in the aetiology of depression. In F. Flash & S. Draghi (Eds.), *The nature and treatment of depression* (pp. 102–119). New York: Wiley.

Pearlin, L. (1985). Social structure and processes of support. In S. Cohen & L. Syme (Eds.), *Social support and health.* New York: Academic Press.

Pearlin, L., & Schooler, C. (1978). The structure of coping. *Journal of Health and Social Behavior, 19*, 2–21.

Pearlin, L., Lieberman, M., Menaghan, E., & Mullan, J. (1981). The stress process. *Journal of Health and Social Behavior, 22*, 337–356.

Pinneau, S. (1975). *Effects of social support on psychological and physiological strain.* Doctoral dissertation, University of Michigan, Ann Arbor.

Rose, R., Hurst, M., & Herd, A. (1979). Cardiovascular and endocrine responses to work and the risk of psychiatric symptoms among air traffic controllers. In J. Barrett (Ed.), *Stress and mental disorder.* New York: Raven.

Sandberg, A. (Ed.). (1979). *Computers dividing man and work.* Stockholm: Arbetslivscentrum

Sandberg, T. (1982). *Work organization and autonomous groups.* Lund, Sweden: CWK Gleerup.

Sauter, S., Gottlieb, M., Jones, C., Dondson, V., & Rohreer, K. (1983). Job and health implications of VDT use: initial results of the Wisconsin-NIOSH study. *Communications of the ACM, 26*, 784–794.

Schoenbach, V., Kaplan, B. H., Fredman, L., & Kleinbaum, D. (1986). Social ties and mortality in Evans County, Georgia. *American Journal of Epidemiology, 123*, 577–591.

Tagliacozzo, R., & Vaughn, S. (1982). Stress and smoking in hospital nurses. *American Journal of Public Health, 72*, 441–448.

Theorell, T. (1974). Life events before and after the onset of a premature myocardial infarction. In B. Dohrenwend & B. Dohrenwend (Eds.), *Stressful life events: Their nature and effects* (pp. 101–118). New York: Wiley.

Theorell, T. (1986). Stress at work and risk of myocardial infarction. *Postgraduate Medical Journal, 62*, 791–795.

Theorell, T., Alfredsson, L., Knox, S., Perski, A., Svensson, J., & Waller, D. (1984). On the interplay between socioeconomic factors, personality and work environment in the pathogenesis of cardiovascular disease. *Scandinavian Journal of Work Environment and Health, 10*, 373–380.

Theorell, T., Knox, S., Svensson, J., & Waller, D. (1985, Spring). Blood pressure variations during a working day at age 28: Effects of different types of work and blood pressure level at age 18. *Journal of Human Stress*, 36–41.

Van Dijkhuizen, N., & Reiche, H. (1980). Psychosocial stress in industry: A heartache for middle management? *Psychotherapy and Psychosomatics, 34*, 124–134.

Wallin, L., & Wright, I. (1986). Psychosocial aspects of the work environment: A group approach. *Journal of Occupational Medicine, 28*, 384–393.

Wurmser, L. (1981). *The mask of shame.* Baltimore: Johns Hopkins University Press.

CHAPTER 8

Cross-Cultural Differences and Social Influences in Social Support and Cardiovascular Disease

William W. Dressler

Disease has been a continuous feature of life throughout human biological and cultural evolution. It has served as a selective pressure, influencing the relative reproductive success of individuals, and it has shaped the development of behaviors to reduce disease risks. The types of disease prevalent within a population have in turn been influenced by a variety of ecological, social, and cultural parameters of human systems. For most of human biocultural evolution, infectious and parasitic diseases have contributed disproportionately to morbidity and mortality patterns within populations; chronic and degenerative diseases have either been unimportant or have been limited to specific kinds of ecological systems. Within this century, however, disease patterns have changed substantially throughout the world. Technological advances (especially in what we generally think of as public health, but also in terms of medical means for preventing and treating diseases) have meant that mortality from specific infectious and parasitic diseases has been substantially reduced. Concomitantly, the prevalence and incidence of chronic diseases—especially cardiovascular diseases—have increased markedly. Some have been moved to refer to these as "diseases of civilization" (Burkitt, 1973), ignoring the fact that civilization long antedates the contemporary study of cardiovascular disease.

What factors in modern society increase the risk of cardiovascular

WILLIAM W. DRESSLER • Department of Behavioral and Community Medicine, University of Alabama School of Medicine, Tuscaloosa, Alabama 35487.

Social Support and Cardiovascular Disease, edited by Sally A. Shumaker and Susan M. Czajkowski. Plenum Press, New York, 1994.

disease? Many have suggested that dietary factors are of primary importance (Burkitt, 1973), that in the process of modernization an increase in fat intake and sodium intake leads to increases in cardiovascular disease risk factors (serum cholesterol and high blood pressure) and higher rates of coronary heart disease. Undoubtedly this is a part of the process; however, there is good evidence that other factors play a role as well. An interesting example of this comes from the comparison of coronary heart disease mortality rates in the Puerto Rico, Honolulu, and Framingham studies. It was found that after adjusting for age, serum cholesterol, smoking, and blood pressure, persons in Framingham were more than twice as likely to develop heart disease than persons in Puerto Rico or Honolulu (Gordon et al., 1974). A contrast such as this is often attributed to genetic differences between populations, but there are substantial cultural differences among these populations that might account for these findings. It therefore seems logical to look to these cultural and socioeconomic contrasts to explain differences in disease rates.

This serves to exemplify what could be termed an anthropological approach to the study of cardiovascular disease. Anthropology developed as a discipline in the 19th century, in an intellectual climate in which differences of all sorts between populations were routinely attributed to biological differences. By taking to the field a different set of conceptual tools, including the concepts of culture and social organization, ethnographers demonstrated that the dissimilarities between populations in beliefs, attitudes, and socially patterned behaviors were greater than the apparent biological differences. A similar orientation can be applied in the cross-cultural study of diseases. Disease distributions within and between populations are embedded in these population differences in social and economic organization. By tracing the links between social and cultural factors and disease, new insights and explanations in the epidemiology of cardiovascular disease can be developed.

When sociocultural factors are taken into account, cardiovascular disease is often attributed to the "stress" of modern society. Unfortunately, for the most part this notion of stress is vague, simplistic, and contaminated with a "mentalistic bias" (Dressler, Santos, Gallagher, & Viteri, 1987). By that I mean that stress is conceived of in terms synonymous with worry, anxiety, tension, anger, hostility, and similar mental states. This notion is problematic in two ways. First, there is no evidence to suppose that these kinds of stresses are absent in traditional non-Western societies (Murphy, 1982). Second, this very general hypothesis fails to consider the substantial structural changes that occur in a modernizing society. For the most part, the structural changes that have been examined have been factors primarily associated with economic systems (wage-labor occupations, increasing education, material life-styles); differential adoption of (or exposure to) these traits have been found to be related to increased levels of cardiovascular disease risk factors (McGarvey & Baker, 1979; Dressler, Mata, Chavez, & Viteri, 1987) and cardiovascular disease mortality (P. Baker & Crews, 1986). Evidence is accumulating, however, that structural changes in *social* systems also play a role in this process (Dressler, 1984). Consideration of these latter changes in human populations has been neglected.

In this chapter, my aim is to review cross-cultural studies that emphasize the role of social relationships in the disease process. First, societal differences in patterns of morbidity and mortality are examined, emphasizing the "epidemiological transition" that occurs in the process of economic development and modernization. Second, the nature of non-Western social structures are briefly reviewed, with a special focus on how systems of social support are organized within different social structures. Third, specific studies of disease and illness in different societies are reviewed from a social structural perspective. Fourth, implications for future research are offered.

It is unfortunate, but hardly surprising, that there are few cross-cultural studies specifically of cardiovascular diseases. Most studies of cardiovascular disease that traverse linguistic or ethnic boundaries are cross-national studies of societies within a particular mode of economic organization—that of advanced industrial society. These are useful studies and are reviewed elsewhere in this volume. There is, however, a uniformity in social organization within this level of societal complexity that is determined by the level of economic development. My emphasis is on a broader range of cultural diversity, but the research is thin. Fortunately there have been a number of cross-cultural studies of arterial blood pressure, and a number of studies of (broadly speaking) psychosomatic symptoms. Mostly this review will focus on these studies, which will illuminate the issues and suggest avenues for further study.

The Epidemiological Transition

Cross-cultural researchers are in general agreement on a broad taxonomy of human societies, that is based on different ways of exploiting the physical environment and systems of social relationships to organize those productive capacities. Ranging from lower to higher levels of energy capture and environmental modification, these categories include (a) hunting-gathering, (b) horticultural/pastoral, (c) subsistence agricultural, (d) peasant agricultural, and (e) industrial societies. Along with differences in energy capture, these types of societies are characterized by varying social structures. Hunting-gathering societies are distinguished by fluid social structures organized through networks of nuclear families. Horticultural/pastoral societies and societies with agricultural ecologies tend to have larger, more formal tribal social structures with extensive lineage systems. As agricultural production becomes more oriented toward market production, social stratification emerges as a nonkin system for structuring social relationships. Finally, in the emergence of the urban industrial state, the focus of kinship returns to smaller families, both nuclear and extended.

Patterns of morbidity and mortality vary considerably between societies. The specific types of infectious and parasitic diseases, as well as the prevalences of those diseases, depend primarily on specific ecologies. Ample research has shown that cardiovascular disease is essentially absent in societies until the stage of peasant agriculture. Cardiovascular disease then emerges as the primary cause of mortality in industrial societies.

Although this taxonomy of societies is useful theoretically, it does not completely account for current realities. Most of the population of the world lives in neither a peasant nor an industrial society; rather, it lives in what we refer to as the Third World, not fully industrialized but not in the smaller-scale, face-to-face communities of peasant society. These societies are undergoing *economic development* or *modernization*; this liminal state with respect to technoeconomic development is reflected in the mortality profile of the populations as well. Within many developing societies, cardiovascular diseases and infectious and parasitic diseases (mainly as evidenced in high infant mortality rates) are combined among the five leading causes of death (Dressler, 1982).

It is this mixed pattern of diseases—or, more specifically, the emergence of cardiovascular disease—that has stimulated research in the cross-cultural epidemiology of cardiovascular disease. The best systematic documentation of this pattern is the survey carried out by Waldron et al. (1982). In the cross-cultural survey method, individual societies are treated as units of analysis; this is logically equivalent to the epidemiological survey that takes a political unit (like a county or city) as the unit of analysis. Cultural characteristics have been coded for approximately 3,000 societies. Waldron et al. merged data on cultural characteristics with epidemiological survey data on blood pressure for 84 societies. When societies were ranked on type of economy, from hunter-gatherers to urban industrial, there was a significant increase in mean population blood pressures with type of economy. The main increase occurred at the transition from "nonmechanized family agriculture" to "large-scale unmechanized agriculture" (i.e., Third World economies; p. 422).

I take some pains to point this out because it appears not to be simply changes in societal scale or complexity that lead to an increase in cardio-vascular disease, but rather social change of the specific kind that we label economic development or modernization. The precise meaning of these terms is not unproblematic, and an exhaustive review is beyond the scope of this chapter; however, it is important to distinguish among the various ways in which the terms are employed. Many cross-cultural epidemiologists work at least implicitly from a unidimensional theoretical orientation on modernization (Labarthe et al., 1973; P. Baker, 1986). In such models, ideals of so-called traditional societies are those in which most individuals participate in a subsistence (or at least precapitalist) economy; literacy rates and amounts of formal education are low; kinship predominates in social relationships; strong religious orientations structure value systems; and modal personality traits include a high need for affiliation. The development of an industrial economy then leads to most individuals involved in wage-labor (especially factory) work; formal education and literacy; an emphasis on voluntary associations over kinship; science and rationality supplanting religious belief; and the emergence of such modern personality traits as a high need for achievement and an internal locus of control (Inkeles & Smith, 1974). Also modernization in this sense is believed to lead to dietary changes relevant to cardiovascular disease.

It has become increasingly clear that this unidimensional model fails to account adequately for what is occurring in contemporary Third World societies. Many societies have been unable to develop any sort of meaningful industrial economy. In societies that have developed substantial industrial economies (e.g., Brazil), staggering foreign debts and high rates of unemployment and inflation have also been created. This has led many theorists to emphasize the "dependency" of developing societies on fully industrialized nations and the interlocking, systemic nature of development and underdevelopment (Worsley, 1981).

Any research that attempts to examine individual-level characteristics and behaviors related to the risk of cardiovascular disease must acknowledge that individual modernization occurs in these contexts of societal economic development. A research approach that treats particular traits as "modern" and distinguishes among individuals only as having few or many of these traits is unlikely identify accurately more than a small portion of individual variability in cardiovascular risk. More useful would be the adoption of social epidemiological models that have been developed for disease in industrialized societies, and the application of those models (correctly specified) to developing societies. As Cassel (1976) pointed out, a useful model is one that distinguishes those social and behavioral factors that increase the risk of disease from those that increase the individual's resistance to disease.

With respect to those factors reducing the risk of disease, studies of systems of social support have increased in industrialized nations (Cohen & Syme, 1985). It seems likely that social supports are important in the contexts of developing societies as well. But these social networks are organized within the contexts of differing social structures and cultural expectations, expectations that vary within as well as between societies. It is therefore important to consider, at least in a general way, how systems of social relationships vary with social structure.

Social Structure and Social Change

Social structure refers to the norms that govern social interaction. These norms, learned in childhood, identify the range of persons with whom social interaction is permissible, prohibited, or prescribed, and what form that interaction should take. These norms determine relationships ranging from the choice of marriage partners to the etiquette of the corporate boardroom. Social structural norms are rarely realized in their cultural ideal but rather are limited in their actual performance by a variety of constraints; *social organization* refers to the empirically observable performance of interactions defined by social structure. Structure and organization often diverge substantially. For example, cross-culturally the proportion of societies favoring polygynous marriages (one male having multiple wives) is about 75%, but within any one society, constraints on the accumulation of resources usually means that monogamous marriages actually outnumber the culturally preferred polygynous type (Murdock, 1965).

Social structural norms thus interact with other (chiefly economic) factors to generate particular patterns of social organization. Within those patterns of social organization, there are more specific patterns of social interaction that can be usefully centered around specific individuals. Each individual stands at the center of a social network of other individuals with whom he or she interacts on a regular basis. This is a specific kind of social network, the ego-centered social network. Finally, within the social network there is a subset of persons upon whom the individual relies for emotional support, information, and tangible resources. This is a person's social support system. Viewed from this perspective, social support refers to the individual's *perception* that these resources are available from particular persons.

Although these concepts have been introduced as if they formed a taxonomy, these factors intersect at different points. For example, throughout most of human history kinship, gender, and age have been the main principles defining social structural norms. When an individual's social network is composed of persons of appropriate consanguinity, sex, and age, then social norms and the individual's frequent interactions are congruent; if, however, the individual's social network is not composed of appropriate persons, then social norms and interactions have failed to intersect.

As noted above, societies vary systematically in the organization of social relationships. A classic example of this cross-cultural variation comes from Nimkoff and Middleton's (1960) paper on family and economy. Using the cross-cultural survey method, they found that domestic group organization (defined as a dichotomy between "independent" versus "extended" families) significantly covaried with the major economic base of the society. Overall, extended families (defined as families containing at least one nuclear family with additional relatives) were found in societies in which the economy required relatively large work groups, such as pastoral-horticultural societies and societies with a great deal of labor-intensive agriculture. Independent families (defined as families consisting of a single nuclear family) were found in societies in which the economy required small, mobile families, such as hunter-harvesters and industrial societies. Hunters are mobile to follow game, whereas workers in industrial societies are mobile to follow jobs.

Not surprisingly, the reciprocal rights and obligations entailed by kinship vary with the size and complexity of families and larger kin groups. Societies with independent families predominating tend to have a looser organization, with fewer formal requirements in terms of postmarital residence rules, prescription or proscription of certain kinds of relationships, extensiveness of kin terminology, or requirements for the contribution of resources to kin groups. Societies with extended families predominating tend toward a tighter organization, with formal requirements governing a whole variety of behaviors, especially those involving the contribution of resources to larger kin groups (Pelto, 1968). Another important factor to consider in the analysis of social relationships is asymmetry. Whereas in industrial societies stratification is based primarily on economic differences, in other cultures differential status and power within a kin group is often ascribed rather than achieved, and it is often allocated on the basis of age and sex (Morsy, 1978). Finally, in a traditional society, the relationships of kinship are of such importance that fictional kinship relationships often are created to sanction social connections actually based on other considerations.

These variations in kinship and social organization are intended to emphasize two issues of relevance to the study of social support. First, kinship provides a means of structuring social relationships that are adaptive in human populations. The adaptation of any human group requires that effective means for solving basic problems of survival be discovered, and that in turn these become institutionalized within a society. Kinship provides a means for organizing and transmitting adaptive patterns of behavior, especially those that enable individuals to pool or trade resources.

Second, outside of industrial societies, the cultural expectations for the supportive transactions that have been hypothesized to contribute to lowered disease risk may apply only to certain categories of individuals, usually (but not always) defined as kin. In other words, one can seek emotional support or material assistance from certain persons in a culturally appropriate way only if one stands in a particular relationship to that person. This, of course, raises the question of what happens when an individual seeks support outside of culturally sanctioned sources. Seeking support in this way certainly raises the potential for conflict, and hence the possibility that seeking social support can be a psychoculturally negative experience, with concomitant implications for health.

Not surprisingly, issues of social organization become more complicated in situations of modernization. Throughout the Third World modernization has a variety of effects that complicate patterns of kinship. An obvious example is the migration of families to the squatter settlements surrounding major cities. People in these settlements rely on social networks for a variety of resources, networks that are usually formed in an ad hoc manner and often involve multiple female-headed households (Bartolomé, 1984; Lomnitz, 1977). The ability of these networks to absorb new migrants from rural areas is not without limits; however, a rural migrant's best bet is to seek out a relative and to try to integrate himself or herself into that network. This situation can create considerable incongruence between cultural expectations and economic realities. But sometimes cultural expectations themselves will evolve under the influence of mass media from developed societies. This can lead to persons occupying certain social roles to seek or demand a new status for themselves, an obvious example of which would be changing sex role expectations.

Waldron et al. (1982) present evidence that these specific considerations of social organization are relevant. They found population mean blood pressures to vary in association with family type (specifically, the dichotomy between extended and independent families). But this evidence is limited by the design of that study. In the remainder of this chapter, more specific studies of health, including arterial blood pressure and reported symptoms, will be reviewed. General studies of modernization and health will be reviewed first, followed by a review of more focused studies of social organization and health.

Modernization and Cardiovascular Disease

The study of modernization and health has been approached in two ways. Investigators have either compared samples living in communities varying in level or degree of development, or they have studied the migration of persons from traditional to modern communities. Prior (1973) presented data on rates of coronary heart disease and hypertension for a number of societies at different levels of modernization in the Pacific region. Rates of hypertension ranged from less than 5% on Pukapuka, the least modernized island in his sample, to over 20% on Rarotonga, the most modernized. Page, Damon, and Moellering (1974) and Zimmet, Jackson and Whitehouse (1980) demonstrated this same relationship in more focused studies.

The most extensive study of migration and blood pressure is the Tokelau migrant study (Prior et al., 1974). Before the mid-1960s there was no significant out-migration from Tokelau, but following a devastating hurricane, a program was instituted to relocate islanders to New Zealand. Individuals were identified prior to migration and were followed in New Zealand. It was found that migrants had higher blood pressures at all ages than those who stayed, and that rates of hypertension were four times higher among migrants independently of premigrant obesity or changes in fatness accompanying migration (Joseph et al., 1983; Salmond, Joseph, Prior, Stanley, & Wessen, 1985).

A number of studies have combined the strategies of studying modernization and migration. McGarvey and Baker (1979) studied three communities varying in modernization in Samoa, as well as a sample of Samoan migrants to Hawaii. Research subjects were sampled from the commercial center of Pago Pago, an intermediate area connected to Pago Pago by a paved road, and a traditional area; these three areas were then each contrasted with migrants to Hawaii. Overall, migrants in Hawaii had higher blood pressures only if they originated in the most traditional area of Samoa. Within Samoa, persons residing in modern and intermediate areas had higher blood pressures than persons in the traditional area.

A similar strategy contrasting rural versus urban residence, and migrants versus nonmigrants in each area, was employed by Hackenburg, Hackenburg, Magality, Cabral, and Guzman (1983). In this study, conducted in the Philippines, migrants had higher blood pressure irrespective of the end point of their migration; that is, rural-to-rural migration was problematic, as was rural-to-urban migration. Surprisingly, however, rural residents had consistently higher blood pressures than urban residents, who presumably had greater exposure to modernizing influences.

Labarthe et al. (1973) combined ecological comparisons of samples from communities differing in modernization with the measurement of modernization at the level of individuals in order to study several cardio-vascular disease risk factors in Belau in the western Pacific. Blood pres-sure, serum cholesterol, triglyceride, glucose, and ECG abnormality levels were all highest in the most modernized of the communities studied. The individual-level indicators of modernization included a history of changes in residence, occupation, and religious preference; these indicators were strongly correlated with blood pressure for males, but not for females, and they were uncorrelated with other cardiovascular disease risk factors.

Patrick et al. (1983) examined blood pressure in Ponape in the Western Pacific, again combining the comparison of three communities with individual-level measurements. The latter included an index of modern-ization that combined occupation, education, income, and English lan-guage proficiency. Male diastolic blood pressure rose with increasing modernization scores; when community comparisons were carried out, however, the remote or least modernized communities had the highest average blood pressures, and for male systolic pressures and for female systolic and diastolic pressures the slope of blood pressure with age was greatest in the rural area.

Although the relationship between modernization and cardiovascular disease has been studied in diverse parts of the world (see Dressler, 1984, for other examples), it is useful to focus on these studies from the specific cultural region of Oceania. These studies actually present a rather confus-ing pattern of results. Where very broad comparisons of entire social systems—or communities with considerable and demonstrable contrasts in modernization—are made, there is an association of development and disease within the limits of a cross-sectional design. Other studies, though, are neither as consistent nor as strong in demonstrating that relationship, especially when intracultural comparisons are made.

I would argue that a problem here is the failure of cross-cultural researchers to distinguish carefully between sociocultural risk factors and resources for resisting those risks, one of which is social support. Further-more, as the theoretical perspective on modernization spelled out above implies, the risks or stressors associated with modernization are likely to be quite similar across diverse settings. The modernization process in-volves an evolving dependency of the developing society on the economics of the developed societies; the developing society depends on the devel-oped world for capital investment (e.g., factories), manufactured goods (or material life-styles), and information. In terms of individual behavior in the developing society, this translates into wage-labor occupations and the pursuit of higher-status life-styles, or just those changes in behaviors found to be related to an increased disease risk in diverse settings (Dressler, Mata, et al., 1987).

Left out of the equation, however, are the more culturally variable social resources brought to the context of modernization by individuals. The Pacific region is interesting in this respect, because some studies of health outcomes have addressed this question. Traditional social structure throughout Polynesia is centered on extended kinship systems, which also function as political systems (Hecht, Orans, & Janes, 1986). These extended family groups hold property in common (ranging from land to trucks and canoes); members of the extended family are selected to assume titles and authority in the allocation of resources and tasks. The titles held by different extended families are in turn ranked among villages, and "high chiefs" and "orators" assume precedence in supravillage political activity. Not surprisingly, two essential elements in the socialization of children in such a society are (a) learning to be cooperative and communal in orientation and (b) learning one's status in the larger social system (T. Baker, 1986).

Graves and Graves (1979) studied this social group orientation in relation to individual modernization and reported psychosomatic symptoms in a traditional village in the Cook Islands. Persons reporting the fewest number of symptoms were those with greater adoption of modern behaviors, but who simultaneously retained a traditional group orientation. In a study of hormone secretion in American Samoa, Hanna, James, and Martz (1986) found a significant association with social group orientation. Individuals in a group with higher overnight excretion levels of epinephrine and cortisol were most self-reliant in their attitudes and perceived friends and neighbors as least helpful, indicating the importance of a feeling of affiliation to the larger group in mediating the stress effects of modernization.

It is not clear, however, that this mediating effect will generalize to other contexts of social change. Graves and Graves (1980) point out that there is a diversity of opinion in the literature regarding the beneficial or deleterious effects of extended kinship in the adaptation of migrants to new urban settings. They argue that it is useful to distinguish among a variety of adaptive strategies employed by migrants, which they distinguish as reliance on kin, peers, and self. Operationally these strategies distinguish such factors as living with older kin versus siblings or an independent conjugal family; spending time with kin, with friends, or alone or with conjugal family members; and having obtained a job through relatives, friends, or one's own efforts. In a study of workers in New Zealand, Graves and Graves found modal strategies to differ among ethnic groups: Pacific Island immigrants tended to be kin reliant, New Zealand–educated islanders tended to be peer reliant, and European New Zealanders tended to be self-reliant. There was, of course, considerable intraethnic diversity as well.

Different patterns of results were obtained for different ethnic groups when these social group orientations were examined in relation to reported psychosomatic symptoms (Graves & Graves, 1985). Europeans reported fewer symptoms if they also reported having more friends resident in the community. For Pacific Islanders, however, the effects of social relationships depended on the specific society from which they migrated. Samoan migrants' reports of symptoms were positively correlated with the number of friends and relatives in the community, whereas Cook Islanders' symptoms were inversely correlated with friends and relatives in the community. It is worth noting, too, that situational stressors were equally correlated with more psychosomatic symptoms for each of the ethnic groups in New Zealand.

Howard's (1986) analysis of Samoan coping behavior helps to place these results in context. He emphasizes again the social group orientation of Samoans, and notes also the potential problems with this kin involvement:

> The fact is that perpetual involvement with kin networks can become enormously burdensome, especially for an upwardly mobile couple. The obligations of committing income to a broad range of relationships, or supporting the church, of sending remittances back home, make it difficult to save for investments in future socioeconomic advancements. (p. 415)

It is not surprising that greater social group involvement would be related differently to health indicators in Samoa (as found by Hanna et al., 1986) versus New Zealand (as found by Graves & Graves, 1985). The pressures for upward mobility in a European society are likely to be much greater than those in even the most modernized area of Samoa, where the overall cultural context is more socially oriented. But this fails to account for the Cook Islanders and their differences from Samoans in New Zealand. Graves and Graves (1985, p. 16) suggest that Cook Islanders are more acculturated to European society and are thus less pressured to contribute to their kin groups; they report that the average Cook Islander contributes only one third of the amount in cash to his or her kin group that Samoans contribute. Kinship relationships appear simply to be less costly, in both an economic and psychosocial sense, for some groups than others.

Clearly it is not possible to account for all of these findings on the basis of existing literature. The major point here is that theoretical orientations guiding studies of modernization and disease have been inadequate for a refined understanding of this process. The studies reviewed above provide some rationale for the hypothesis that variation in the availability of social resources for adapting to situations of social change would help to account for some of the inconsistencies in results. The formulation of adequate hypotheses relating modernization, social support, and cardiovascular disease requires an understanding of traditional social structure and the nature of social relationships in different contexts of change. The overall pattern of results suggests that traditional kinship orientations are adaptive in the context of social change occurring in relatively isolated communities; among migrants to more urbanized areas, however, the maintenance of traditional kinship orientations may be problematic and hence of less adaptive value.

Cross-Cultural Studies of Social Support

A number of studies of social relationships and health status, including several specifically of cardiovascular disease and its risk factors, have been conducted either in non-Western settings or in communities in developed countries, but with an emphasis placed on the culturally unique structuring of social relationships. It should be recognized at the outset that each of these studies suffers from methodological weaknesses. Notable among these is that there are no true prospective studies. Also, given the kinds of populations studied, it is often difficult to assess the representativeness of the samples. Many of these studies employ only rudimentary controls either for known risk factors or correlates of disease, or for risk factors that might serve as competing hypotheses (e.g., diet). Health outcomes and social supports are often defined in different and noncomparable ways. Nevertheless, as Cassel (1976) noted, if there emerges an interpretable pattern of results from the review of these studies, then it is likely that there are important biocultural processes operating. This review is best regarded as an exercise in hypothesis development and theory building, to suggest new avenues for empirical exploration.

Scotch's (1963) classic study of hypertension among rural and urban Zulus in South Africa examined a number of social factors. He found extended family structure—the traditional form—to be related to hypertension in the urban (but not in the rural) community studied. Extended family households are difficult to maintain in urban areas with limited availability of housing and employment and low incomes, and hence they represent a constraint as opposed to an adaptive strategy in that environment. Church involvement was related to less hypertension in the rural area for both sexes; church involvement was related to less hypertension for women in the urban area, but for urban males it was related to more hypertension. Scotch attributes this to differing sex role expectations in rural versus urban areas: In rural areas, church involvement performs the function of a resistance resource for both sexes, but in the urban area, men involved in churches are seen to be deviant. Men in urban areas are expected to be more involved in secular (sports and drinking) than in sacred activities. These cultural expectations thus alter the meaning of this particular factor and its relationship to cardiovascular response.

The effects of differing expectations, and of the individual's place in the social system, is particularly evident in Scotch's study in the relationship between menopause and hypertension in the two samples. As in many traditional societies, a woman's status in the rural community is very much a function of her role in bearing and rearing children. Women gain in prestige as they progress through the lifecycle and are successful in this role. In the rural area, menopause is associated with hypertension, but having more children in a household is not; in the urban area, more children in a household is associated with hypertension, and menopause is associated with normal blood pressure. Scotch argues that in the city, the end of childbearing actually frees a women from a problematic constraint, given low wages and the problems of caring for many children. Menopause in the rural area means an end to higher social status that is only partly compensated for by the generally higher status of old age. This analysis points to the diversity of social structural dimensions that may relate to health, and to the need for specifying the cultural context of the sample. It also suggests that what seems to be a simple biological fact (menopause) can vary considerably in terms of social meaning.

Bruhn and Wolf (1979) examined the incidence of coronary heart disease in two adjacent communities in eastern Pennsylvania. Roseto, an Italian-American community established in the late 19th century, maintained a very low rate of coronary heart disease through the 1970s despite average to high rates of elevated serum cholesterol, blood pressure, obesity, and smoking. Neighboring communities of mixed ethnicity had rates of heart disease comparable to overall U.S. rates. Roseto was different in that it had maintained a strong ethnic identity, a commitment to traditional values, and a social organization characterized by strong mutual support. As this social organization began to change in the 1970s, rates of coronary heart disease began to increase, especially among younger persons. This study is an example of the beneficial effects of the maintenance of a traditional social organization under changing circumstances.

Another example of this is a study (Dressler, 1979) of family and household organization, modernization, and blood pressure on the West Indian island of St. Lucia. Marriage, household, and family formation do not necessarily overlap in Afro-Caribbean cultures. Although cultural norms place great value on the usual European pattern, low social class and the need for geographic mobility constrain this ideal pattern of family formation; typically, family formation precedes the establishment of an independent household, which in turn precedes marriage. It is common for a man and woman to begin to have children while each still resides in his or her parental household. The children stay with their mothers, while fathers contribute materially and affectively to their support; people may have children with more than one partner at this stage. At the second stage, a conjugal household is established by a male and female, their common children, and the woman's children from other relationships; they may marry at this point, or marriage may be postponed for several years. The man's "outside" children remain with their mother(s). In a sample of middle-aged adults from one community, about half had borne children with two or more partners.

This pattern of relationships can be interpreted either as evidence of social disorganization or as an adaptation to two centuries of economic marginality. Because men are expected to and do support their outside children, this means that material resources flow into a household from multiple sources. For women who never marry this material support is essential, but it is useful for married women as well. Men are provided with options in this system, because if one conjugal relationship dissolves, they often have others to choose from. Finally, for both sexes it increases the number of children available to care for them in their old age. The number of multiple matings is related to lower systolic ($r = -.20$, $p < .05$) and diastolic ($r = -.22$, $p < .01$) blood pressure for both males and females, controlling for age and obesity. The network of relationships formed in this way represents a culturally specific support system in this West Indian society.

The importance of specifying social relationships in culturally appro-priate ways is exemplified in a recent study of Samoan migrants to the San Francisco area (Janes & Pawson, 1986). As noted earlier, Samoans can be constrained by a strong set of obligations, often material in nature, to their extended families. Janes and Pawson contrasted this set of obligations with what they refer to as "core social networks." This latter concept identifies a much smaller set of kin, primarily adult siblings, with whom Samoans will often maintain lifelong, affectively close relationships. In Janes and Pawson's study, individuals who simultaneously had a high involvement in the larger extended kin group and low economic resources had higher blood pressures, whereas Samoans with larger core social networks had lower blood pressures (again independent of age and obesity). It is useful to contrast these findings with those of Graves and Graves (1985), who found a number of measures of kin group involvement to be related to more reported psychosomatic symptoms. Janes and Pawson's (1986) results indicate that different types of kin involvement have different health implications.

Social interaction was examined in relation to blood pressure in the study of Tokelau Island migrants to New Zealand (Beaglehole, Salmond, & Hooper, 1977). An index of social interaction included items reflecting interaction with Tokelauan or non-Tokelauan persons, such as ethnic affiliation of workmates, ethnic affiliation of friends, commitment to Tokelauan activities, ethnic affiliation in church membership, and others. Higher scores on this index assessed greater non-Tokelauan social interaction and were associated with higher blood pressure. Unfortunately, variables were assessed in such a way that Tokelauan versus non-Tokelauan social involvement was contrasted, with no consideration given to the possibility that different kinds of social interaction *within* the Tokelauan migrant community might have different health effects.

Kunitz and Levy (1986) examined diagnosed hypertension in relation to a variety of sociocultural factors among elderly Navajo living on a reservation in the U.S. Southwest. Traditionally Navajo have lived in matrilineal, matrilocal extended kin groups (parents with their daughters, their daughter's husbands and children) in livestock herding camps dispersed throughout their arid territory. The investigators developed a social isolation/integration index based on the degree to which camp living arrangements diverged from the traditional pattern. For women, the prevalence of hypertension was five times greater among those not living in the most traditional extended kin groups; there was no effect for men.

Frate (1978) studied the prevalence of hypertension in extended kin groups in a rural black community in the southern United States. He found that persons within this community referred to extended families as "strong" or "weak." A strong family was characterized by traits such as high religiosity, leadership in the community, strength of character attributed to family elders, and patterns of strong mutual support; weak families were characterized by deficits on these and related traits. In a sample of 16 extended families totaling 266 individuals, 49.4% of members of weak families had hypertension, whereas only 14.6% of strong family members had hypertension. He concluded that strong extended families provide greater social and emotional support for their members, thus buffering the effects of hypertension risk factors.

Thus far, all studies reviewed have employed structural measures of social support; these are measures that assess support in terms of the presence, absence, or numbers of social relationships in which the individual is engaged (Cohen, 1988). There is some evidence to indicate, however, that measures assessing kinds of support or the functions provided by social relationships may be more important in predicting health outcomes (Kessler & McLeod, 1985). Another way of contrasting these approaches is to use the terminology introduced above: Social network measures are structural measures, whereas social support measures are functional measures. These latter measures specifically assess the extent to which an individual *perceives* particular types of resources (material support, information, emotional support) as being available within his or her network.

Social support and arterial blood pressure in a Mexican community were examined using this strategy (Dressler, Mata, Chavez, Viteri, & Gallagher, 1986). The study community was a small provincial marketing and official center serving a region dominated by peasant agriculture. The assessment of social support was based on existing ethnographic analyses of traditional Mexican family structure. Family relationships are strongly patrilocal (male dominated); preferred residence after marriage is in an independent household located next to the household of the man's parents, so that a series of seemingly independent households actually combine to form an extended family that pools resources with respect to labor, child care, and food. Relationships within the family are stratified by age and gender; women are expected to be self-effacing and submissive. Men are authoritarian and represent the family to the outside world. Male sons are subordinate to their father, and wives are subordinate to their husband's mother. A woman gradually gains status within the family as she grows older and has children, and a close affective bond develops between her and her children, especially her sons.

Relationships outside the family are generally restrained, as nonkin bonds could threaten the ties of kinship. One set of nonkin bonds are of sufficient importance, however, to be elevated through fictive kinship to the level of family relationships. These are ties established through the system of *compadrazgo*. A *compadre* ("coparent") is selected for a child at critical junctures (e.g., baptism, marriage). The ostensible reason for the *compadre* is to oversee the moral education and uprightness of the child (who addresses him as *padrino*, or godfather); perhaps more importantly, this establishes a formal, kinshiplike relationship between the coparents. This important dimension of the system enables individuals to extend formal relationships vertically in the status hierarchy. One attempts to gain through one's *compadres* more resources (economic, social, and political).

Social support was assessed using a 24-item function-by-relationship matrix; for each of four social relationships (relatives, friends, neighbors, *compadres*), respondents were asked six questions concerning the availability of support from that person (e.g., "If you needed to borrow money, could you ask your _____?"). When factor analyzed, each of the social relationships formed its own factor on which problems where the respondent would ask that type of individual for help loaded.

Each of the four social support factors was inversely correlated with blood pressure for males; the correlations for *compadre* support were largest ($r = -.39$, $p < .01$ for systolic pressure; $r = -.26$, $p < .05$ for diastolic pressure). The only significant correlation for females was friend support with higher diastolic blood pressure. When the subsample of women was broken down by age, relative support was related to lower blood pressure for older women, but not younger women. For younger women, higher blood pressure was related to more friend support. All correlations were calculated controlling for age and obesity.

This seemingly complex pattern of results is consistent with ethnographic analyses of traditional Mexican village social structure. *Compadrazgo* is a system of social relationships, dating back centuries, that enables individuals to gain access to greater resources of all kinds. Men in this patrilocal culture have a freedom of movement in the social sphere that allows them to establish many different kinds of supportive relationships. Overall there were no effects for women; but for older women, support from relatives (probably their adult children) was a significant factor. Younger women have the lowest status of all, being dominated by the husband and his family. These women are expected to provide support, not receive it. If under the duress of these conditions they seek out support outside the family, this could be seen as threatening to the integrity of the kin group and be negatively sanctioned, thus reversing the role of that relationship.

A related study was conducted in an urban area of Brazil (Dressler, 1986). That research provided an interesting contrast with the Mexican study, especially with respect to family structure. Although traditional family structure in Brazil is very much like that of Mexico, both being southern Iberian in origin, the Brazil study was conducted among diverse occupational groups in a major urban center. The role of extended kinship, though still present, is reduced in such areas, and independent conjugal families are more the norm. Also, sex roles are rapidly changing, with a substantial mix of feminist and more traditional beliefs regarding women's roles. Finally, the institution of *compadrazgo* has been altered to the extent that it more closely resembles the middle-class American notion of godparenthood than it resembles the traditional Mexican institution.

Factor analysis also returned four support factors in that study; however, the pattern of loadings was such that the rank of the measurement model could be further reduced to two factors: relative (or kin) support and nonkin support. Differences in the effects of support for males and females were again explored. Higher kin support was related to lower blood pressure for males, but higher blood pressure for females. Higher nonkin support was related to lower blood pressure for females, but higher blood pressure for males (all correlations controlled for age, obesity, and ethnicity). These results are consistent with a model of a patrilocal family system undergoing modernization, in which males still receive substantial benefits from their role within the family; women, although still seemingly constrained to perform a particular supportive role within the family, are nevertheless free to move into the larger social milieu and establish supportive relationships outside the family.

More recently, this distinction between support from kin and nonkin has been explored in research on depression (Dressler, 1991a) and arterial blood pressure (Dressler, 1991b) in an African-American community in the rural South. Traditionally, the extended family was the primary source of social support within American black communities; throughout the long period of social and economic marginality following emancipation, and continuing well into the period of the civil rights movement, one's kin were the only social safety net. The reciprocal rights and obligations to demand and provide support were reinforced by bonds of consanguinity. With the advent of the struggle for civil rights, however, the world has changed for a generation of African Americans. Younger black people have been thrust into new occupational and educational settings as they aspire to the social mobility that is a primary collective motive in American culture. The obstacles and barriers faced in these settings may or may not have been faced by extended kin, but they certainly are being faced by peers: friends, coworkers, and members of voluntary associations. It was therefore hypothesized that among younger African Americans, nonkin had become the culturally meaningful source of social support. For older members of the community, it was hypothesized that extended kin would have retained their traditional cultural salience and would be the meaningful source of social support.

These hypotheses were tested in two separate samples, each having somewhat different characteristics. Social support was assessed using an expanded function-by-relationship matrix that was scaled using factor analysis into two independent dimensions, one measuring kin support and one measuring nonkin support. In each sample, social support had no independent effect, but rather moderated or buffered the effect of social stressors (i.e., individuals who perceived higher levels of support showed no increased risk of adverse outcomes in relation to higher stressor levels, whereas among persons who perceived little social support, the effects of stressors on outcomes were exacerbated). Among persons age 39 or younger, the effects of social stressors were moderated by nonkin support in relation both to depression and arterial blood pressure; among persons age 40 or older, the effects of social stressors were buffered by kin support (Dressler, 1991a, b). It is important to note, too, that younger and older persons did not differ with respect to the perceived level of support from kin or nonkin. Therefore it was the cultural salience of the support that made the difference, not the amount.

A recent paper has explored the hypothesis, posed earlier in this chapter, that the health effects of social supports are likely to be more culturally variable than the effects of social stressors. Using data on blood pressure from communities in Brazil, Mexico, and Jamaica—where comparable data on stressors and social supports had been collected—Dressler, Viteri, Grell, Chavez, and Santos (1991) found that the effect of one stressor (status incongruence) on blood pressure was invariant across the three field sites. There were, however, significant statistical interaction effects between community of residence (or culture) and measures of social support, indicating that the relationship between social support and blood pressure could only be anticipated on the basis of the knowledge of cultural context.

Discussion

The focus in this chapter has been on the cross-cultural distribution of cardiovascular disease, and on the ways in which differences in social relationships within and between societies influence the distribution of disease. It was argued that in the process of social change in worldwide perspective, societies undergoing economic development or modernization experience an epidemiological transition. In this transition, higher rates of cardiovascular disease and high rates of infectious and parasitic diseases account for most morbidity. The task becomes one of explaining the emergence of cardiovascular diseases (Henry & Cassel, 1969).

Changes in diet, including increased intake of fats and sodium and higher rates of obesity, certainly account for a portion of this increase. Similarly, differences within populations in terms of a genetic predisposition to cardiovascular disease may influence the response of a group to changes in diet. It is unlikely, however, that these factors could account for the social patterning of blood pressure, symptoms, or cardiovascular disease observed in these studies.

Most research in cross-cultural epidemiology has been conducted from a narrow and unidimensional perspective on modernization in which societies are viewed as slowly evolving toward industrial development, and in which individual modernization can be described as the progressive assimilation of "modern" traits (or what we have elsewhere termed the "accretion" model of modernization; Dressler, Mata, et al., 1987). This model is faulty on two grounds. First, it fails to recognize that developing societies are locked into states of dependency in the larger world system. Second, it fails to recognize that counterbalancing the risks associated with the modernization process are resistance resources extant within cultures that, under certain circumstances, reduce the risk of disease and buffer the stressors associated with culture change.

Any analysis of social support as a resistance resource must begin with an understanding of traditional social structure and especially of kinship systems, which serve an important function in organizing social relationships. Culture modifies the social support–disease relationship in two ways. First, the content of social support varies across cultural systems. In other cultures, the social world is delimited by reciprocal rights and obligations (usually defined by kinship) such that social support is appropriately only sought from or provided to certain individuals who stand in a particular relationship to the seeker or provider. This does not mean that support functions—both material and emotional—are not provided through relationships other than those deemed culturally appropriate; however, it does lead to the second modifying influence of culture: Culture (or, more specifically, cultural context) modifies the relationship between social support and disease, depending on the meanings and expectations surrounding the transaction.

Both of these propositions are exemplified by the study in Mexico (Dressler, Mata, et al., 1986). Males benefit from support perceived to be available from all sources, but especially through the *compadrazgo* system of fictive kinship. Females, on the other hand, benefit (in terms of lower blood pressure) only from support within the kinship system, and only if they have achieved the status of older age. Young women do not benefit from support, and indeed their blood pressures are higher if they perceive available support outside the family. Does this mean that young women do not receive the nonkin support they perceive to be available? I would argue that they probably do receive such support in the sense that information, material assistance, and even emotional supports are exchanged, but because these exchanges occur outside the normative context of culture, the beneficial effects of social support are not realized or are confounded by the nonnormative relationships.

There are several ways in which this might occur. First, the seeking of support outside of the family by a young woman may lead to an increase in negative social interactions with her husband or mother-in-law, who could perceive this to be a threat to the integrity of the family. Second, because supportive interactions among young peers are not consistent with traditional social structural norms, the supportive exchanges may not be effectively accomplished. Shumaker and Brownell (1984), for example, have argued that a variety of situational variables may interfere with the supportive transactions: Providers and recipients of support may perceive transactions differently, persons may seek support but providers may not recognize it, or persons may need support but not seek it out. All of these situational factors may create a circumstance in which an individual could perceive support to be available, but that perception would end up being related to a worse health outcome.

A third reason why beneficial effects of social support may not be realized, or why seemingly supportive transactions might be deleterious, relates to the socially patterned meanings surrounding social interaction. It was argued earlier that within traditional societies, supportive transactions could only be anticipated if one stood in a particular relationship (governed by the relations of kinship) to another individual. Empirical studies bear out this proposition, although it is clearly complicated by other factors. It is useful to conceive of these relationships as having a meaning that causes supportive transactions to be of particular emotional and physiological significance to the recipient. It is entirely possible that precisely the same supportive transactions could occur in two different relationships, but that only one of those relationships would have this meaning; hence only transactions in the latter would have the beneficial social, emotional, and physiological effects associated with social support.

In Western (and especially American) society, with the ever-increasing emphasis placed on individualism, this dimension of social relationships is almost completely divorced from specific relationships. For example, in an extensive study of depressive affect among Anglos in northern California, Phillips and Fischer (1981) found interaction with kin to be unrelated to affect, and interaction with nonkin to be related to positive affect. Shumaker and Brownell (1984) suggest that short-term supportive interactions with strangers might be particularly effective precisely because of the anonymity involved. These arguments suggest that in modern society the meaning of a relationship is established solely by the participants, and that cultural expectations combining this meaning with specific relationships are absent. The one relationship where this is not true in Western society is marriage; Brown and Harris (1978) argue that a close and confiding relationship of a woman and her husband (or boyfriend) carries a particular meaning such that it should be considered apart from other sorts of social ties as a risk reduction factor for depression.

In non-Western societies, and within specific subcultural groups in Western society, this significance of specific relationships is culturally defined as belonging to particular kinds of (mainly kinship) relationships. A careful analysis of social structure should tell us which kinds of relationships are likely to be culturally significant with respect to support and which are not (e.g., Janes & Pawson, 1986). This hypothesis squares with laboratory research showing that the definition of a social situation alters the psychophysiological reactivity of participants. Long, Lynch, Machiran, Thomas, and Manilow (1982) found that normotensive college students evidenced larger blood pressure increases when speaking in the presence of an experimenter of higher social status than themselves, as opposed to one of equal social status. By experimentally altering the *meaning* of the social interaction, blood pressure responses to the inter- action were also altered. Here I am suggesting that socially patterned meanings, derived from local culture, surrounding social support trans- actions can alter pressor responses in the same way.

This notion may better help to explain discrepancies in findings from other research on social relationships and cardiovascular disease. For example, Reed, McGhee, Yano, and Feinleib (1983) found measures of social networks to be prospectively unrelated to cardiovascular disease among Japanese men in Hawaii (see Chapter 6). Although there was some attempt to take cultural context into account in developing an index of social networks for that study, given that traditional Japanese social struc- ture is very complex (with considerable stratification within families ac- cording to various roles), it is difficult to say whether the measure of networks captures social relationships that carry such cultural meaning. Similarly, simply asking respondents if they receive support from anyone, as others have attempted to do in non-Western settings (Hackenburg et al., 1983), is unlikely to assess relevant dimensions. If the hypothesis offered here has any merit, then support from "anyone" cannot be considered meaningful; rather, it must be support from *someone*, whose identity is defined by culture and social structure.

The hypothesis has been put forth that satisfaction with support is an important dimension (Stokes, 1983). The concept offered here is however, quite different from "satisfaction." An individual may be very satisfied with his or her transactions with other individuals, but if those individuals do not stand in a particularly meaningful relationship to the person seeking support, then the affective feedback and information provided by the supporter is unlikely to carry the positive emotional impact required to activate the physiological pathways necessary to ameliorate the cardio- vascular diseases process. What I am arguing for here is an analysis of meaning in social relationships, just as Brown (Brown & Harris, 1978) has argued for meaning in the study of life event stressors and Eckenrode and Gore (1981) have argued for in the study of social support. The evidence reviewed here is consistent with the notion that meanings of social support relationships can be understood in terms of the cultural (rather than biographical) context of individuals, based on an ethnographic analysis of social structure.

Future research in diverse cultures is required to develop a better understanding of social support processes. Insights regarding these processes from studying industrialized nations cannot be generalized to non-Western, or even modernizing, social groups. Rather, research is needed that is precise with respect to an understanding of the cultural context studied, and sophisticated with respect to epidemiological methods. In this way general theories of social relationships and disease processes can be developed and tested.

References

Baker, P. T. (1986). Rationale and research design. In P. T. Baker, J. M. Hanna, & T. S. Baker (Eds.), *The changing Samoans: Behavior and health in transition* (pp. 3–18). New York: Oxford University Press.

Baker, P. T., & Crews, D. E. (1986). Mortality patterns and some biological predictors. In P. T. Baker, J. M. Hanna, & T. S. Baker (Eds.), *The changing Samoans: Behavior and health in transition* (pp. 93–122). New York: Oxford University Press.

Baker, T. S. (1986). Changing socialization patterns of contemporary Samoans. In P. T. Baker, J. M. Hanna, & T. S. Baker (Eds.), *The changing Samoans: Behavior and health in transition* (pp. 146–173). New York: Oxford University Press.

Bartolomé, L. J. (1984). Forced resettlement and the survival systems of the urban poor. *Ethnology, 23,* 177–192.

Beaglehole, R. C., Salmond, E., & Hooper, A. (1977). Blood pressure and social interaction in Tokelau migrants in New Zealand. *Journal of Chronic Diseases, 29,* 371–380.

Brown, G. W., & Harris, T. (1978). *Social origins of depression.* New York: Free Press.

Bruhn, J. G., & Wolf, S. (1979). *The Roseto story: An anatomy of health.* Norman: University of Oklahoma Press.

Burkitt, D. P. (1973). Some diseases characteristic of modern Western civilization. *British Medical Journal, 1,* 274–278.,

Cassel, J. (1976). The contribution of the social environment to host resistance. *American Journal of Epidemiology, 104,* 107–123.

Cohen, S. (1988). Psychosocial models of the role of social support in the etiology of physical disease. *Health Psychology, 7,* 269–297.

Cohen, S., & Syme, S. L. (Eds.) (1985). *Social support and health.* Orlando, FL: Academic Press.

Dressler, W. W. (1979). "Disorganization," adaptation, and arterial blood pressure. *Medical Anthropology, 3,* 225–248.

Dressler, W. W. (1982). *Hypertension and culture change: Acculturation and disease in the West Indies.* South Salem, NY: Redgrave.

Dressler, W. W. (1984). Social and cultural influences in cardiovascular disease: A review. *Transcultural Psychiatric Research Review, 21,* 5–42.

Dressler, W. W. (1985). Psychosomatic symptoms, stress, and modernization: A model. *Culture, Medicine, and Psychiatry, 9,* 257–286.

Dressler, W. W. (1986, December). *Blood pressure, sex roles, and social support.* Paper presented at the 85th annual meeting of the American Anthropological Association, Philadelphia.

Dressler, W. W. (1991a). *Stress and adaptation in the context of culture: Depression in a southern black community.* Albany: State University of New York Press.

Dressler, W. W. (1991b). Social support, lifestyle incongruity, and arterial blood pressure in a southern black community. *Psychosomatic Medicine, 53,* 608–620.

Dressler, W. W., Mata, A., Chavez, A., & Viteri, F. E. (1987). Arterial blood pressure and individual modernization in a Mexican community. *Social Science and Medicine, 24,* 679–687.

Dressler, W. W., Mata, A., Chavez, A., Viteri, F. E., & Gallagher, P. N. (1986). Social support and arterial blood pressure in a central Mexican community. *Psychosomatic Medicine, 48,* 338–350.

Dressler, W. W., Santos, J. E. D., Gallagher, P. N., Jr., & Viteri, F. E. (1987). Arterial blood pressure and modernization in Brazil. *American Anthropologist, 89,* 389–409.

Dressler, W. W., Viteri, F. E., Grell, G. A. C., Chavez, A., & Santos, J. E. D. (1991). Comparative research in social epidemiology: Measurement issues. *Ethnicity and Disease, 1,* 379–393.

Eckenrode, J., & Gore, S. (1981). Stressful events and social supports: The significance of context. In B. H. Gottlieb (Ed.), *Social networks and social support* (pp. 43–68). Beverly Hills, CA: Sage.

Frate, D. A. (1978). *Family functioning and hypertension in a black population.* Unpublished doctoral dissertation, Department of Anthropology, University of Illinois.

Gordon, T., Garcia-Palmieri, M. R., Kagan, A., et al. (1974). Differences in coronary heart disease in Framingham, Honolulu, and Puerto Rico. *Journal of Chronic Diseases, 27,* 329–344.

Graves, T. D., & Graves, N. B. (1979). Stress and health: Modernization in a traditional Polynesian society. *Medical Anthropology, 3,* 23–59.

Graves, T. D., & Graves, N. B. (1980). Kinship ties and the preferred adaptive strategies of urban migrants. In L. S. Cordell & S. J. Beckerman (Eds.), *The versatility of kinship* (pp. 195–217). New York: Academic Press.

Graves, T. D., & Graves, N. B. (1985). Stress and health among Polynesian migrants to New Zealand. *Journal of Behavioral Medicine, 8*(1), 1–19.

Hackenburg, R. A., Hackenburg, B. H., Magalit, H. F., Cabral, E. I., & Guzman, S. V. (1983). Migration, modernization and hypertension. *Medical Anthropology, 7,* 45–71.

Hanna, J. M., James, J. D., & Martz, J. M. (1986). Hormonal measures of stress. In P. T. Baker, J. M. Hanna, & T. S. Baker (Eds.), *The changing Samoans: Behavior and health in transition* (pp. 203–221). New York: Oxford University Press.

Hecht, J. A., Orans, M., & Janes, C. R. (1986). Social settings of contemporary Samoans. In P. T. Baker, J. M. Hanna, & T. S. Baker (Eds.), *The changing Samoans: Behavior and health in transition* (pp. 39–62). New York: Oxford University Press.

Henry, J. P., & Cassel, J. C. (1969). Psychosocial factors in essential hypertension. *American Journal of Epidemiology, 90,* 171–200.

Howard, A. (1986). Questions and answers: Samoans talk about happiness, distress, and other life experiences. In P. T. Baker, J. M. Hanna, & T. S. Baker (Eds.), *The changing Samoans: Behavior and health in transition* (pp. 174–202). New York: Oxford University Press.

Inkeles, A., & Smith, D. H. (1974). *Becoming modern.* Cambridge, MA: Harvard University Press.

Janes, C. R., & Pawson, I. G. (1986). Migration and biocultural adaptation: Samoans in California. *Social Science and Medicine, 22,* 821–834.

Joseph, J. G., Prior, I. A. M., Salmond, C. E., et al. (1983). Elevation of systolic and diastolic blood pressure associated with migration: The Tokelau Island migrant study. *Journal of Chronic Diseases, 36,* 507–516.

Kessler, R. C., & McLeod, J. D. (1985). Social support and mental health in community samples. In S. Cohen & S. L. Syme (Eds.), *Social support and health* (pp. 219–240). Orlando, FL: Academic Press.

Kunitz, S. J., & Levy, J. E. (1986). The prevalence of hypertension among elderly Navajos: A
   test of the acculturative stress hypothesis. *Culture, Medicine and Psychiatry, 10,* 97–121.
Labarthe, D., Reed, D., Brody, J., et al. (1973). Health effects of modernization in Palau.
   American Journal of Epidemiology, 98, 161–174.
Lomintz, L. (1977). *Networks and marginality: Life in a Mexican shantytown.* New York: Aca-
   demic Press.
Long, J. M., Lynch, J. J., Machiran, N. M., Thomas, S. A., & Malinow, K. L. (1982). The effects
   of status on blood pressure during verbal communication. *Journal of Behavioral Medicine,
   5,* 165–172.
McGarvey, S. T., & Baker, P. T. (1979). The effects of modernization and migration on Samoan
   blood pressure. *Human Biology, 51,* 467–479.
Morsy, S. (1978). Sex roles, power, and illness in an Egyptian village. *American Ethnologist, 5,*
   137–150.
Murdock, G. P. (1965). *Social structure.* New York: Free Press.
Murphy, H. B. M. (1982). Blood pressure and culture: The contribution of cross-cultural
   comparisons to psychosomatics. *Psychotherapeutics and Psychosomatics, 38,* 244–255.
Nimkoff, M. F., & Middleton, R. (1960). Types of family and types of economy. *American
   Journal of Sociology, 66,* 215–224.
Page, L., Damon, A., & Moellering, R. C. (1974). Antecedents of cardiovascular disease in six
   Solomon Island societies. *Circulation, 49,* 1132–1146.
Patrick, R. C., Prior, I. M., Smith, J. C., et al. (1983). Relationship between blood pressure and
   modernity among Panopeans. *International Journal of Epidemiology, 12,* 36–44.
Pelto, P. J. (1968). The difference between "tight" and "loose" societies. *Transaction, 5,* 37–40.
Phillips, S. L., & Fischer, C. S. (1981). Measuring social support networks in general
   populations. In B. S. Dohrenwend & B. P. Dohrenwend (Eds.), *Stressful life events and their
   contexts.* New York: Prodist.
Prior, I. (1973). Epidemiology of cardiovascular diseases in Asian-Pacific region. *Singapore
   Medical Journal, 14,* 223–227.
Prior, I. A. M., Stanhope, J. M., Evans, J. G., et al. (1974). The Tokelau Island migrant study.
   International Journal of Epidemiology, 3, 225.
Reed, D., McGhee, D., Yano, K., & Feinleib, M. (1983). Social networks and coronary heart
   disease among Japanese men in Hawaii. *American Journal of Epidemiology, 117,* 384–396.
Salmond, C. E., Joseph, J. G., Prior, I. M., Stanley, D. G., & Wessen, A. F. (1985). Longitudinal
   analysis of the relationship between blood pressure and migration: The Tokelau Island
   migrant study. *American Journal of Epidemiology, 122,* 291–301.
Scotch, N. A. (1963). Sociocultural factors in the epidemiology of Zulu hypertension.
   American Journal of Public Health, 53, 1205–1213.
Shumaker, S. A., & Brownell, A. (1984). Toward a theory of social support: Closing conceptual
   gaps. *Journal of Social Issues, 40,* 11–36.
Stokes, J. P. (1983). Predicting satisfaction with social support from social network structure.
   American Journal of Community Psychology, 11, 141–152.
Waldron, I., Nowotaksi, M., Freimer, M., et al. (1982). Cross-cultural variation in blood
   pressure: A quantitative analysis of the relationships of blood pressure to cultural
   characteristics, salt consumption, and body weight. *Social Science and Medicine, 16,*
   419–430.
Worsley, P. (1981). Social class and development. In G. D. Berreman (Ed.), *Social inequality:
   Comparative and developmental approaches* (pp. 221–225). New York: Academic Press.
Zimmet, P., Jackson, L., & Whitehouse, S. (1980). Blood pressure studies in two Pacific
   populations with varying degrees of modernization. *New Zealand Medical Journal, 91,*
   249–252.

PART IV

The Development of Cardiovascular Disease

CHAPTER 9

Social Support and Coronary Heart Disease

Underlying Psychological and Biological Mechanisms

Sheldon Cohen, Jay R. Kaplan, and Stephen B. Manuck

Social support has been prospectively associated with mortality and implicated in the etiology of coronary heart disease (CHD; see reviews by Berkman, 1985; Broadhead et al., 1983; Cohen, 1988; House, Landis, & Umberson, 1988; Wallston, Alagna, DeVellis, & DeVellis, 1983). Although there has been a tremendous effort to establish a relation between support and CHD, relatively little work has focused on how social support influences CHD pathogenesis. We feel that differentiation between conceptions of social support and specification of pathways through which each type of support influences CHD are requisite for understanding the role of support in the prevention of disease. In service of this goal, we review studies of the role of social support in the etiology of CHD, suggest some distinctions in social support based on existing research, argue for functionally

SHELDON COHEN • Department of Psychology, Carnegie-Mellon University, Pittsburgh, Pennsylvania 15213.   *JAY R. KAPLAN* • Bowman Gray School of Medicine, Wake Forest University, Winston-Salem, North Carolina 27157-1040.   *STEPHEN B. MANUCK* • Department of Psychology, University of Pittsburgh, Pittsburgh, Pennsylvania 15260.

Social Support and Cardiovascular Disease, edited by Sally A. Shumaker and Susan M. Czajkowski. Plenum Press, New York, 1994.

distinct stages of CHD pathogenesis, and propose a series of psychological and biological models linking different conceptualizations of social support to CHD. Our discussion is limited to the etiology of disease (onset and progression, but not recovery) and focuses on disease end points (morbidity and mortality) rather than illness behaviors such as symptom reporting and use of medical services.

The major thrust of our argument is that in order to understand the influence of social support on CHD, we must take into account both how we conceptualize social support and the stage of disease under consideration. The development of CHD subsumes numerous stages, each accompanied by a somewhat different set of pathophysiological processes. Conditions that influence coronary artery atherogenesis, for instance, may not be the same as those responsible for the various functional and clinical expressions of CHD. Moreover, various conceptualizations of social networks and supports vary widely, and individual concepts may be plausible predictors of some stages of disease but not of others.

Differentiating Social Support

There is little agreement among the scientific community in regard to a precise definition of social support (Cohen & Syme, 1985; Shumaker & Brownell, 1984; Wilcox & Vernberg, 1985). Moreover, existing studies apply the term to a broad range of conceptualizations of social networks and the functions that they provide. Rather than attempt an all-encompassing definition, we propose broad categorical classifications of the concepts commonly included under the social support rubric, and we define some specific concepts that we feel may be linked with physical disease. Cohen and his colleagues (Cohen & Syme, 1985; Cohen & Wills, 1985) proposed a distinction between *structural* and *functional* support measures. Structural measures describe the existence of and interconnections between social ties; functional measures assess whether interpersonal relationships serve particular functions (e.g., provide affection).

Only a small sample of possible conceptions of social support have been used with any frequency in studies of CHD morbidity and mortality. The most common measure is a structural index of social ties that is often termed *social integration* (SI). A prototypical SI index includes marital status, closeness of family and friends, participation in group activities, and church and religious affiliations. Functional measures used in the physical disease literature include network satisfaction and perceived availability of material aid or psychological support.

Differentiating Stages of CHD

The Natural History of CHD

Available research reveals much about the course of development of coronary disease and about the risk factors that contribute to it. CHD is usually the clinical manifestation of an underlying pathological process, coronary artery atherosclerosis. Atherosclerosis refers to the development of fibrofatty plaques (atheromas) within the inner lining, or intima, of the artery. With the progression of atherosclerosis, plaques frequently change in composition as well as size; other changes include calcification and, later, ulceration and hemorrhage (McGill, 1972). The progressive enlargement and complication of atherosclerotic plaques may narrow the arteries and eventually obstruct blood flow to the heart, resulting in cardiac electrical instability, damage or death of the heart tissue, or both. These sequelae of coronary artery atherosclerosis ultimately affect the ability of the heart to maintain its normal rhythmicity and essential function as a pump. The usual clinical expressions of CHD include angina pectoris and its variants (chest pain, generally resulting from insufficient coronary blood flow), acute myocardial infarction (death of the heart tissue as a result of interrupted coronary blood flow), cardiac arrhythmias (electrical instability) and sudden death (often the consequence of arrhythmia; Sokolow & McIlroy, 1987).

Epidemiological and experimental studies of the origins of CHD have advanced vigorously over the past several decades, and a variety of physiological and environmental variables are clearly of etiological significance. Elevated serum lipid concentrations, arterial hypertension, and cigarette smoking account for much of the geographic distribution of CHD, and within geographic areas, these variables act as risk factors for extent and severity of the disease (Keys et al., 1972; McGill, 1968). There is evidence that the behavioral characteristics of individuals (e.g., coronary-prone behavior) also modulate risk for CHD, as do several attributes of social support summarized elsewhere in this chapter (Manuck, Kaplan, & Matthews, 1986). The mechanism(s) by which psychosocial variables contribute to coronary disease risk remain unclear, however, and (unlike such established risk factors as hypertension and elevated serum lipids) have only recently become a subject of intensive investigation. Nevertheless, a review of the sequence of events leading from development of the atherosclerotic lesion to the clinical manifestations of CHD helps identify a group of biologic processes upon which psychosocial factors could exert significant influence.

Biological Processes underlying CHD

The first lesion usually observed in the arterial intima is the fatty streak (Figure 1). Universally observed in children, such lesions are believed to be reversible and to have no physiological consequences (McGill, 1972). Although the process by which nonreversible, fibrous plaques develop is not known with certainty, injury (or possibly repeated injury) to the endothelial lining of the artery is believed to play an important initiating role (Ross, 1981). Such injury may lead to the local adherence of platelets and subsequent release of mitogenic (growth) substances, an

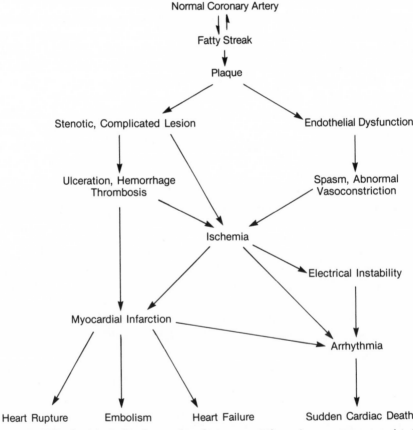

Figure 1. Pathophysiological pathways thought to connect the various processes associated with coronary artery atherogenesis and coronary heart disease.

increased infiltration of lipids into the artery wall, and intimal smooth muscle cell proliferation, all of which are aspects of plaque formation (Davies, 1986; Schwartz, Campbell, & Campbell, 1986).

Once formed, a progressing plaque may interfere with the ability of the artery wall (particularly the endothelial lining) to dilate in response to hemodynamic demands or to the presence of endogenous vasoactive substances. Such vascular dysfunction may result in arterial spasm, possibly contributing to myocardial ischemia—an inadequate supply of oxygen to the muscular tissue of the heart (Furchgott, 1983; Sokolow & McIlroy, 1987). The plaque may also induce aggregation and activation of platelets and the release by platelets of thomboxane A_2, a potent vasoconstrictor (Neri-Serneri et al., 1981). Independently of effects on endothelial or platelet function, the atherosclerotic plaque may progress through various stages of complication. An enlarging plaque can impede blood flow through the artery and thus cause ischemia, especially if myocardial oxygen demand should increase (e.g., during exercise). Finally, the plaque may also hemorrhage within itself (or rupture), resulting in thrombus formation, an interruption of blood flow to the heart, and ischemia (Sokolow & McIlroy, 1987).

Myocardial ischemia can have a number of consequences. If severe, ischemia may result in myocardial infarction and perhaps death of the individual. When death occurs quickly, it is generally because the infarction has triggered a fatal arrhythmia (Segal, Kotler, & Iskandrian, 1985). Post-infarction events include heart failure (impaired ability of the heart to function as a pump because of muscle death), embolization of such organs as the brain or gut (by thrombi found within the left ventricular cavity), and heart rupture. Even if not severe, myocardial ischemia may disrupt the electrical stability of the heart, thereby heightening its vulnerability to arrhythmias (Lown, 1987), which may then be triggered independently of such anatomical events as thrombosis, hemorrhage, and myocardial infarction. Arrhythmias triggered by ischemia-induced electrical instability, often ventricular tachycardia or fibrillation, are believed to be a major cause of sudden cardiac death (SCD; Segal, Kotler, & Iskandrian, 1985).

Research Suggesting a Link between Social Support and the Etiology of Physical Disease

Below we present a select review of the studies linking various conceptions of social support to the etiology of CHD. We focus on conceptions of social support that are examined across several studies.

Mortality Studies

The best documented effects in this literature are the role of social integration (SI) on all-cause mortality. In general, after controlling for traditional risk factors such as blood pressure, cigarette smoking, and serum cholesterol levels, healthy persons with higher SI scores are at lower risk for all-cause mortality than their more isolated counterparts (Berkman & Syme, 1979; House, Robbins, & Metzner, 1982; G. Kaplan, Cohn, Cohen, & Guralnik, 1988; G. Kaplan, Salonen, et al., 1988; Orth-Gomér & Johnson, 1987; Schoenbach, Kaplan, Fredman, & Kleinbaum, 1986; Seeman, Kaplan, Knudsen, Cohen, & Guralnik, 1987; Welin et al., 1985). SI deterioration (loss of network contacts) has also been associated with higher all-cause mortality risk (G. Kaplan & Hahn, 1989). Associations of SI and mortality in this literature are generally weaker for women and nonwhites than for white men (Berkman, 1986). Although there are also data on the role of satisfaction with social support in total mortality, the limited number of studies and lack of conceptual consistency across studies makes it difficult to draw conclusions (see Berkman & Syme, 1979; Blazer, 1982; House et al., 1982).

Data on the role of SI in mortality attributable to CHD are most relevant to this discussion. The studies that provided these data report beneficial effects of SI similar to those found in all-cause analyses (House et al., 1982; G. Kaplan, 1985, for Alameda County data originally reported by Berkman & Syme, 1979; G. Kaplan, Cohn, et al., 1988; G. Kaplan, Salonen, et al., 1988; Orth-Gomér & Johnson, 1987; Orth-Gomér, Undén, & Edwards, 1988; Vogt, Mullooly, Ernst, Pope, & Hollis, 1992). There is also evidence that SI predicts CHD mortality for persons who are unhealthy at the onset of the study—specifically, male survivors of acute myocardial infarction (MI; Ruberman, Weinblatt, Goldberg, & Chaudhary, 1984). These men were followed for 1 to 3 years after their MI. After controlling for traditional risk factors, relatively isolated survivors with low levels of education were found to have more total deaths and more sudden cardiac deaths than their less isolated, more educated counterparts.

Mortality studies of initially healthy persons do not clarify the stage of the disease process at which support acts. Hence greater CHD mortality for those with fewer social contacts may be accounted for by SI influences on the development of early lesions, lesion progression, or functional expressions of CHD such as MI. These studies also fail to indicate when in the course of diagnosed disease death occurs. Some specificity is provided by the single study reporting SI prediction of mortality for persons with serious disease (Ruberman et al., 1984). Because this study predicts CHD mortality after an initial event, it suggests that support plays a role in processes involved in triggering MI, or possibly in processes leading to alterations in the rate of progression of coronary artery occlusion. These results do not, however, eliminate the possibility of SI influences on early disease onset or progression.

Morbidity Studies

Although there are strong suggestions that various conceptions of social support are associated with the onset of CHD, the results of the morbidity studies are less consistent and generally more difficult to interpret. There is evidence from two studies of Japanese-American men that SI is associated with decreased prevalence of MI, angina pectoris (AP), and total coronary heart disease (Joseph, 1980; Reed, McGee, Yano, & Feinlieb, 1983). A recent study of Swedish men similarly indicates an association between SI and decreased incidence of CHD (Orth-Gomér, Rosengren, & Wilhelmsen, 1993).

Evidence from three angiography studies, however, is less clear. In the first, British valvular heart disease patients who felt they could rely on family and friends were less likely to have histories of hypertension and myocardial infarction, as well as ECG evidence of myocardial infarction (Cooper, Faragher, Bray, & Ramsdale, 1985). Perceptions of support were not, however, related to signs of peripheral vascular disease, mitral valve disease, angina, or number of vessels with significant narrowing. In the second, patients in six San Francisco Bay Area hospitals who reported greater availability of instrumental support or feeling loved had less coronary occlusion than their unsupported counterparts (Seeman & Syme, 1987). Coronary occlusion was unrelated to SI, its structural components, or emotional support from family or friends. In the third study, a group at Duke University found that coronary occlusion was related to less emotional support among Type A individuals, but to more emotional support among Type Bs (Blumenthal et al., 1987). Although Seeman and Syme also tested the Type A behavior pattern by emotional support interaction, they did not find this effect.

Sample biases in angiography studies also suggest cautious interpretation. Because angiography study samples are limited to symptomatic and other high-risk patients, these investigations attempt to discriminate between high-risk persons who have CAD and those who do not, which differs substantially from distinguishing between the diseased and healthy in the general population (Cohen & Matthews, 1987).

One of the studies of CHD in Japanese-American men, the Honolulu Heart Study, examined SI as a predictor of the onset (incidence) of CHD, as well as the concurrent (prevalence) relations between SI and disease (Reed, McGee, & Yano, 1984; Reed et al., 1983). Total CHD rates were higher among more isolated men when a SI scale developed through factor analysis was used. This effect was accounted for primarily through the prediction of nonfatal MI. This scale was not associated with the incidence of angina or of fatal MI, however, and a conceptually developed SI scale failed to predict any of these outcomes.

Several morbidity studies that examine the possible role of social support as a buffer (or moderator) of the increased risk of CHD associated with high levels of stress are also relevant. Johnson and Hall (1988) found that degree of interaction with coworkers buffered work stress against CHD prevalence for both males and females. Medalie and Goldbourt (1976) found that men who reported that their wives loved and supported them were buffered from the effects of high anxiety on the incidence of angina pectoris. In contrast, the Honolulu Heart Study (Reed et al., 1984) found no stress-buffering effect of an SI-like index for men in predicting CHD incidence.

Psychosocial Models Linking Social Support to CHD

At the most elementary level, it can be posited that social networks and social supports are linked to CHD either through their influence on behavioral patterns that decrease risk for disease or through effects on biological responses that influence disease onset and progression. In the following section, we discuss possible psychological and behavioral pathways through which social networks and supports could influence behavioral and biological risk for CHD.

We alluded earlier to two generic models of the influence of social support on CHD. The *stress-buffering* model proposes that support operates by protecting people from the potentially pathogenic influence of stressful events. The *main effect* model suggests that support has a beneficial influence irrespective of whether persons are under stress. The epidemiological data we reviewed are consistent with research on other health outcomes indicating that social integration is the primary cause of main effects of social support, and perceived availability of support is the primary cause of stress-buffering effects (see Cohen & Wills, 1985; Kessler & McLeod, 1985).

Social Integration and the Main Effect Model

Social integration has been conceptualized by Thoits (1983) as having multiple identities or ties to members of the network with different roles. Summaries of a number of psychological pathways through which social integration may influence the susceptibility to disease follow.

Information-Based Models

Having a wide range of network ties presumably provides multiple sources of information and hence an increased probability of having access to an appropriate information source. Information could influence health-relevant behaviors or help one to avoid stressful or other high-risk situations. For example, network members could provide information regarding access to medical services or regarding the benefits of behaviors that positively influence health and well-being. It is noteworthy, however, that integration in a social network could also operate to the detriment of health: discouraging use of medical services, providing inadequate alternative care, or influencing people to adopt behaviors inimical to health (e.g., McKinlay, 1973; Sanders, 1982; Seeman, Seeman, & Sayles, 1985).

Identity- and Self-Esteem-Based Models

There are several theoretical perspectives suggesting that social integration increases feelings of self-esteem, of self-identity, and of control over one's environment that result in better health. Social integration is presumed to provide a source of generalized positive affect, a sense of predictability and stability in one's life situation, and a recognition of self-worth because of demonstrated ability to meet normative role expectations (Cassel, 1976; Hammer, 1981; Thoits, 1983; Wills, 1985). These positive psychological states are presumed to be facilitative because they lessen psychological despair (Thoits, 1985), result in greater motivation to care for oneself (Cohen & Syme, 1985), or result in a benign neuroendocrine response (Bovard, 1959; Cassel, 1976).

A popular model in this category assumes that it is isolation that causes disease, rather than social integration that enhances health. This approach assumes that isolation increases negative affect and sense of alienation, and decreases a sense of control. Alternatively, one can merely view isolation as a stressor.

Social Influence Models

A socially integrated person is subject to social controls and peer pressures that influence normative health behaviors. To the extent that these pressures promote healthful behaviors (e.g., exercise, better diet, not smoking, moderating alcohol intake), social integration would promote better health. To the extent that normative behaviors within a social network promote behaviors that are deleterious to health, social integration would result in poorer health and well-being.

Tangible Resource-Based Models

A network may operate to prevent disease by providing aid and tangible and economic services that result in better health and better health care for network members. For example, network members could provide food, clothing, and housing that operate to prevent disease and limit exposure to risk factors. Networks may also provide nonprofessional health care that prevents minor illness from developing into more serious disease.

Perceived Social Support and the Stress-Buffering Models

The stress-buffering model posits that support protects persons from the potentially pathogenic influence of stressful events. The following models focus on the *perceived* availability of social support because this conception has been found to result in stress-buffering effects. We (Cohen & McKay, 1984; Cohen & Wills, 1985) have also proposed that stress buffering occurs only when there is a match between the needs elicited by the stressful event and the functions of support that are perceived to be available. For example, having someone who would loan you money may be useful in the event of a temporary job loss but useless when facing the death of a friend. A matching of support with need is implied, although not specified, in many of the models discussed below. We have also argued that certain types of support may be useful in coping with all or many stressors. Specifically, having people to talk to about problems (appraisal support) and having people who make you feel better about yourself (self-esteem support) may be generally useful, because these are coping requirements elicited by most stressors.

All of the stress-buffering models we discuss assume that stress puts persons under risk for CHD. This risk is presumed to occur either because stress triggers neuroendocrine response or arterial flow disturbances, or because behavioral adaptations to stress often include detrimental health practices like smoking and poor diet. Perceived social support operates in these models by decreasing the probability that situations will be appraised as stressful, by directly dampening neuroendocrine responses to stress, or by preventing persons from adopting unhealthy behaviors.

Information-Based Models

Stress may elicit network provision of information about the nature of the potential stressful events or about ways of coping with those events (see discussion of social comparison under stress by Cohen & McKay, 1984; Wills, 1983). To the extent that this information reduces the evaluation of potential threat or harm in the context of existing coping resources, the event would be appraised as less threatening and/or harmful, and hence the risk of illness would be decreased (Lazarus & Folkman, 1984). It is also likely that in many cases the perception of available support operates *without any actual support being provided*, that is, believing that others will provide needed information if it becomes necessary can similarly result in potentially stressful events being appraised as benign (e.g., Wethington & Kessler, 1986). In both cases, a reduction in stress appraisal would be presumed to reduce negative affect, negative health behaviors, and concomitant physiological reactivity.

Identity- and Self-Esteem-Based Models

These models are minor twists on the information models described above. They suggest that others' willingness to help and/or the enhanced ability to cope that results from receiving help increase feelings of personal control and self-esteem. Such feelings may influence health through increased motivation to perform health behaviors or through suppression of neuroendocrine responses. Again, the mere perception that help is available may similarly trigger these processes.

Social Influence Models

Social controls and peer pressures could influence persons to cope with stressors in particular normative manners. Such influence processes would promote health to the extent that the normative coping behaviors were effective in reducing perceptions of stress, nonadjustive behavioral adaptations, and negative affective responses. Inappropriate norms, however, could lead to less effective coping and hence greater risk of stress-elicited CHD. To the extent that social coping norms were internalized, or that persons expect others to pressure them to cope in a particular manner, the mere perception of availability could influence the stress–disease process in the same manner as actually receiving support.

Tangible Resource-Based Models

Network contribution of aid or of tangible or economic services could reduce the probability of potentially stressful events being appraised as threatening or harmful and hence reduce the behavioral and affective concomitants of such an appraisal. Again, the mere perception of the availability of aid may operate without actual receipt of help. Tangible resources could also help resolve specific tangible problems after a stress appraisal is made.

Biological Models Linking Social Support to CHD

The models discussed above link social support to CHD either through influences on health practices or through neuroendocrine or hemodynamic response. The stress-buffering models generally address how perceived availability of support short-circuits the potential behavioral, hemodynamic, and neuroendocrine pathways that link stress to CHD pathogenesis, and the main effect models suggest direct influences of social integration on behavioral, neuroendocrine, and hemodynamic pathways. We alluded to evidence of increased risk for CHD among those with poor health practices (e.g., smoking), and these risks are discussed in detail elsewhere in this volume (see Chapters 10 and 11). In this section, we address the role that hemodynamic and neuroendocrine alterations accompanying or resulting from behavioral responses to provocative psychosocial stimuli may play in various stages of disease progression.

Central to our analysis is the argument that to understand the role of social support in CHD, it is necessary to consider the temporal courses of both the support concept and the disease stage under investigation. In short, some stages of the development of CHD extend over many years; to influence these stages, a psychosocial factor must endure over a similar period. Other stages of CHD develop very quickly, and as a consequence, a presumption of support endurance is not necessary for support to influence such a stage. In general, we argue that temporally stable concepts of support are plausible predictors of long-term stages of disease development (e.g., lesion formation and progression), and that both stable and unstable support concepts are plausibly involved in short-term stages of disease expression (e.g., myocardial infarction or arrhythmia).

We assume that social integration is a relatively stable support concept because it involves the existence of relationships (e.g., marriage and friendship) that tend to last for prolonged periods. We also assume that perceived availability of support is a relatively unstable concept because it is responsive to changes in the quality of relationships and in social and physical contexts. There is, however, little existing evidence on the stability of these or other social support concepts, and we accept the possibility that these stability assumptions may prove wholly or partly incorrect (see conflicting evidence on the stability of perceived support in Cohen, Sherrod, & Clark, 1986; Sarason, Sarason, & Shearin, 1986). For example, it is likely that the relative stability of support concepts vary across the life course (see Chapters 2 and 11). The correctness of our current assumptions about the stabilities of SI and perceived support, though, is not central to our premise that temporal stability is a key issue in proposing plausible models of the relations between social support and CHD.

Behavioral Stimuli and Coronary Risk

Current speculation regarding the biological mediation of behavioral influences on CHD is of a rather general nature, typically emphasizing the potential effects that acute cardiovascular and neuroendocrine reactions to stress might have on either atherogenesis or the precipitation of acute clinical events (Manuck et al., 1986). This focus on hemodynamic and neuroendocrine parameters derives in large measure from the frequent observation that Type A individuals respond to diverse psychomotor, cognitive, and interpersonal challenges with larger blood pressure and catecholamine reactions than do their more placid Type B counterparts (Houston, 1986; Wright, Contrada, & Glass, 1985). Additionally, there are several reports that patients with histories of angina pectoris or previous infarction show greater blood pressure responses to common laboratory stressors than patients without CHD or nonpatient controls (Corse, Manuck, Cantwell, Giordani, & Matthews, 1982; Dembroski, MacDougall, & Lushene, 1979; Shiffer, Hartley, Schulman, & Abelmann, 1976). In one prospective investigation of initially healthy men, large diastolic blood pressure reactions to cold immersion (the cold pressor test) predicted the 23-year incidence of CHD (Keys et al., 1971). Similarly, studies in cynomolgus monkeys show a significant positive association between the magnitude of animals' heart rate responses to an experimental stressor and extent of diet-induced coronary artery atherosclerosis (Manuck, Kaplan, & Clarkson, 1983, 1985). Together these findings suggest that recurrent episodes of acute cardiovascular and neuroendocrine reactivity evoked by behavioral stimuli may contribute to risk for coronary disease, and that such risk may be greatest among those individuals who exhibit the largest magnitude of psychophysiological response.

It is unclear when in the natural history of coronary disease these stress-induced cardiovascular or neuroendocrine adjustments would most likely contribute to pathogenesis. Nevertheless, it may be useful to consider what role such factors might play at successive stages in disease progression and to summarize the relevant evidence that currently exists.

Influences on Atherogenesis

Early Lesion Development

We hypothesized previously that arterial flow disturbances (turbulence, shear stress) that accompany marked cardiovascular reactions to behavioral stimuli promote injury to arterial endothelium (Manuck et al., 1986). Consistent with this hypothesis are experimental studies showing that exposure to behavioral stressors (e.g., physical restraint, tail shock) produces several effects compatible with the development of early athero-sclerotic lesions; these include structural changes in the arterial intima, subendothelial accumulation of mononuclear leukocytes, and the rapid turnover of endothelial cells in rat aorta (Gordon, Guyton, & Karnovsky, 1981; Hirsch Maksem, & Gagen, 1984). The further observation that beta-adrenergic receptor blockade mitigates both the endothelial changes and hemodynamic responses evoked by stress suggests that behaviorally induced endothelial injury may stem in part from acute cardiovascular adjustments associated with sympathetic nervous system activation (Hirsch et al., 1984). Unfortunately the arterial endothelium is not directly observable or amenable to imaging at the cellular level, and hence the forgoing results of animal experiments are not currently confirmed by in vivo studies of human beings.

Because stress is associated with biological responses that promote the development of early lesions, it is possible that support concepts that buffer stress might also enter into this phase of pathogenesis. This prem-ise, however, is subject to several qualifications. Atherogenesis usually proceeds slowly, with significant lesions developing during early adult-hood but generally not culminating in clinical events until the fifth decade of life. In order for a psychosocial factor to influence its development, we must assume either that short-term exposure to the psychosocial factor is sufficient to trigger a biological process with long-term implications or that the psychosocial factor endures and actively influences the pathogenic process over the course of the disease stage. The latter assumption is usually thought to be reasonable for the various behavioral dispositions previously implicated in coronary disease, such as Type A behavior and personality traits relating to hostility and the expression of anger. Hence it can be assumed that in order to buffer the influences of chronic stress or recurring acute stress, one would need to have perceptions of support that endure over many years. Although there is little known about the stability of support concepts, perceived support is generally thought to be only moderately stable and would not meet the above criterion. The implica-tions of this work for social integration are less ambiguous: Because SI is considered quite stable and has been found to be negatively associated with negative affect and psychological distress, we expect that persons with lower SI are at greater risk for early lesion development.

Lesion Progression

Beyond the initiating events in atherogenesis, the progressing lesions of atherosclerosis also appear to be influenced by behavioral factors. For instance, there are now several demonstrations that Type A behavior, as well as aspects of anger and its expression, are correlated significantly with coronary artery atherosclerosis in patients undergoing diagnostic cineangiography (Dembroski, MacDougall, Williams, Haney, & Blumenthal, 1985; Frank, Heller, Kornfeld, Sporn, & Weiss, 1978; MacDougall, Dembroski, Dimsdale, & Hackett, 1985; Williams et al., 1988; Williams et al., 1980). Yet there is no evidence that these associations are mediated by hemodynamic or neuroendocrine mechanisms. In fact, in the one published study germane to this question, no significant relationship was observed between extent of angiographically documented atherosclerosis and the magnitude of patients' cardiovascular reactions to mental stress (Krantz et al., 1981). Studies employing animal models, in contrast, offer some support for the hypothesis that sympathetic nervous system arousal (or its hemodynamic manifestations) underlie behavioral influences on plaque development. We noted earlier that the coronary atherosclerosis of cholesterol-fed cynomolgus monkeys was found, in two investigations, to be greatest among animals that exhibited the largest cardiac responsivity to a common laboratory stressor (Manuck et al., 1983, 1985). When males of the same species are housed in small social groups subject to periodic reorganization (i.e., an unstable social environment), the more dominant animals develop more extensive coronary atherosclerosis than their less competitive, subordinate counterparts (J. Kaplan, Manuck, Clarkson, Lusso, & Taub, 1982). Moreover, the worsened atherosclerosis of socially dominant monkeys can be prevented by long-term administration of a beta receptor blocking agent (propranolol hydrochloride), further indicating that sympathetic activation contributes to the behavioral exacerbation of atherogenesis in this animal model (J. Kaplan, Manuck, Adams, Weingand, & Clarkson, 1987).

Whether elevations in sympathetic-adrenal medullary activity potentiate atherogenesis through associated cardiovascular adjustments (e.g., turbulence accompanying an increased heart rate and blood pressure) or via effects attributable to increased levels of circulating catecholamines is a matter of some debate. Fluid dynamics are often invoked as contributing factors in atherogenesis because of the nonuniform (or focal) distribution of lesions within arteries. Atherosclerosis tends to predominate within large arteries and in close proximity to bifurcations or bends in the vessels—the same areas where flow disturbances (as might occur under stress) are most readily propagated (Manuck, Muldoon, Kaplan, Adams, & Polefrone, 1989). Elevated catecholamine concentrations have also been implicated in the development of arterial lesions. Such associations could reflect effects directly on the artery wall or influences of the catecholamines on such other pathogenic processes as alterations in lipid metabolism and platelet aggregation (Herd, 1983; Schneiderman, 1977). Other neuroendocrine substances may play a role in atherogenesis as well. For instance, the release of corticosteroids is increased under stress. In one investigation with coronary angiography, arterial occlusion was found to be greatest among men having high plasma cortisol concentrations (Troxler, Sprague, Albanese, Fuchs, & Thompson, 1977). The reproductive hormones are similarly reactive to disruptions of the social environment. In animal studies, impaired female reproductive function potentiates atherogenesis. In cynomolgus monkeys, for instance, loss of ovarian function following surgical ovariectomy produces a corresponding loss of female "protection" against diet-induced coronary artery atherosclerosis (Adams, Kaplan, Clarkson, & Koritnik, 1985). Interestingly, social subordination among reproductively intact female cynomolgus monkeys is also associated with impaired ovarian function (as evidenced by anovulation and low luteal-phase progesterone concentrations) and, in the presence of a cholesterol-containing diet, with an increased severity of coronary artery athero-sclerosis (Kaplan, Adams, Clarkson, & Koritnik, 1984).

The preceding paragraphs enumerate some of the ways that behav-ioral variables might foster atherosclerosis. If perceived social supports protect individuals against coronary disease by ameliorating the athero-genic influences of predisposing psychosocial factors (e.g., Type A behav-ior or stress), this protection might be achieved by modulation of the same hemodynamic or neuroendocrine mechanisms that underlie the behav-ioral exacerbation of atherosclerosis. To the extent that the direct influence of SI is mediated by decreases in chronic emotional distress, the neuro-endocrine mechanisms outlined earlier may similarly provide indirect evidence for the plausibility of the main effects of SI on lesion progression. Because of the stability of SI, we would expect that it could play a role in the long-term development of lesion progression. Again, it is somewhat unclear what duration of stress (or support) exposure is required to influence lesion progression, and hence it is difficult to assess the potential roles of stress and perceived support in these stages.

It should be cautioned that there is still little evidence that behav-iorally evoked physiological reactions of any kind, whether cardiovascular or neuroendocrine, contribute to atherogenesis. Additionally, what data do support such an association are derived largely from experimental studies employing animal models.

Functional Expressions of CHD

Several investigators have demonstrated that emotional arousal and exposure to behavioral stressors can provoke transient and often painless (or silent) myocardial ischemia in individuals with existing coronary artery disease (Sigler, 1967; Taggart, Gibbons, & Somnerville, 1969; Selwyn et al., 1986; Rozanski et al., 1988). It is noteworthy that the ischemia induced by emotional factors typically occurs at substantially lower heart rates than those associated with exercise-induced ischemia in these same individuals (Selwyn et al., 1986; Rozanski et al., 1988; Sung, Wilson, Robinson, Thadani, & Lovallo, 1988). This observation suggests that exercise and emotional factors may produce ischemia by somewhat different mechanisms (Sung et al., 1988). It is most likely that exercise causes ischemia in coronary patients by increasing myocardial oxygen demand to a level that cannot be supplied by the individual's atherosclerosis-laden (and hence occluded or stenotic) arteries (Sokolow & McIlroy, 1987). Emotional arousal or stress, in contrast, may induce coronary artery vasospasm or rapid thrombus formation within the artery, thereby reducing the supply of blood to the myocardium and creating an oxygen deficit (and thus ischemia) in the absence of an increased myocardial oxygen demand (Selwyn et al., 1986; Rozanski et al., 1988). An additional possibility is that behavioral factors raise myocardial oxygen demand beyond the individual's threshold for ischemia, but do so by increasing myocardial *contractility* in the absence of a corresponding rise in heart rate (Sung et al., 1988). Whatever the exact mechanism(s) of behaviorally induced ischemia, this functional manifestation of CHD (unlike patients' underlying atherosclerosis) is highly amenable to investigation because of the wide availability of portable EKG monitoring devices and software for detection of ischemic events, as well as the recent development of instrumentation permitting ambulatory radionuclide ventriculography (for measurement of left ventricular performance).

Myocardial infarction and electrical instability of the heart represent further escalations in CHD severity (Sokolow & McIlroy, 1987). It is generally accepted that thrombosis in a stenotic coronary artery (possibly associated with plaque rupture and hemorrhage) is a major cause of myocardial infarction (Segal et al., 1985; Sokolow & McIlroy, 1987). Although behavioral stimuli have been shown to trigger myocardial ischemia in individuals with existing coronary artery disease, it is not clear that psychosocial factors similarly potentiate the anatomical events immediately preceding myocardial infarction. Rather, it is likely that such events are related more closely to slow developmental processes operating within plaques (Bracket & Powell, 1988). Additionally, the occurrence and timing of heart rupture, myocardial thrombotic embolism, and heart failure (all of which are potential consequences of myocardial infarction and generally result in death) appear to reflect the condition of the anatomical substrate more than they do the prevailing hemodynamic and metabolic (i.e., neurogenic) milieu.

Unlike myocardial infarction, which is usually associated with acute anatomical changes, electrical instability of the heart represents an electrophysiological abnormality (Lown, 1987). This instability predisposes to arrhythmia and SCD (Segal et al., 1985). It is difficult to overestimate the importance of SCD (often defined as death occurring within 24 hours of the onset of initial symptoms), as it accounts for 50% to 65% of all mortality associated with CHD (Sokolow & McIlroy, 1987). The terminal event in most SCD cases is thought to be an arrhythmia that has degenerated to ventricular fibrillation, and a large proportion of SCD appears not to be associated with acute infarction or thrombosis (Friedman et al., 1973; Segal et al., 1985). The hallmark of SCD is its occurrence without warning or prodromal signs; thus there is no history of CHD in approximately half of SCD cases, and most patients having a previous history evidence no signs of worsening prior to their sudden demise (Lown, 1987; Segal et al., 1985).

Although the role of behavioral factors in myocardial infarction remain unclear, there is evidence linking emotional arousal and stress to both electrical instability of the heart and its sequelae, arrhythmia and SCD (Lown, 1987). It should be noted that the most common autopsy finding in cases of SCD is severe, multifocal coronary artery atherosclerosis (Friedman et al., 1973; Segal et al., 1985). This underlying atherosclerosis probably creates the ischemic environment within which electrical instability develops. But although such instability may have an atherosclerotic origin, once present the electrophysiologic abnormality is apparently independent of its anatomical substrate (Lown, 1987).

It has been hypothesized that in the electrically unstable heart, momentary changes in myocardial excitability caused by transient stimuli (e.g., neural traffic triggered by emotional arousal) provoke ventricular fibrillation (Kuller, Talbott, & Robinson, 1987; Lown, 1987; Verrier, 1987). Experimental studies in dogs have shown that various behavioral stimuli (aversive stimulation, avoidance conditioning, and induced rage) reduce thresholds for ventricular fibrillation (Verrier, 1987). Related experimental work indicates that similar behavioral challenges also alter myocardial perfusion, possibly acting as an arrhythmogenic stimulus (Billman & Randall, 1981; Vatner et al., 1971). In human beings, it is known that ventricular premature beats (VPBs) can initiate ventricular fibrillation and that frequent or complex VPBs are associated with an increased risk of SCD (Segal et al., 1985). Importantly, the incidence of VPBs in both cardiac patients and normal individuals can be increased with exposure to a variety of psychological challenges, including standard laboratory stressors, public speaking, and automobile driving (Lown, 1987; Taggart, Carruthers, & Sommerville, 1973; Taggart et al., 1969).

Among epidemiological evidence pertinent to the role of social supports in SCD are results of the Health Insurance Plan ancillary study of the Beta Blocker Heart Attack Trial (Ruberman et al., 1984). Here, a 3-year follow-up of individuals with previous myocardial infarction and complex VPBs revealed that both stress and isolation were independently related to elevated risk for SCD. A further and particularly striking example of sudden death potentially associated with behaviorally induced arrhythmia is that observed among young male Hmongs (members of a Laotian mountain tribe) who recently emigrated to large cities in the United States. Upward of 100 instances of unexplained nocturnal death have occurred among this population since the early 1980s. These deaths are thought to be the result of ventricular fibrillation (Baron et al., 1983; Otto, Janxe, & Cobb, 1984) and have been linked to stress arising from the clash between life in a primitive mountain culture and the demands of adapting to a modern urban environment.

The mechanism(s) mediating behavioral influences on VPBs, ventricular tachycardia, ventricular fibrillation, and SCD remain uncertain. These effects could be attributable to such factors as acute stimulation of the myocardium, alterations in coronary artery tone (and thus blood flow), platelet activation (with consequent effects on blood flow), or modification of the electrophysiological properties of the Purkinje fibers (Lown, 1987). Whatever the exact mechanism, it is likely that sympathetic nervous system stimulation plays a role. It has been shown experimentally, for example, that surgical sympathectomy, beta-adrenergic blockade, and relaxation can all reduce the profibrillatory effects of stress (Verrier, 1987) and that beta antagonists reduce the incidence of arrhythmia in CHD patients (Podrid & Lown, 1982). Moreover, the balance between vagal and sympathetic tone also affects the cardiac predisposition to arrhythmia. Hence the deleterious effects of stress on vulnerability to ventricular fibrillation can be reduced by enhancement of vagal tone (as with morphine); conversely, administration of the vagal antagonist atropine can increase vulnerability to ventricular fibrillation in stressed animals (Kuller et al., 1987; Lown, DeSilva, & Lenson, 1978).

We noted the distinction between sudden and nonsudden cardiac death. This distinction is more than heuristic and may relate importantly to behavioral influences in CHD (Friedman et al., 1973; Segal et al., 1985). Relevant here is a prospective study of post-MI pati ents in which SCD was found to be predicted predominantly by psychosocial factors (e.g., Type A behavior, low socioeconomic status, lack of a college education), whereas nonsudden cardiac death was produced by biological characteristics of the patients (e.g., severity of preexisting disease, location of infarction; Brackett & Powell, 1988). These findings are consistent with our understanding of the biological processes underlying sudden and nonsudden cardiac death, inasmuch as the former is probably associated with arrhythmia (and therefore subject to neurogenic influences) and the latter more strongly related to acute anatomical alterations (which may be less susceptible to autonomic and neuroendocrine reactions induced by behavioral stimuli).

We have already suggested that only those dimensions of social support that are stable over long periods of time are likely to affect the decades-long processes of atherogenesis. The acute clinical manifestations of coronary disease (e.g., myocardial ischemia and ventricular arrhythmia), though, might be triggered by autonomic nervous system responses associated with transient episodes of emotional arousal. Because perceived social support has been found to operate as a stress buffer, and because its modest temporal stability would probably be sufficient to protect persons from transient stress-triggered events, we expect that perceived support is an important predictor of arrhythmia and SCD. Although social integration's stability is sufficient to operate in this context, there is little empirical reason at this point to believe that SI operates to protect persons from stress-induced coronary events.

Discussion and Summary

We provided evidence that different conceptions of social networks and supports are related to CHD morbidity and mortality, and we discussed the psychological and behavioral underpinning of such relations. The development of CHD, however, subsumes numerous stages, each accompanied by a somewhat different set of pathophysiological processes. Conditions that provoke endothelial injury and early plaque development, for instance, may not be the same as those responsible for plaque rupture and hemorrhage, outcomes associated with tissue necrosis, or the initiation of ischemic events and precipitation of myocardial infarction or SCD. It is plausible (and there is initial experimental evidence) that acute hemodynamic or neuroendocrine responses to stress contribute to coronary artery atherosclerosis and at least some of the functional expressions of CHD, such as cardiac arrhythmia and SCD. In turn, these relationships may mediate psychosocial influences on the development of CHD. Because of the differing temporal parameters that define events at each stage of pathogenesis, though, the types of behavioral factors that may either predispose or protect against coronary disease might also differ at varying points in the natural history of CHD.

The primary characteristic in relating a support concept to a pathophysiological process is the *stability of the support concept over time*. Plausible models assume either that (a) the support conception under examination is relatively stable over the period of development of a disease stage, or (b) a short-term exposure to a particular level of social support is sufficient to influence the process underlying the disease stage. Social integration is a temporally stable conceptualization of social support; hence it is plausible that it could influence a process (e.g., development of atherosclerotic plaques) that has a very long and slow course of development. Thus there is a reasonable match here between stability of the support measure and the temporal characteristics of a pathogenic process (i.e., exposure to relatively lower levels of social integration lasts over the period of disease stage development).

Conceptualizations of social support with much shorter temporal stabilities, such as support satisfaction or perceived availability, would *not* be plausible predictors of atherosclerosis (see Cohen & Matthews, 1987). It is possible, however, to propose plausible models of CHD pathogenesis that focus on support measures with shorter stabilities. Consider, for example, modeling sudden cardiac death incidence. Assume that persons with undetected coronary artery disease (CAD) are more likely to suffer SCD if they experience stress (e.g., Glass, 1977). A severe stressor might trigger onset of the event. In this case, perceived available support may be important if it is stable over the course of stressor exposure and operates to buffer persons from stress *at the trigger point.*

In sum, the question of whether a particular stage of disease is susceptible to support influence depends on (a) whether the conceptualization of support under consideration affects processes that influence disease pathogenesis, (b) the temporal stability of the support concept, and (c) the nature and time course of the disease stage. The issue of temporal stability is important methodologically as well as conceptually. Consider a prospective study in which perceived support is measured at the onset in healthy individuals who are followed for 10 years. Because perceived support may not be a highly stable concept, the measure taken at onset may provide a poor estimate of the level of support at a later point when an acute stressor triggers an event. Hence, in order to study prospectively the role of an unstable support concept, it is necessary to repeatedly measure the concept over the course of the study at intervals that guarantee stability. A similar problem applies to retrospective studies. Consider, for example, the research on the relation between support and coronary artery occlusion in persons undergoing angiography. Because atherosclerosis emerges gradually over a lifetime, behavioral factors assessed at the time of angiographic evaluation could only have contributed to lesion development if the same factor also characterized that individual over a substantial portion of his or her life. Again, an unstable measure may provide a poor estimate of the level of support over the course of atherogenesis.

Our general message is to enter this work with clear hypotheses regarding both the psychosocial and biological processes by which specific conceptualizations of support influence specific stages of coronary heart disease. Choices of social support concepts and of disease stages should be driven by theory specifying the psychological and biological pathways by which such outcomes could occur. These choices must consider the temporal parameters of both social and biological variables in forming plausible hypotheses and designing valid tests of these hypotheses.

ACKNOWLEDGMENTS. Preparation of this chapter was supported in part by an NIMH Research Scientist Development Award (K02 MH00721) to the first author and grants from the National Heart Lung and Blood Institute to the second (HL35121 & HL14164) and third (HL26561) authors. Parts of this chapter are adapted from Cohen, S. (1988), Psychosocial models of the role of social support in the etiology of physical disease, *Health Psychology*, and are reprinted with the permission of the publisher, Lawrence Erlbaum Associates, Hillsdale, New Jersey.

References

Adams, M. R., Kaplan, J. R., Clarkson, T. B., & Koritnik, D. R. (1985). Ovariectomy, social status, and atherosclerosis in cynomolgus monkeys. *Arteriosclerosis, 53*, 192–200.

Baron, R. C., Thacker, C. O., Gorelkin, L., Vernon, A. A., Taylor, W. R., & Choi, K. (1983). Sudden death among Southeast Asian refugees: An unexplained nocturnal phenomenon. *Journal of the American Medical Association, 250*, 2947.

Berkman, L. F. (1985). The relationship of social networks and social support to morbidity and mortality. In S. Cohen & S. L. Syme (Eds.), *Social support and health*. New York: Academic Press.

Berkman, L. F. (1986). Social networks, support, and health: Taking the next step forward. *American Journal of Epidemiology, 123*, 559–562.

Berkman, L. F., & Syme, S. L. (1979). Social networks, host resistance, and mortality: A nine-year follow-up study of Alameda County residents. *American Journal of Epidemiology, 109*, 186–204.

Billman, G. E., & Randall, D. C. (1981). Mechanisms mediating the coronary vascular response to behavioral stress in the dog. *Circulation Research, 48*, 214.

Blazer, D. G. (1982). Social support and mortality in an elderly community population. *American Journal of Epidemiology, 115*, 684–694.

Blumenthal, J. A., Burg, M. M., Barefoot, J., Williams, R. B., Haney, T., & Zimet, G. (1987). Social support, Type A behavior, and coronary artery disease. *Psychosomatic Medicine, 49*, 331–339.

Bovard, E. (1959). The effects of social stimuli on the response to stress. *Psychology Reviews, 66*, 267–277.

Brackett, C. D., & Powell, L. H. (1988). Psychosocial and physiological predictors of sudden cardiac death after healing of acute myocardial infarction. *American Journal of Cardiology*, *61*, 979–983.

Broadhead, W. E., Kaplan, B. H., James, S. A., Wagner, E. H., Schoenbach, V. J., Grimson, R., Heyden, S., Tibblin, G., & Gehlbach, S. H. (1983). The epidemiologic evidence for a relationship between social support and health. *American Journal of Epidemiology*, *117*, 521–537.

Cassel, J. C. (1976). The contribution of the social environment to host resistance. *American Journal of Epidemiology*, *104*, 107–123.

Cohen, S. (1988). Psychosocial models of the role of social support in the etiology of physical disease. *Health Psychology*, *7*(3), 269–297.

Cohen, S., & Matthews, K. A. (1987). Editorial: Social support, Type A behavior and coronary artery disease. *Psychosomatic Medicine*, *49*, 325–330.

Cohen, S., & McKay, G. (1984). Social support, stress and the buffering hypothesis: A theoretical analysis. In A. Baum, S. E. Taylor, & J. E. Singer (Eds.), *Handbook of psychology and health*. Hillsdale, NJ: Erlbaum.

Cohen, S., Sherrod, D. R., & Clark, M. S. (1986). Social skills and the stress protective role of social support. *Journal of Personality and Social Psychology*, *50*, 963–973.

Cohen, S., & Syme, S. L. (1985). Issues in the study and application of social support. In S. Cohen & S. L. Syme (Eds.), *Social support and health*. New York: Academic Press.

Cohen, S., & Wills, T. A. (1985). Stress, social support, and the buffering hypothesis. *Psychological Bulletin*, *98*, 310–357.

Cooper, C. L., Faragher, E. B., Bray, C. L., & Ramsdale, D. R. (1985). The significance of psychosocial factors in predicting coronary disease in patients with valvular heart disease. *Social Science and Medicine*, *20*, 315–318.

Corse, C. D., Manuck, S. B., Cantwell, J. D., Giordani, B., & Matthews, K. A. (1982). Coronary-prone behavior pattern and cardiovascular response in persons with and without coronary heart disease. *Psychosomatic Medicine*, *44*, 449–459.

Davies, P. F. (1986). Vascular cell interactions with special reference to the pathogenesis of atherosclerosis. *Laboratory Investigation*, *55*, 5–24.

Dembroski, T. M., MacDougall, J. M., & Lushene, R. (1979). Interpersonal interaction and cardiovascular response in type A subjects and coronary patients. *Journal of Human Stress*, *5*, 28–36.

Dembroski, T. M., MacDougall, J. M., Williams, R. B., Haney, T., & Blumenthal, J. A. (1985). Components of Type A, hostility, and anger-in: Relationship to angiographic findings. *Psychosomatic Medicine*, *47*, 219–233.

Frank, K. A., Heller, S. S., Kornfeld, D. S., Sporn, A. A., & Weiss, M. B. (1978). Type A behavior pattern and coronary angiographic findings. *Journal of the American Medical Association*, *240*, 761–763.

Friedman, M., Manwaring, J. H., Rosenman, R. H., Donlon, G., Ortega, P., & Grube, S. M. (1973). Instantaneous and sudden deaths, clinical and pathological differentiation in coronary artery disease. *Journal of the American Medical Association*, *225*, 1319–1328.

Furchgott, R. F. (1983). Role of endothelium in responses of vascular smooth muscle. *Circulation Research*, *58*, 373–376.

Glass, D. C. (1977). *Behavior patterns, stress, and coronary disease*. Hillsdale, NJ: Erlbaum.

Gordon, D., Guyton, J. R., & Karnovsky, M. J. (1981). Intimal alterations in rat aorta induced by stressful stimuli. *Laboratory Investigation*, *45*, 14–27.

Hammer, M. (1981). "Core" and "extended" social networks in relation to health and illness. *Social Science and Medicine*, *17*, 405–411.

Haynes, S., & Feinleib, M. (1980). Women, work and coronary heart disease: Prospective findings from the Framingham Heart Study. *American Journal of Public Health, 70,* 133–141.

Herd, J. A. (1983). Physiological basis for behavioral influences in atherosclerosis. In T. M. Dembroski, T. H. Schmidt, & G. Blumchen (Eds.), *Biobehavioral bases of coronary heart disease* (pp. 248–256). Basel, Switzerland: Karger.

Hirsch, E. Z., Maksem, J. A., & Gagen, D. (1984). Effects of stress and propanolol on the aortic intima of rats [Abstract]. *Arteriosclerosis, 4,* 526.

House, J. S., & Kahn, R. L. (1985). Measures and concepts of social support. In S. Cohen & S. L. Syme (Eds.), *Social support and health.* New York: Academic Press.

House, J. S., Landis, K. R., & Umberson, D. (1988). Social relationships and health. *Science, 241,* 540–545.

House, J. S., Robbins, C., & Metzner, H. L. (1982). The association of social relationships and activities with mortality: Prospective evidence from the Tecumseh Community Health Study. *American Journal of Epidemiology, 116,* 123–140.

Houston, B. K. (1986). Psychological variables and cardiovascular and neuroendocrine reactivity. In K. A. Matthews, S. M. Weiss, T. Detre, T. M. Dembroski, B. Falkner, S. B. Manuck, R. B. Williams (Eds.), *Handbook of stress, reactivity, and cardiovascular disease* (pp. 207–230). New York: Wiley.

Johnson, J. V., & Hall, E. M. (1988). Job strain, work place social support, and cardiovascular disease: A cross-sectional study of a random sample of the Swedish working population. *American Journal of Public Health, 76,* 1336–1342.

Joseph, J. (1980). *Social affiliation, risk factor status, and coronary heart disease: A cross-sectional study of Japanese-American men.* Unpublished doctoral dissertation, University of California, Berkeley.

Kaplan, G. A. (1985). Psychosocial aspects of chronic illness: Direct and indirect associations with ischemic heart disease mortality. In R. M. Kaplan & M. H. Criqui (Eds.), *Behavioral epidemiology and disease prevention* (pp. 237–269). New York: Plenum.

Kaplan, G. A., Cohn, B. A., Cohen, R. D., & Guralnik, J. (1988). The decline in ischemic heart disease mortality: Prospective evidence from the Alameda County study. *American Journal of Epidemiology, 127,* 1131–1142.

Kaplan, G. A., & Hahn, M. N. (1989). Is there a role for prevention among the elderly? Epidemiologic evidence from the Alameda County study. In M. G. Ory & K. Bond (Eds.), *Aging and health care: Social science and policy perspectives* (pp. 27–55). London: Tavistock.

Kaplan, G. A., Salonen, I. T., Cohen, R. D., et al. (1988). Social connections and mortality from all causes and cardiovascular disease: Prospective evidence from eastern Finland. *American Journal of Epidemiology, 128,* 370–380.

Kaplan, J. R., Adams, M. R., Clarkson, T. B., & Koritnik, D. R. (1984). Psychosocial influences on female "protection" among cynomolgus macques. *Atherosclerosis, 53,* 283–295.

Kaplan, J. R., Manuck, S. B., Adams, M. R., Weingand, K. W., & Clarkson, T. B. (1987). Propanolol inhibits coronary atherosclerosis in behaviorally predisposed monkeys fed an atherogenic diet. *Circulation, 76,* 1364–1373.

Kaplan, J. R., Manuck, S. B., Clarkson, T. B., Lusso, F. M., & Taub, D. B. (1982). Social status, environment, and atherosclerosis in cynomolgus monkeys. *Arteriosclerosis, 2,* 359–368.

Keys, A., Aravnis, C., Blackburn, H., Van Bucham, F. S., Bezina, R., Djordjevic, B. S., Fidanza, F., Karkonen, M., Menotti, A., Puddu, V., & Taylor, H. L. (1972). Probability of middle-aged men developing coronary heart disease in five years. *Circulation, 45,* 815–828.

Keys, A., Taylro, H. L., Blackburn, J., Brozek, J., Anderson, J. T., & Somonson, E. (1971). Mortality and coronary heart disease among men studied for 23 years. *Archives of Internal Medicine, 128,* 201–214.

Kessler, R. C., & McLeod, J. D. (1985). Social support and mental health in community samples. In S. Cohen & S. L. Syme (Eds.), *Social support and health*. New York: Academic Press.

Krantz, D. S., Schaeffer, M. A., Davis, J. E., Dembroski, T. M., MacDougall, J. M., & Shaffer, R. T. (1981). Extent of coronary atherosclerosis, Type A behavior, and cardiovascular response to social interaction. *Psychophysiology, 18*, 654–664.

Kuller, L. H., Talbott, E. O., & Robinson, C. (1987). Environmental and psychosocial determinants of sudden death. *Circulation, 76*(Suppl. I), 48–56.

Lazarus, R. S., & Folkman, S. (1984). *Stress, appraisal and coping*. New York: Springer.

Lown, B. (1987). Sudden cardiac death: Biobehavioral perspective. *Circulation, 76*(Suppl. I), 186–196.

Lown, B., DeSilva, R. A., & Lenson, R. (1978). Roles of psychologic stress and autonomic nervous system changes in provocation of ventricular premature complexes. *The American Journal of Cardiology, 41*, 979–985.

MacDougall, J. M., Dembroski, T. M., Dimsdale, J. E., & Hackett, T. P. (1985). Components of Type A, hostility, and anger-in: Further relationships to angiographic findings. *Health Psychology, 4*, 137–152.

Manuck, S. B., Kaplan, J. R., & Clarkson, T. B. (1983). Social instability and coronary artery atherosclerosis in cynomolgus monkeys. *Neuroscience and Behavioral Reviews, 7*, 485–491.

Manuck, S. B., Kaplan, J. R., & Clarkson, T. B. (1985). Stress-induced heart rate reactivity and atherosclerosis in female macaques [Abstract]. *Psychosomatic Medicine, 47*, 90.

Manuck, S. B., Kaplan, J. R., & Matthews, K. A. (1986). Behavioral antecedents of coronary heart disease and atherosclerosis. *Arteriosclerosis, 6*, 2–14.

Manuck, S. B., Muldoon, M. F., Kaplan, J. R., Adams, M. R., & Polefrone, J. M. (1989). Coronary artery atherosclerosis and cardiac response to stress in cynomolgus monkeys. In A. W. Siegman & T. M. Dembroski (Eds.), *In search of coronary prone behavior* (pp. 207–227). Hillsdale, NJ: Erlbaum.

McGill, J. C. (1968). *The geographic pathology of atherosclerosis*. Baltimore: Williams & Wilkins.

McGill, J. C. (1972). Atherosclerosis: Problems in pathogenesis. *Atherosclerosis Reviews, 2*, 27–66.

McKinlay, J. B. (1973). Social networks, lay consultation and help-seeking behavior. *Social Forces, 51*, 275–292.

Medalie, J. H., & Goldbourt, U. (1976). Angina pectoris among 10,000 men: II. Psychosocial and other risk factors as evidenced by a multivariate analysis of a five year incidence study. *American Journal of Medicine, 60*, 910–921.

Neri-Serneri, G. G., Masotti, G., Gensini, G. F., Abbate, R., Poggessi, L., Galanti, G., & Favilla, S. (1981). Prostacyclin thromboxane and ischemic heart disease. *Atherosclerosis Reviews, 8*, 139–157.

Orth-Gomér, K., & Johnson, J. V. (1987). Social network interaction and mortality: A six year follow-up study of a random sample of the Swedish population. *Journal of Chronic Disease, 40*, 949–957.

Orth-Gomér, K., Rosengren, A., & Wilhelmsen, L. (1993). Lack of social support and incidence of coronary heart disease in middle-aged Swedish men. *Psychosomatic Medicine, 55*, 37–43.

Orth-Gomér, K., Undén, A. L., & Edwards, M. E. (1988). Social isolation and mortality in ischemic heart disease. *Acta Medica Scandanavica, 224*, 205–215.

Otto, C. M., Janxe, R. V., & Cobb, L. A. (1984). Ventricular fibrillation causes sudden death among Southeast Asian immigrants. *Annals of Internal Medicine, 100*, 45.

Podrid, P. J., & Lown, B. (1982). Pindolol for ventricular arrhythmias. *American Heart Journal*, 491–496.

Reed, D., McGee, D., & Yano, K. (1984). Psychosocial processes and general susceptibility to chronic disease. *American Journal of Epidemiology, 119,* 356–370.

Reed, D., McGee, D., Yano, K., & Feinleib, M. (1983). Social networks and coronary heart disease among Japanese men in Hawaii. *American Journal of Epidemiology, 117,* 384–396.

Ross, R. (1981). Atherosclerosis: A problem of the biology of arterial cell walls and their interactions with blood components. *Arteriosclerosis, 1,* 293–311.

Rozanski, A., Bairey, C. N., Krantz, D. S., Friedman, J., Resser, K. L., Morell, M., Hilton-Chalfen, S., Hestrin, L., Bietendorf, J., & Berman, D. S. (1988). Mental stress and the induction of silent myocardial ischemia in patients with coronary artery disease. *New England Journal of Medicine, 318,* 1005–1012.

Ruberman, W., Weinblatt, E., Goldberg, J., & Chaudhary, B. S. (1984). Psychosocial influences on mortality after myocardial infarction. *New England Journal of Medicine, 311,* 552–559.

Sanders, G. S. (1982). Social comparison and perceptions of health and illness. In G. S. Sanders & J. Suls (Eds.), *The social psychology of health and illness.* Hillsdale, NJ: Erlbaum.

Sarason, I. G., Sarason, B. R., & Shearin, E. N. (1986). Social support as an individual difference variable: Its stability, origins, and relational aspects. *Journal of Personality and Social Psychology, 50,* 845–855.

Schneiderman, N. (1977). Animal models relating behavioral stress and cardiovascular pathology. In T. M. Dembroski, S. M. Weiss, J. L. Shields, S. G. Haynes, & M. Feinleib (Eds.), *Coronary-prone behavior* (pp. 155–182). New York: Springer-Verlag.

Schoenbach, V. J., Kaplan, B. H., Fredman, L., & Kleinbaum, D. G. (1986). Social ties and mortality in Evans County, Georgia. *American Journal of Epidemiology, 123,* 577–591.

Schwartz, S. M., Campbell, G. R., & Campbell, J. H. (1986). Replication of smooth muscle cells in vascular disease. *Circulation Research, 58,* 427–444.

Seeman, M., Seeman, T. E., & Sayles, M. (1985). Social networks and health status: A longitudinal analysis. *Social Psychology Quarterly, 48,* 237–248.

Seeman, T. E., Kaplan, G. A., Knudsen, L., Cohen, R., & Guralnik, J. (1987). Social network ties and mortality among the elderly in the Alameda County study. *American Journal of Epidemiology, 126,* 714–723.

Seeman, T. E., & Syme, S. L. (1987). Social networks and coronary artery disease: A comparison of the structure and function of social relations as predictors of disease. *Psychosomatic Medicine, 49,* 340–353.

Segal, B. L., Kotler, M. N., & Iskandrian, A. S. (1985). Sudden cardiac death. In J. Morganroth & L. N. Horowitz (Eds.), *Sudden cardiac death* (pp. 1–21). Philadelphia: Grune & Stratton.

Selwyn, A. P., Sheal, M., Deanfield, J. E., Wilson, R., Horlock, P., & O'Brien, H. A. (1986). Character of transient ischemia in angina pectoris. *American Journal of Cardiology, 58,* 21B–25B.

Shiffer, F., Hartley, L. H., Schulman, C. L., & Abelmann, W. H. (1976). The quiz electrocardiogram: A new diagnostic and research technique for evaluating the relation between emotional stress and ischemic heart disease. *Journal of Human Stress, 6,* 39–46.

Shumaker, S. A., & Brownell, A. (1984). Toward a theory of social support: Closing conceptual gaps. *Journal of Social Issues, 40,* 11–36.

Sigler, L. (1967). EKG changes observed on the recall of past emotional disturbances. *British Journal of Medical Psychology, 40,* 55–64.

Sokolow, M., & McIlroy, M. B. (1987). *Clinical cardiology* (4th ed.), Los Altos, CA: Lange Medical Publications.

Sung, B. H., Wilson, M. F., Robinson, C., Thadani, U., & Lovallo, W. R. (1988). Mechanisms of myocardial ischemia induced by epinephrine: Comparison with exercise-induced ischemia. *Psychosomatic Medicine, 50,* 381–393.

Taggart, P., Carruthers, M., & Somnerville, W. (1973). Electrocardiogram, plasma cate-cholamines and lipids and their modification by oxprenolol when speaking before an audience. *Lancet, 2,* 311.

Taggart, P., Gibbons, D., & Somnerville, W. (1969). Some effects of motor-car driving on the normal and abnormal heart. *British Medical Journal, 4,* 130–134.

Thoits, P. A. (1983). Multiple identities and psychological well-being: A reformulation and test of the social isolation hypothesis. *American Sociological Review, 48,* 174–187.

Thoits, P. A. (1985). Social support processes and psychological well-being: Theoretical possibilities. In I. G. Sarason & B. R. Sarason (Eds.), *Social support: Theory, research and applications.* The Hague, Netherlands: Martinus Nijhoff.

Troxler, R. G., Sprague, E. A., Albanese, R. A., Fuchs, R., & Thompson, A. J. (1977). The association of elevated plasma cortisol and early atherosclerosis as demonstrated by coronary angiography. *Atherosclerosis, 26,* 151–162.

Turner, R. J. (1983). Direct, indirect and moderating effects of social support upon psychologi-cal distress and associated conditions. In H. B. Kaplan (Ed.), *Psychosocial stress: Trends in theory and research* (pp. 105–156). New York: Academic Press.

Vatner, S. F., Franklin, D., Higgins, C. B., Detrick, T., White, S., & VanCitters, R. L. (1971). Coronary dynamics in unrestrained conscious baboons. *American Journal of Physiology, 221,* 1369.

Verrier, R. L. (1987). Mechanisms of behaviorally induced arrhythmias. *Circulation, 76*(Suppl. I), 48–56.

Vogt, T. M., Mullooly, J. P., Ernst, D., Pope, C. R., & Hollis, J. F. (1992). Social networks as predictors of ischemic heart disease, cancer, stroke, and hypertension: Incidence, survival and mortality. *Journal of Clinical Epidemiology, 45,* 659–666.

Wallston, B. S., Alagna, S. W., DeVellis, B. M., & DeVellis, R. F. (1983). Social support and physical health. *Health Psychology, 4,* 367–391.

Welin, L., Tibbin, G., Svardsudd, K., Tibbin, B., Ander-Peciva, S., Larsson, B., & Wilhelm-sen, L. (1985). Prospective study of social influences on mortality. *Lancet, 1,* 915–918.

Wethington, E., & Kessler, R. C. (1986). Perceived support, received support, and adjustment to stressful events. *Journal of Health and Social Behavior, 27,* 78–89.

Wilcox, B. L., & Vernberg, E. (1985). Conceptual and theoretical dilemmas facing social support research. In I. G. Sarason & B. R. Sarason (Eds.), *Social support: Theory, research and application.* The Hague, Netherlands: Martinus Nijhoff.

Williams, R. B., Barefoot, J. C., Haney, T. L., Harrell, F. E., Blumenthal, J. A., Pryor, D. B., & Peterson, B. (1988). Type A behavior and angiographically documented coronary athero-sclerosis in a sample of 2,289 patients. *Psychosomatic Medicine, 50,* 139–152.

Williams, R. B., Haney, T. L., Lee, K. L., Kong, Y. H., Blumenthal, J. A., & Whalen, R. E. (1980). Type A behavior, hostility, and coronary atherosclerosis. *Psychosomatic Medicine, 42,* 539–546.

Wills, T. A. (1983). Social comparison in coping and help-seeking. In B. M. DePaulo, A. Nadler, & J. D. Fisher (Eds.), *New directions in help seeking, vol. 2.* New York: Academic Press.

Wills, T. A. (1985). Supportive functions of interpersonal relationships. In S. Cohen & S. L. Syme (Eds.), *Social support and health.* New York: Academic Press.

Wright, R. A., Contrada, R. J., & Glass, D. C. (1985). Psychophysiologic correlates of Type A behavior. In E. D. Katkin & S. B. Manuck (Eds.), *Advances in behavioral medicine* (pp. 39–88). Greenwich, CT: JAI Press.

CHAPTER 10

Social Influences on the Development of Cardiovascular Risk during Childhood and Adolescence

Carol K. Whalen and Wendy Kliewer

Cardiovascular Risk during Childhood and Adolescence: The Case for Concern

It has been estimated that more than half of today's youths are predestined to cardiovascular disease (CVD) morbidity and mortality (Frank, Webber, & Berenson, 1982). Because cardiovascular diseases are usually considered adult maladies, some readers may ask why risk factors should be a cause for concern during childhood and adolescence. Autopsy studies of youths provide a compelling answer to this question: Although signs of disease are rarely obvious before midlife, atherosclerosis begins in infancy, with fatty streaks evident by age 3 and fibrous plaques appearing during adolescence (Cresanta et al., 1986). Behavioral indicators further underscore the importance of childhood and adolescence to CVD risk, given evidence of a gradual and consistent decline in health behaviors from the early primary to high school years (Leventhal, Prohaska, & Hirschman, 1985). As Berenson (1986) asserts, "Maximum potential for prevention occurs in early life, especially for high-risk individuals" (p. 21). In the following paragraphs, we consider four fundamental indications for a focus on CV risk in youth: risk factor tracking or continuity, the clustering

CAROL K. WHALEN • Department of Psychology and Social Behavior, School of Social Ecology, University of California, Irvine, Irvine, California 92717.   WENDY KLIEWER • Department of Psychology, Virginia Commonwealth University, Richmond, Virginia 23284.

Social Support and Cardiovascular Disease, edited by Sally A. Shumaker and Susan M. Czajkowski. Plenum Press, New York, 1994.

of health risk indicators and behaviors, the preferability of prevention to intervention, and natural developmental windows or sensitive periods.

Risk Factors Track across the Life Span

Emerging evidence of progressive subclinical disease in youth has been accompanied by increased empirical attention to the CVD risk factors most relevant during childhood: elevated serum lipids and lipoproteins, hypertension, smoking, obesity, and sedentary habits combined with lack of exercise. These risk factors show tracking across the life span, beginning during childhood. Several independent studies have provided strong evidence of continuity in blood pressure, with children maintaining their relative rank with respect to their peers over extended time periods. The evidence for tracking of cholesterol levels seems even more robust than that for blood pressure. In the longitudinal Bogalusa studies, for example, correlations of low-density lipoprotein cholesterol (LDL-C) levels over a 5-year period ranged from 0.62 to 0.78 (Cresanta et al., 1986). Moreover, of the children whose LDL-C levels reached the 90th percentile during their first examination, 80% were at the 80th percentile or above 5 years later.

Continuity of cigarette smoking and weight status have also been documented repeatedly. Johnston (1986) reported that of those adolescents who smoked daily during their high school years, 73% were still daily smokers 8 years later. An obese preschooler has about a 25% chance of becoming an obese adult, and the figure increases to between 70% and 75% by ages 10 to 13 (Epstein, Wing, & Valoski, 1985; Garn & LaVelle, 1985). Clarke, Woolson, and Lauer (1986) found that a child between the ages of 5 and 8 who is in the upper quintile (20%) of his or her age group for ponderosity has a 55% chance of being in the upper quintile 10 years later. In contrast, a child in one of the bottom four quintiles has only one chance in eight of rising to the top quintile over the next 10 years.

Thus there seems to be no doubt either about the presence of CVD risk factors during childhood or about their relative stability over the years. Despite significant developmental changes and individual differences, people tend to maintain their ranks relative to their peers, and this continuity is particularly apparent at the health-endangering extreme of each factor.

Risk Factors and Risky Behaviors Tend to Cluster

It is no longer appropriate to treat individual risk factors in isolation, describing etiology and prescribing treatment as though each dimension had a distinct course and consequence. Risk factors show robust patterns of intraindividual linkages (e.g., Gortmaker, Dietz, Sobol, & Wehler, 1987; Task Force on Blood Pressure Control in Children, 1987). Heavier children are more likely than their lighter peers to have high blood pressure and elevated cholesterol levels, and cigarette-smoking youths also tend to have elevated cholesterol levels. Moreover, the interactions of individual risk factors such as hypertension and cholesterol significantly elevate overall CVD risk (Perkins, 1989). The good news is that clustering maintains with change, as illustrated by the fact that weight loss is typically accompanied by meaningful decreases in blood pressure (Clarke et al., 1986).

There are also interrelations among risk-related behavior patterns. Youths who smoke are more likely to abuse alcohol and drugs and to exhibit other health-compromising behaviors (Jessor, 1984; Johnston, 1986), and they are less likely to engage in positive diet, nutrition, and hygiene practices (Balding & Macgregor, 1987). In studies of such adolescent problem behaviors as drug and alcohol use, Jessor and his colleagues (Jessor, 1984) have documented a pattern of psychosocial risk or "proneness," raising the possibility of an analogous "health-risk behavior syndrome." Although only modest intercorrelations among behaviors conducive to health have emerged to date (Leventhal et al., 1985), effective risk-reduction programs may help shape intraindividual linkages, laying the foundation for a generalized disposition toward health-promoting actions.

Learning Is Often Easier than Unlearning:
Indications for Prevention

A strong case can be made for early efforts at behavioral risk reduction, rather than merely attempting to contain the damage when disease seems imminent, evident, or irreversible. Many unhealthy habits are well established by adulthood and notoriously intractable. For example, approximately one third of all smokers attempt to quit each year, and among those who succeed the relapse rate is disconcertingly high, often reaching 80% within the first year (Klesges, Meyers, Klesges, & LaVasque, 1989). Obesity is a similarly intractable problem, particularly in terms of long-term maintenance of weight loss. Although there are always individual success stories, it is exceedingly difficult for healthy adults to modify unhealthy patterns once these patterns become firmly entrenched. There seems to be little question not only that learning is easier than unlearning, but also that many behaviors are more malleable during childhood than adulthood.

Recent studies of children's health habits and status provide disquieting confirmation of the need for early prevention. The numbers of overweight children and adolescents have increased approximately 54% and

39%, respectively, in the past two decades (Gortmaker et al., 1987), and the vast majority of American youths exceed recommended blood cholesterol levels (Walter, Hofman, Vaughan, & Wynder, 1988). A substantial proportion of children consume far more food than their bodies need for energy or sustenance. In the ongoing Bogalusa studies of cardiovascular (CV) status in children, it was found that 80% to 90% of each age group consumes more than 100% of the recommended dietary allowance for protein and as much as twice the daily level for sodium estimated to be safe and adequate (Frank et al., 1982). The diets of most children and adolescents include excessive levels of fats, salts, and sugars, and deficient quantities of fruits, vegetables, and fiber (Cresanta et al., 1986). Moreover, the high heritability and limited modifiability of adiposity (Jeffery, 1988; Stunkard et al., 1986) underscore the wisdom of early dietary interventions.

Nor does the picture change when we turn to findings on smoking or physical fitness. Each year 2 million children begin to smoke (Tye, Warner, & Glantz, 1987), and recent surveys indicate that children are starting to smoke at progressively earlier ages despite massive public health and education campaigns (Bell & Levy, 1984). In a recent large-scale fitness study it was found that 50% of today's youths do not engage in appropriate physical activity and that 74% do not meet the standards set for their age and sex in such activities as bent-knee sit-ups, pull-ups, and sprints (Brandt & McGinnis, 1985; Iverson, Fielding, Crow, & Christenson, 1985). These investigators also reported that typical school physical education programs are not the type to maintain CV fitness, and that participation in even the limited programs that are available drops steeply from 98% in grade 5 to only 50% in grade 12. Thus many schoolchildren are receiving neither adequate fitness training nor the message that exercise is an important component of everyday life.

Natural Temporal Windows for Health Promotion

Childhood and adolescence are important not only because the early signs of CVD are already appearing, but also because these ages may be particularly sensitive developmental periods for both biological influences and the acquisition of lifelong habits. As part of their natural developmental work, children are acquiring and refining health beliefs and attitudes, dietary preferences and practices, and patterns of activity and stress management. While adolescents are establishing autonomy, consolidating their identities, and exploring life options, they are also shaping lifelong health-related behaviors. Moreover, adolescence is a period of heightened health risk, given increased access to health-compromising role models and materials and, for many, tendencies toward experimentation and unconventionality (Jessor, 1984). Thus these early phases may be the most natural times during the life cycle to foster the information, skills, and values needed to develop salutary life-style practices.

The concept of "sensitive period" is brought into sharp relief by the data on cigarette smoking. Smoking rates escalate dramatically beginning in junior high school, with the highest-risk period for the initiation of smoking behavior thought to be the 12–14 age range (Johnston, 1986). Sixty percent of smokers start by age 13, and 90% before age 20 (Tye et al., 1987). As Strasser (1980) astutely notes, "While the smoking habit is usually formed in childhood and adolescence, by the same token, the nonsmoking attitude is established early in life, too" (p. 82). Another example of the primacy of youth stems from recent indications that regular exercise during the teenage years may produce not only immediate but also lifelong health benefits (Frisch, Wyshak, Albright, Albright, & Schiff, 1986).

Summary

School-age children, already, are beginning to behave in health-promoting or health-endangering ways. The cumulative CV impact of these behaviors begins in the earliest years. Youngsters are also laying the foundations for lifelong health habits—practices and routines that will become increasingly resistant to change over the years. Moreover, risk factors tend to cluster, and clustering compounds risk. Thus there are pressing short-term as well as long-term needs for a focus on the CV health of nonsymptomatic youth.

Social Influences on Cardiovascular Risk in Youths

Although it has long been recognized that the human being is a social animal and that development occurs in interpersonal contexts, only recently have health specialists accepted the direct role that human contact plays in health and illness. As documented throughout this volume, there are multiple threads of evidence that social support can facilitate disease resistance and amelioration in adults. For children, it is more difficult than for adults to separate the role of social support (in the narrow sense of exchanges intended to provide help or companionship) from broader social influences that are the natural concomitants and outcomes of the child's immature and dependent status. Moreover, although there is extensive literature on the contributions of families and peers to health-related behaviors in youth, there is little direct information about potential health-enhancing or disease-ameliorating effects of social support per se during childhood or adolescence. For these reasons, the following discussion expands the focus beyond social support to include diverse interpersonal experiences that may contribute during the early years to long-term CV health.

Rather than attempt a comprehensive review of each risk factor, we present selected risk factor research as a means of illustrating basic psychosocial processes in the development and modification of life-style health behaviors. We will focus on two broad risk factor domains, diet and cigarette smoking, and then briefly consider the role of anger and the Type A behavior pattern (TABP). Diet and smoking were selected because each is molded and modulated by social factors, and together they illustrate the differential roles played by families and peers during progressive developmental phases. Weight control problems often surface during middle childhood, when families are the prepotent influences, whereas cigarette smoking emerges during late childhood and early adolescence, encouraged by peer cultures as well as by family and media influences. The importance of these two domains is underscored by estimates that cigarette smoking contributes to about 22% and dietary excess to another 22% of total mortality (Perry, Klepp, & Schultz, 1988). Anger and childhood TABP are included not because of demonstrated links to CVD, but rather to illustrate current controversies and highlight research needs. Space constraints prevent discussion of links between childhood TABP and cardiovascular reactivity, but this promising research area is reviewed by Matthews and Woodall (1988). For comprehensive coverage of the broader array of CV risk factors during the early years, interested readers are referred to Coates, Perry, Killen, and Slinkard (1981) and Cresanta et al. (1986).

Diet, Nutrition, and Obesity

Social Influences on the Development of Dietary Practices

Children acquire eating preferences, styles, and habits in interpersonal contexts, first within the family and later in peer cultures and society at large. For better or worse, family members select and prepare foods, model eating patterns and styles, structure eating cues and environments, and embed food and eating in psychologically meaningful space for children. Families differ in the types, amounts, and varieties of food provided; the extent to which food is used as a reinforcer and associated with giving or withdrawing parental love and attention; and the vigor with which eating and nutrition are promoted. Each of these factors has been shown to influence dietary patterns and preferences. Behavioral studies demonstrate that parents who repeatedly prompt and encourage their infants to eat tend to have heavier infants than do parents who make fewer food-related bids (Klesges et al., 1983), and there is also some evidence that overweight children receive less parental encouragement to be active than do normal-weight age-mates (Klesges et al., 1984).

Another important social environmental influence is television. It has been estimated that while watching an average of 28 hours of television each week, children see more than 11,000 low-nutrition ("junk") food ads a year. Many youngsters tend to believe such ads and to actively seek highly advertised foods (Jeffrey, McLellarn, & Fox, 1982). Galst and White (1976), for example, reported a relationship between the amount of commercial television a child watched at home and the number of purchase-influencing attempts he or she made at the supermarket. Given that most advertisements are for low-nutrition foods, television has been dubbed the "unhealthy persuader." Attempts to counteract such media messages have had disappointing results to date; children exposed to pronutrition television programs do indeed learn the information conveyed, but their food preferences and choices remain unchanged (Peterson, Jeffrey, Bridgwater, & Dawson, 1984).

Thus it comes as no surprise that television viewing is a strong predictor of future obesity in children—second only to prior obesity in one study, with the prevalence of obesity increasing between 1% and 3% for each additional hour of television watched per day (Dietz & Gortmaker, 1985). There are several likely reasons for this relationship, including the facts that (a) television viewing is a sedentary activity accompanied by large drops in basal metabolic rate; (b) children tend to eat junk food while watching television; and (c) foods consumed are likely to be those advertised on television.

We should not end a section of this type without a methodological caveat. Correlations are correlations. Obviously, many of the ones we have presented here are compelling, but causality remains unspecified. At times the causal arrows might be pointed in directions opposite to those assumed, and in most cases there are third variables that could account for the associations. For example, the link between television and supermarket behaviors may be attributable to a "pushover parent" effect: Children with overly permissive parents may be allowed both to watch more television and to make more purchase-influence bids than their peers. Similarly, many of the other correlations cited here and throughout this chapter are open to alternative interpretations and should be subject to the same cautions.

Social Influences on the Modification of Dietary Practices

As illustrated above, a consistent theme is emerging from attempts to modify diverse health-related behaviors: Knowledge can be increased and attitudes (at least those that are expressed) changed with relative ease, but it is exceedingly difficult to effect enduring modifications of habitual behaviors. It is also the case that habit changes are difficult to document objectively and reliably. One comprehensive school-based program designed to enhance heart-healthy eating and exercise included behavioral measures rather than relying exclusively on equivocal self-report or parent-report inventories (Coates, Jeffery, & Slinkard, 1981). To rule out the possibility of illusory rather than actual changes in consumption, these investigators surreptitiously checked the contents of lunch bags brought from home and playground trash cans after lunch periods. Happily, these counts indicated both program-related increases in the number of heart-healthy foods brought to school and parallel decreases in the number of heart-healthy foods discarded, and these positive changes in food consumption survived a 4-month follow-up period that spanned summer vacation. (Unfortunately, observed changes in exercise patterns did not parallel those for diet.)

Coates et al. (1981) concluded that family involvement seemed essential for the success of this program, and that families reported consuming increased amounts of heart-healthy foods at home. No measures of actual family involvement were available, however, and reports of home eating practices were not verified, so it is difficult to separate actual behavior changes from reported changes that may result merely from increased parental knowledge of sound nutritional practices. Answers to questions about the optimal role of family members in such school-based programs, as well as the likelihood of positive ripple effects in nonparticipant family members, must await further study. Indeed, some encouraging findings are emerging from more recent cardiovascular risk reduction programs, suggesting modest family aggregation of behavioral changes (Patterson et al., 1989).

Several school-based demonstration projects designed to improve normal children's heart-healthy behaviors have been implemented, including "Go For Health" (Simons-Morton, Parcel, & O'Hara, 1988), "Heart Smart" (e.g., Downey et al., 1987), and "Slice of Life" (Perry et al., 1988). These multifaceted programs focus on improving school lunches, enhancing physical education activities, and teaching normal-weight children to manage diet, exercise, smoking, and stress. Whether such comprehensive efforts will succeed not only in increasing knowledge and improving behavior in the short term but also in reducing long-term risk behaviors is not yet known. To date, large-scale programs for modifying cardiovascular risk have had only modest success (Walter et al., 1988).

Substantially more information is available about the outcomes of treatment programs for overweight youths than about attempts to change dietary practices in normal-weight children. These multifaceted clinical packages typically involve nutrition and exercise education; goal setting regarding decreased caloric intake and increased exercise; training in self-monitoring, self-regulation, and self-reinforcement; stimulus control and cue elimination (e.g., removing stimuli that prompt eating); and habit changes (e.g., slowing down the rate of eating). Many programs also use external reinforcement (e.g., money or lottery tickets), and some include training in social problem solving.

Weight control is one of the few areas in which social support, most frequently operationalized as parental involvement, has been incorporated and tested systematically as a component of the treatment package. The data on short-term effects are contradictory, with some investigators reporting clear superiority when parents are involved with their children, and others finding no differences as long as a solid behavioral program is implemented. When we turn to long-term maintenance, however, the value of parental involvement has been documented in a compelling fashion. Epstein, Wing, Koeske, and Valoski (1987) evaluated 77 children and their parents 5 years after participation in an 8-month behavioral program to combat obesity. One group of children was treated with their parents (Group P-C), a second group was treated alone (Group C-A), and a third group received "nonspecific target treatment" (Group N-T) intended to control for education and attention. At the end of the program and again at a 21-month follow-up assessment, there were no between-group differences in child weight status. After 5 years, however, only Group P-C had maintained treatment losses, whereas children in the other two groups had returned to baseline relative weights. The percentage overweight figure was -12.7% for Group P-C, in contrast to $+4.3\%$ and $+8.2\%$ for Groups C-A and N-T, respectively. According to their self-reports, children in Group P-C differed from the other children in three behaviors during the follow-up period: They continued selecting lower-calorie foods, graphing their weight, and keeping high-calorie foods out of their vicinity.

The reasons for these intriguing findings are unclear. Parental modeling is not a sufficient explanation, given that parents from all three groups had returned to baseline weight levels themselves and there were no group differences in parental weight loss at the end of 5 years. The parents in Group P-C may have been more knowledgeable about and more supportive of the child's own weight-control attempts, however, even if they did not succeed in maintaining their own weight losses. It would be worthwhile to study actual parent-child interactions revolving around food in order to detect behavioral differences that may have important treatment and maintenance implications.

Obesity is often a shared family problem, a fact that raises questions about possible spillover effects from treated to nontreated family members. Addressing this question as part of a 5-year follow-up assessment, Epstein, Nudelman, and Wing (1987) found that the effects on nontreated obese siblings were in fact comparable to those for treated siblings. There were no significant differences in percent of weight loss, and the same relative superiority of the parent-child condition emerged with the siblings as with the children targeted for treatment. Interestingly, nontreated obese parents (fathers) did not enjoy such positive ripple effects. Because they are based on small samples and unconfirmed assessments, these findings invite replication. If substantiated, they raise multiple empirical questions concerning treatment effects on family dynamics and household eating patterns. The cost-effectiveness of intensive treatments will also need reconsideration, given the positive effects on nontreated siblings.

The importance of developmental differences is highlighted by findings from a weight loss program for young adolescents (ages 12 to 16). Brownell, Kelman, and Stunkard (1983) focused on the nature, rather than merely the fact, of parent involvement, comparing the relative efficacy of the same behavioral treatment program under three parent-child conditions: child alone (C-A), child and mother meeting in separate groups (MC-S), and child and mother meeting together (MC-T). The MC-S condition resulted in more weight loss during treatment (-8.4 kg) than either the MC-T (-5.3 kg) or the C-A (-3.3 kg) conditions. The differences were even more striking at 1-year follow-up, with the MC-S group maintaining weight loss (-7.7 kg) and the other two groups gaining to approximately 3 kg above baseline.

These findings indicate that it is not just the fact of parental involvement that is important, but also its timing and quality. Conventional wisdom casts early adolescence as a time for developing autonomy, and thus as a time when parental involvement may be experienced as overly intrusive or restrictive. Parallel participation in a weight-reduction program may be ideal, providing an adequate amount of support, facilitation, modeling, and perceived similarity while leaving the adolescent's needs for autonomy and self-regulation relatively unconstrained. It should also be noted that social support was an integral component of this treatment program, and group meetings were included in all conditions. For adolescents, social support generated by peers with similar problems may be more relevant and efficacious than that generated by groups of parent-child dyads.

Age, of course, is only one factor to consider in this complex social support matrix. Another is individual differences in parental style and competence. Studies demonstrate greater or more durable success when parents are trained not only in weight control but also in child management and social problem-solving skills (Graves, Meyers, & Clark, 1988; Israel, Stolmaker, & Andrian, 1985). Parents with effective problem-solving skills may have the competence and flexibility needed to generalize specific strategies across problem settings and domains, and to adjust their involvement in an optimal fashion from one treatment phase or developmental level to the next.

Social support has also been incorporated into a school-based program that emphasized social networks and provided specific instruction in emotional support for overweight children (Brownell & Kaye, 1982). A wide net of social support was developed, one that included parents, teachers, and peers as well as school personnel. Physical education instructors shifted the emphasis from competitive to noncompetitive athletic activities so that the overweight children would not be embarrassed or excluded. Peer support was sought by encouraging participants to help each other with food choices and physical activities. Teachers attempted to channel the reactions of normal-weight, nonparticipating peers by discouraging ridicule and encouraging positive feedback for behavior and weight changes. Participation in this program was presented by school personnel as an honor rather than a stigmatic sign of deficit or defeat. The success of this message was indicated by the requests of some nonobese children to join the program!

Ninety-five percent of the program children lost weight, with a mean weight loss of 4.4 kg and a decrease in percentage overweight of 15.4%. For the control children, there was a mean weight *gain* of 1.2 kg and an increase of 2.8% in percentage overweight, with 71% increasing their weight and percentage overweight (and only 21% losing weight) during this 10-week period. A partial replication yielded positive but less robust results, and a disconcerting lack of maintenance over an 18-week follow-up period, again indicating the limits of our knowledge about key treatment ingredients (Foster, Wadden, & Brownell, 1985).

The studies described above yield hints and hypotheses rather than intervention directives. Many questions remain about the optimal balance between child and parental control and responsibility, and about how families and schools may best be involved in the treatment of childhood obesity. Complex questions surface about the role, quality, and timing of child self-control strategies in weight control programs, as demonstrated by a recent failure to find any differences in weight loss over a 5-year period between a parent-managed and a child-managed treatment program (Epstein, Wing, Valoski, & Gooding, 1987). Although suggestive, available findings are still sparse, contradictory, and difficult to integrate given broad variations in samples, settings, and strategies.

Summary and Future Directions

The most successful behavioral weight control programs for overweight children involve families in the treatment program. These programs have demonstrated impressive short-term successes and, under some conditions, even long-term maintenance. The comforting success rates tend to obscure the fact, however, that substantial proportions of overweight children (perhaps one third to one half) make no progress, even in the most effective programs (Israel et al., 1985). The long-term maintenance statistics are even more disconcerting. Epstein, Wing, Valoski, and Gooding (1987) reported that only 31% of children with nonobese parents, and only 15% of those with one or two obese parents, were considered nonobese 5 years following treatment. Research is needed on individual differences, family factors, and environmental dimensions that facilitate or impede specific approaches. The nature of home and school involvement in a child's treatment program needs to be matched not only to the child's developmental level but also to the individual temperaments, proclivities, and competencies of all participants, as well as to the characteristics and resources of the environment. Also needed is more detailed information about the life course of obesity and about the most potent influences during each stage (from initial weight gain through treatment-related weight loss to long-term maintenance or relapse).

Finally, the most intensive research to date has focused primarily on a small number of children, those at greatest risk in terms of the single factor of obesity. It is well-known that unhealthy dietary practices can have insalubrious effects on cardiovascular status even in people who maintain optimal weights, as illustrated by the link between sodium intake and blood pressure. Thus far the effects of interventions aimed at improving the dietary practices of normal-weight children and adolescents have been far less compelling in terms of actual behavior changes. The successes of the clinical treatment programs may provide both the challenge and the means for enhancing lifelong dietary practices in healthy children.

Cigarette Smoking

Social Influences on the Initiation of Smoking Behavior

The psychosocial correlates of smoking have been studied extensively. Although the results vary according to gender, age, ethnicity, and stage of smoking, certain trends are apparent. The strongest predictors of adolescent smoking seem to be family and peer smoking, with the risk growing as the number of smoking models in a child's environment increases. The importance of the social environment is highlighted by indications that when both parents smoke, 35% of the offspring are experimenting with cigarettes by the sixth grade (Flay, d'Avernas, Best, Kersell, & Ryan, 1983). If both a parent and a sibling smoke, a child is four times more likely to begin smoking than if no one in the family smokes (Hamburg, Elliott, & Parron, 1982).

We also know that peers exert strong influences; implicitly or explicitly they suggest, model, and enable smoking behavior, and sometimes they directly challenge or coerce youth who refuse. In a 2-year study predicting experimentation with cigarettes, Mittelmark et al. (1987) found that the most pervasive predictor was whether a best friend or several friends smoked. It comes as no surprise that the relative roles of family and peer models seem to vary not only with age of child but also with stage of smoking. Family members play a greater role for younger children and during the early "preparation" stages of smoking, not only through modeling but also by providing access and opportunities. Peer groups and personal experiences with cigarettes exert increasing influences on older adolescents and on youths of any age who have progressed through the experimentation stage (Flay et al., 1983).

The media also exert powerful influences. Twenty years after the ban on television advertising, cigarettes remain the most heavily promoted and advertised product in America. Although the tobacco industry insists that smoking advertisements are aimed at encouraging current smokers to switch brands rather than at recruiting new smokers, economic exigencies, as well as the location and content of many magazine ads, indicate quite clearly that youthful nonsmokers have been targeted (Tye et al., 1987). There has been a dramatic increase in the number of cigarette advertisements appearing in youth-oriented magazines since the late 1960s, and these ads tend to link smoking to conviviality, adventure, risk taking, and prestige, attributes and behaviors valued by many adolescents. The disconcerting increases in relative smoking rates among women—especially young women (Tye et al., 1987)—raise special concerns about a parallel trend toward increased cigarette advertising in women's magazines, where smoking is associated with being slim, fashionable, emancipated, and erotic (Altman, Slater, Albright, & Maccoby, 1987).

Social Influences on Prevention and Smoking Cessation Interventions

As in other areas of health promotion, traditional smoking prevention programs, oriented toward providing information, prove far more effective at increasing knowledge and changing attitudes than in modifying behaviors (Rundall & Bruvold, 1988). A far better track record has been achieved by innovative prevention programs aimed at "social inoculation," not only through antismoking arguments but also by providing youths with the means for justifying and protecting nonsmoking behavior in peer cultures. Typically these school-based programs target seventh-grade students, who are considered to be entering the high-risk period for smoking onset. Because adolescents are thought to be more concerned with immediate than with long-range impact and with social and athletic than with health outcomes, emphasis is placed on the short-term interpersonal and physiological effects of smoking rather than on ultimate medical consequences. Thus discussions tend to focus more on bad breath, discolored teeth, clothing odors, and reduced athletic capacity than on cancer and CVD. Because adolescents tend to overestimate smoking prevalence among peers (Sussman et al., 1988), attempts are made to provide more accurate normative expectations. Nonsmoking, rather than smoking, is promoted as the contemporary adolescent norm, thereby harnessing adolescents' desires to conform to the values and actions of their peer groups.

With teenage participants generating their own material, skits are enacted and role-play exercises presented to teach a behavioral repertoire for resisting cigarette smoking without diminishing social status or alienating peers. Advertising tactics as well as peer pressures are examined, and a public commitment not to smoke may also be included. Some programs incorporate broader domains of personal competence, self-management strategies, and decision-making skills.

What may be a particularly important ingredient in smoking prevention programs is the use of high-status peer models. It is uncertain why peer leaders often prove more effective than adults. Perhaps peers personalize the program and make it more interesting and engaging; they may communicate better and elicit higher levels of involvement, using contemporary vernacular and inserting relevant content into the role-play exercises. High-status peer leaders may also signal the appropriateness and even the desirability of nonsmoking, whereas the absence of adult authority figures may obviate the putative adolescent need to resist or rebel. It is also possible that the continued presence of these peers in the school environment, after the program concludes, provides nonsmoking cues and reminders.

Personality and peer group characteristics may also influence the effectiveness of intervention efforts. In a trenchant analysis of peer group identification, Mosbach and Levanthal (1988) identified two types of students who seemed to be at highest risk for smoking. The "dirts" engaged in problem behaviors, were poor students, and seemed to seek risk and excitement. In contrast, the "hotshots" or "populars" were successful but dissatisfied leaders. These divergent profiles suggest the wisdom of designing alternative smoking intervention programs tailored to differing psychological profiles and environmental contexts. For example, appeals to the macho self-image and social precocity of "dirts" may have optimal impact, whereas enhancing strategies for dealing with anxiety and social pressures may be more effective with "hotshots." Smoking prevention research also underscores the importance of considering the stage of smoking as well as age and personality factors. It is not surprising that smoking behavior has been more readily restrained among nonsmokers and experimenters than in regularly smoking youths (Flay et al., 1985; Murray, Davis-Hearn, Goldman, Pirie, & Luepker, 1988).

Summary and Future Directions

Recent social learning programs to prevent smoking onset have been remarkably successful, demonstrating decreases of 40% to 70% in smoking onset rates. Although the long-term efficacy is unknown, maintenance has been demonstrated between up to 3 and 5 years (Murray et al., 1988; Perry et al., 1988). Even if smoking does begin at a later date for some, a delay of several years may still be beneficial, given indications that the strongest smoking-related predictor of CVD is total life consumption of cigarettes (Perkins, 1989).

Despite the impressive track record, there are remaining questions and research needs. One concern is that current programs may be focused too narrowly on providing inoculations against peer pressure tactics, ignoring other important predisposing and enabling factors, particularly individual characteristics and environmental models and resources (Botvin, 1982). It also seems that insufficient attention is being paid to the two developmental progressions discussed above: the transition from childhood to adulthood, and the progressive stages of becoming a smoker. Different approaches may be needed for these different ages and stages, and some of the apparent contradictions in the literature may be attributable to unreported age or stage variations across studies. Questions are also surfacing about some of the underlying assumptions of social inoculation approaches, including the superiority of peer models, the emphases on immediate rather than future consequences, and the efficacy of public commitments not to smoke (e.g., Flay, 1985). Finally, there are indications that the effects may fade over time (Murray et al., 1988), suggesting the potential benefits of "booster shots" during the high school years.

The heartening successes have also raised questions about implementation on a broader scale, beyond the carefully conducted and specially funded demonstration studies. Given the exigencies of daily life and public policy, the short-term costs of widescale prevention programs must be considered somewhat independently of the long-term savings that will ineluctably accrue as an increasingly nonsmoking society moves toward greater health and productivity. Flay et al. (1985) reported a failure to find positive treatment effects in sixth-grade students who had never smoked or had merely tried smoking once, a failure these investigators attributed to the low rate of exit from these nonsmoking categories in the control group. Moreover, the positive effect on the smoking experimenters was limited primarily to the subgroup considered at high risk because they had at least two smokers in their immediate environment.

These findings lead inescapably to a consideration of the pros and cons of targeting high-risk groups rather than entire age cohorts for preventive interventions. Children who begin experimenting in elementary school and those with smoking models in their daily environments are two such (overlapping) subgroups, and a third may be youths who leave school early, given recent findings that more than 75% of high school dropouts are daily smokers (Pirie, Murray, & Luepker, 1988). Even for younger adolescents still in school, higher smoking rates are associated with academic disinterest or dislike, and lower rates with higher grade point averages (Johnston, 1986). Although it is impossible to disentangle cause from effect in correlational findings of this nature, these associations suggest the value of exploring programs designed to enhance academic experiences, programs that should have effects on health and adjustment that extend far beyond the realm of smoking.

Childhood TABP, Anger, and Hostility

The initial spate of studies of TABP conducted in the 1960s and 1970s provided seemingly unequivocal evidence of an association with CHD. The 1980s, however, brought a steady accumulation of negative evidence (Haynes & Matthews, 1988; Krantz, Contrada, Hill, & Friedler, 1988). Several important large-scale investigations failed to find any relations between TABP and CHD (e.g., Shekelle et al., 1985), and one study suggested that TABP may actually be advantageous in men who have survived an initial heart attack (Ragland & Brand, 1988). What has been described as the topsy-turvy career of TABP (Dimsdale, 1988), including marked divergence between early and more recent findings, has prompted some investigators to challenge the consensus position that TABP is a risk factor auguring unfavorable clinical outcomes for CHD patients (Krantz et al., 1988).

There are additional problems when applying the notion of TABP to children, including limited stability of childhood TABP and the paucity of evidence linking childhood and adult TABP. Repeat administrations of the MYTH, the most widely used measure of TABP in children, reveal significant 2-year and 5-year correlations ranging between .38 and .45 (Visintainer & Matthews, 1987), suggesting moderate continuity at a level that compares favorably with that of other CV risk factors in children (Matthews & Woodall, 1988). Correlations in this range, however, also indicate substantial change even within the childhood period. Other longitudinal studies suggest that there may be some continuity in TABP between adolescence and adulthood, but thus far these associations have not extended to childhood (Bergman & Magnusson, 1986; Steinberg, 1986). In fact, MacEvoy et al. (1988) reported marked discontinuities between childhood and adolescence in the components and correlates of TABP.

Another concern is the lack of congruence among measures of childhood TABP. Not only are the cross-measure associations weak, but examinations of the concordance of Type A-B classifications have revealed that the probability that a child will receive the same classification from two measures is only slightly above chance (Jackson & Levine, 1987). Moreover, contradictory relations between TABP and such phenomena as physiological reactivity, physical symptom reporting, and absenteeism caused by illness are emerging from studies using different measures or indexes to classify children as high or low TABP (e.g., Eagleston et al., 1986; Leikin, Firestone, & McGrath, 1988).

Recent findings suggest the fruitfulness of narrowing the focus by examining the developmental antecedents of anger and hostility. Anger not only appears to be the most stable component of TABP (Steinberg, 1986), but also has demonstrated the clearest relations with hypertension and heart disease (Krantz et al., 1988). In addition to direct links between anger and CVD, elevated or poorly managed anger may have deleterious indirect effects by disrupting healthy life-style behaviors and reducing an individual's social support resources. One indicator of the pivotal role of anger is the robust and stable link between childhood aggression and psychosocial problems during adulthood (e.g., Parker & Asher, 1987). Until recently there was a paucity of research on childhood anger per se— in contrast to overt externalizing behaviors such as aggression—and progress has been hampered by a dearth of adequate measures. High research density in recent years has resulted in significant advances, however, and information is beginning to emerge on both the developmental antecedents of anger and possible links between anger and CVD risk (Finch, Saylor, & Nelson, 1987; Thoresen, Eagleston, Kirmil-Gray, & Wiedenfeld, 1989).

Preventing Program-Generated Problems:
Emanations and Antidotes

Iatrogenic Potential:
Inadvertent Effects of Health Promotion Programs

Many child health promotion programs are based on goals and principles derived from research on adults (following the "stitch in time saves nine" principle) without recognizing that behavior patterns recommended for adults may be irrelevant or perhaps even contraindicated with children. There is a serious need for caution when intervening in the lives of healthy people, using unproven techniques, to alter projected trajectories by changing factors that at best account for small portions of the total variance in health status (Albino, 1984; Coates, Petersen, & Perry, 1982).

The difficulty is that there is no totally benign intervention. Every attempt to teach or change health habits has iatrogenic potential, possible *emanative* effects—inadvertent and often undesirable consequences that may be overlooked (Whalen & Henker, 1980). In this section, we identify some potential emanative effects of intervening in the lives of healthy children and then suggest protective processes (or "antidotes") worthy of examination.

Misguided Diets

There are few if any health specialists who would disagree with the assertion that it is undesirable to be obese; at this point, however, consensus ends. Although many specialists recommend carefully controlled dietary intakes and exercise regimens starting during infancy, there are indications that dietary concerns have been exaggerated, with unsalutary consequences. Some health-conscious parents, for example, are placing their infants on extremely low-fat diets that produce potentially harmful growth retardation (Pugliese, Weyman-Daum, Moses, & Lifshitz, 1987).

Recent surveys provide consistent evidence of societal overconcern with weight and body girth. Drewnowski and Yee (1987) reported that 89% of normal-weight women and 53% of normal-weight men desire to be thinner. A study of high school students revealed that only about one quarter of the women (compared to half of the men) were either maintaining or doing nothing about their weights, even though most were of normal weight (Rosen & Gross, 1987). Still another study found that almost one third of a sample of high school freshmen had misperceptions of their actual weight status, and more than half of those considered normal had been dieting to lose weight in the past 6 months (Desmond, Price, Gray, & O'Connell, 1986).

Particularly striking is the fact that dissatisfaction with body size and weight is surfacing at progressively earlier ages, especially in females (Cohn, Adler, & Irwin, 1987). Mellin, Scully, and Irwin (1986) found that almost half of a sample of 9-year-old girls, and 81% of the 10- and 11-year-olds, reported that they had already dieted to lose weight. These findings heighten concerns not only about the development of eating disorders such as anorexia and bulimia, but also about the possibility that over-zealous dieting may retard normal growth and delay puberty even in youths showing no evidence of psychological disturbance (Pugliese, Lifshitz, Grad, Fort, & Marks-Katz, 1983).

Trends in cigarette smoking among women raise further concerns about excessive worrying over weight. Clear associations—beyond those portrayed in cigarette ads—have been documented between cigarette smoking and slimness, as well as between smoking cessation and weight gain (Klesges et al., 1989). Women are beginning to smoke at increasingly early ages, and the frequency of smoking among girls and young women now exceeds that among boys and young men. Although the 1970s and 1980s witnessed a heartening decrease in smoking prevalence, the rate of decline among women is substantially lower than that among men, and today's female smoker smokes more than yesterday's (Fielding, 1987). These patterns suggest that inordinate weight concerns can have far-reaching health consequences that extend beyond the nutritional realm.

Fortunately, cases of overzealous dieting as drastic as those described by Pugliese et al. (1983) are rare. The concern here is not with the extremes of self-starvation, but rather with what might be considered a subclinical and perhaps pernicious level of weight concern and caloric restriction in youths (and their parents) that may have far-reaching consequences in both physiological and psychological realms. Recent evidence suggesting that repeated "yo-yo" dieting may slow subsequent weight losses and facilitate rapid regaining (as the body becomes more efficient in its use of food) raises additional questions about the wisdom of early dieting (Brownell, Greenwood, Stellar, & Shrager, 1986). The problem is of such concern that dieting, ironically depicted as both normative and pathological, has been identified as a serious health hazard (Mallick, 1983; Polivy & Herman, 1987).

There are, of course, no indications that health promotion efforts have created societal overconcerns with dieting and weight control. The point is that children and adolescents interpret dietary intervention programs within this context of societal overconcern, and this overconcern may exacerbate the effects of such programs far beyond the intended impact. Broad-based health promotion programs may inoculate some normal-weight youth against future weight problems, but they also stand the chance of engendering maladaptive preoccupation and worry, a point to which we return below.

Tempering Type A and its Correlates

Indications that TABP is an independent risk factor for CVD have led many health specialists to recommend that these habits be diverted during childhood, when individuals are presumed to be more malleable. Such recommendations raise several concerns. First, as noted above, only moderate stability of TABP within childhood has been found, and there is as yet no documentation of continuity between childhood and adulthood. Also lacking is direct evidence linking childhood TABP to CVD at any age. Children do, of course, show many of the same behaviors that have been designated as Type A in adults, but topographically similar behaviors do not necessarily have the same causes or consequences. Indeed, recent studies demonstrating strong relationships between problem behaviors (especially hyperactivity) and TABP raise serious questions about the meaning and measurement of childhood TABP (Whalen & Henker, 1986; Whalen, Henker, Hinshaw, & Granger, 1989).

Given these unknowns, it is not yet possible to isolate the most changeworthy childhood behaviors—those that relate to cardiovascular risk in adulthood. Both positive and negative dispositions are subsumed under the TABP rubric, and there is some evidence that the more and less desirable aspects are positively correlated during childhood (Steinberg, 1986). Thus attempts to taper TABP during childhood could succeed in curtailing some correlates that are commonly linked with success and happiness in our culture, such as achievement motivation, persistence, zest and zeal. This concern is buttressed by findings from a study of more than 800 school-age children demonstrating that the Competition subscale of the MYTH proved to be positively related to both academic achievement and sociability and negatively related to depression and inhibition (Bachman, Sines, Watson, Lauer, & Clarke, 1986). Similarly, positive links between TABP and IQ, achievement, and academic grades were reported by Matthews, Stoney, Rakaczky, and Jamison (1986). Emerging data also suggest that Type B (or nonA) behaviors may themselves carry psychosocial costs, at least for some children (Kliewer, Lepore, & Evans, 1990).

Social Ties That Go Awry

Given the demonstrated links between social support and health in adults (e.g., House, Landis, & Umberson, 1988), the recommendation has been made that children be provided with sufficient "doses" of social support to inoculate them against later difficulties. There are several problems with this proposition. First, the construct has experienced such semantic elasticity that it is difficult to know what defines social support and distinguishes it from other aspects of interpersonal functioning. Second, social support sources, processes, and consequences assuredly differ during progressive stages of the life span, but little is known about either age-appropriate support or the long-term effects of different types of social support during various developmental phases. Third, systematically provided social support may differ from naturally occurring social support, with the former likely to be off the mark or to appear artificial and consequently failing to produce any inoculatory effect (e.g., Rook & Dooley, 1985). Fourth, a "prescription" for social support does not consider the possibility that social support—of some types, from some sources, and under some conditions—may have harmful rather than healthful consequences (Rook & Pietromonaco, 1986). Our knowledge of cigarette-smoking initiation provides a singular example, indicating that adolescents who are more involved in social (in contrast to academic or athletic) activities are more likely than their peers to begin smoking (Murray, Swan, Johnson, & Bewley, 1983).

In a different context, an intriguing study of adolescent social support by Hirsch and Reischl (1985) highlights other undesirable possibilities. As expected, higher levels of support were related to better psychosocial adjustment in adolescents with healthy parents. For those with either a depressed or an arthritic parent, however, the opposite pattern emerged: Higher levels of social support were associated with poorer adjustment. There are several plausible explanations of this pattern, including a causal direction opposite to that usually assumed. Perhaps psychosocial difficulties were influencing social support networks rather than (or in addition to) the reverse, with the most troubled adolescents seeking and obtaining high levels of social support. Another possibility is that youngsters with many social ties had more opportunities to compare their parents to others and more stigmatizing experiences because of their parents. This possibility is buttressed by findings from a related study indicating that events usually considered positive were strongly related to decreased psychosocial symptoms in adolescents with normal parents, but to elevated symptom levels in those with depressed or arthritic parents (Hirsch, Moos, & Reischl, 1985).

In summary, the lesson here is that we do not yet know enough about the facets and functions of social support or about developmental and individual differences to design effective support-enhancing programs for youths. Moreover, the potential consequences of artificially induced social support networks range not from positive to neutral, but rather from positive to noxious. Available information about long-term adjustment indicates the wisdom of enhancing social competence so that people will be able to recruit their own social support as needed, a point to which we return below.

Fueling Family Disharmony

A good proportion of the 25% of Americans who continue to smoke, the 15% to 25% who are overweight, and the 70% to 80% who fail to get enough exercise are themselves raising children. Many parents are not ideal models for heart-healthy behaviors, nor do they establish household routines that encourage careful attention to diet and exercise. In fact, consuming cuisines low in fat and high in fiber and engaging in regular aerobic exercise may be viewed as counternormative behaviors that disrupt family plans, routines, and traditions. The few data available suggest that family members tend not to provide much social support to each other for health-enhancing diet and exercise patterns, either in their natural environments or following intervention programs designed specifically to promote such social support (Baranowski, Nader, Dunn, & Vanderpool, 1982).

Thus life-style interventions based exclusively in extrafamilial settings such as schools may place children in direct conflict with their families and cultures. One obvious implication is that school-based health promotion programs may fail unless they involve entire family units. A less obvious, but perhaps more pernicious implication is that such programs may place some children at risk for increased family discord.

Symptom Sensitization and Heightened Health Anxiety

Children may distort or misinterpret prohealth messages and develop an oversensitivity to somatic processes and health such that mundane sensations and discomforts become serious cause for concern, and isolated instances of "food abuse" or other minor transgressions come to elicit disproportionate guilt and anxiety. Nor are teenagers immune to such misinterpretations and exaggerations. Mechanic (1983) has described adolescence as a period of heightened attention to inner feelings and bodily changes, particularly in individuals who are prone to introspection and who have had certain early family experiences with illness. It is not hard to imagine how health promotion efforts, in concert with normal developmental processes, may lead some youth to overattend to somatic cues and become too narrowly centered on their physiological selves.

Rising health care costs have focused increasing attention on people who seek unnecessary medical care, estimated at 7% to 25% of the medical patient population (Wagner & Curran, 1984). Children and adolescents are typically at the opposite end of the "worry scale," notorious for what has been labeled unrealistic optimism concerning health-related morbidity and mortality (Weinstein, 1987). The challenge is to increase self-responsibility for health enhancement and disease prevention without converting youthful optimists into the "worried well." Even more important than unnecessary health care expenditures from symptom over-reporting are the psychic costs, the uncertainty and undue anxiety potentially induced by repeated exposures to the message that "your heart can kill you." Programs that prove effective for youths at known risk for cardiovascular disease may have undesirable consequences for their healthier age-mates; the cost-benefit ratios for these two groups may differ dramatically.

Disease as Failure or Irresponsibility

With the growing success of public health campaigns designed to convince people of linkages between life-style and health outcomes, society may soon be witnessing the reemergence of a blame-the-victim stance, further fueled by burgeoning concerns about the escalating costs of medical care. Given their limited cognitive capacities, children may be especially susceptible to this view, interpreting health promotion messages in ways that lead them to attribute illness to personal transgressions or controllable defects. Such beliefs may in the long run have adverse effects on self-perceptions as children or their significant others experience health problems over which they have no volitional control. It would not be surprising to find this blame-the-victim notion affecting interpersonal competence and social relationships as well, perhaps having its greatest impact on relations with less fortunate peers (e.g., those with chronic illnesses or weight control problems).

Toward Behavioral Health:
Suggested Antidotes and Reformulations

These examples of emanative effects are more accurately considered possible than probable, but their incidence may be amplified as increasing numbers of young people participate in life-style risk-reduction programs. Our knowledge about cognitive and social development, combined with these warning signs, underscores the need for careful attention both to the messages communicated in health promotion programs and to the habit patterns targeted for modification. We now turn to some specific recommendations for youth-oriented health promotion programs.

Reframing and Refocusing Intervention Efforts

The design of prevention and promotion programs can be enhanced by explicit recognition of the diverse messages that may be conveyed inadvertently. Attention to potential sources of distortion can lead to salutary reframing of behavioral recommendations without requiring changes in goals or techniques. In terms of putative coronary-prone behaviors, for example, the focus can be on acquiring optimal stress-management and coping strategies and dealing effectively with anger, rather than on curtailing energy or drive. Fitness programs for normal-weight children can de-emphasize calorie restriction and weight control, focusing instead on exercise enhancement and balanced nutrient intake. Drastic dieting and excessive exercise regimens can be reframed as health endangering rather than as meritorious self-control, and resistance resources and skills can be presented for combating unhealthy peer and societal influences.

The Social-Competence Path to Social Support

Children who are interpersonally inept, intrusive, or disruptive are often excluded from peer cultures and thus deprived both of normal socialization experiences and important sources of support. Social isolation and rejection are also prime sources of stress, and chronic psychosocial stress may elevate CV risk (Perkins, 1989). Moreover, there is substantial evidence that early interpersonal difficulties and peer rejection persist and are related to psychosocial difficulties during adulthood (Parker & Asher, 1987). Rather than artificially crafting social networks, health promotion specialists can work toward enhancing children's social competence, facilitating the acquisition of interpersonal skills that will enable them to recruit their own social support as desired or needed.

Tailoring Treatments to Individuals

Biological heterogeneity is a given, and behavior–risk factor linkages vary in direction and strength across individuals and subgroups. The association between dietary intake of saturated fats and serum cholesterol levels is an instructive case in point. Some people maintain admirably low cholesterol levels without paying particular attention to their dietary intake, whereas others scrutinize every morsel and still hover in the hazardous range.

Individual differences in the personality and psychosocial realms also affect health outcomes. Jessor (1987) and his colleagues have described a dimension of psychosocial unconventionality, involving a generalized skepticism about societal values, that emerges in some adolescents. Such qualities may prevent adoption of behavior patterns prescribed by adults. In fact, when compared to their more conventional counterparts, unconventional adolescents appear to engage less regularly in health-enhancing behaviors such as wholesome dietary intake and more regularly in health-compromising behaviors such as sedentary life-styles and risk taking (Donovan, Jessor, & Costa, 1987). It may be for these adolescents in particular, rather than for teenagers in general, that peers are more powerful persuaders than adults, reminding us once again of the need to tailor treatments to individuals.

In the effort to communicate simply and clearly, health promotion programs may obscure such omnipresent individual differences. Moreover, they may inadvertently encourage a focus on rules and prescribed regimens rather than a more flexible problem-solving approach tailored to individual preferences and proclivities. The value of a flexible approach was demonstrated in a behavioral treatment study for obese children conducted by Epstein, Wing, Koeske, Ossip, and Beck (1982). Children were assigned randomly either to a programmed aerobic exercise condition (in which they earned points for performing specified aerobic exercise at a scheduled time daily) or a life-style condition (where points were based on increasing energy expenditures by engaging in a variety of less intensive, self-selected games and activities each day). Though weight loss in the two groups was equivalent during the 8-week treatment program, the life-style group lost more additional weight and maintained weight loss better during more than a year of maintenance and follow-up. The superior maintenance produced by the life-style program may be attributable to its flexibility, which facilitated matching program requirements to the child's preferences and the family's daily routines.

Enhancing Self-Efficacy Beliefs

Self-perceived efficacy refers to people's beliefs in their capacity to exercise control over their own motivations and behaviors, as well as over environmental phenomena and outcomes (Bandura, 1986). Social influences play a major role in the development of these beliefs. Starting very early, children acquire, validate, and modify their self-judgments on the basis of social comparisons—perceptions of the skills and successes of family members, peers, teachers, and other role models. These self-perceptions in turn influence behavioral choices, effort and persistence, and affective reactions. If children interpret experiences and social comparisons as suggesting that they lack requisite capabilities, or that what happens to them is unrelated to their own efforts, they are unlikely to expend the effort required for new learning and to persist when challenged or frustrated.

Bandura (1986) asserts that people with a low sense of self-efficacy are likely to forgo preventive health practices and even to avoid corrective treatments. Diverse intervention programs have demonstrated how adults' self-efficacy beliefs can foster the achievement of life-style behavior changes in such areas as smoking cessation, weight control, and exercise (Strecher, DeVellis, Becker, & Rosenstock, 1986). Efficacy judgments can also promote or impede recovery from illness. In one study of acute myocardial infarction, patients' perceptions of their own cardiac capability 3 weeks after a heart attack predicted treadmill performance 6 months later. Of particular interest in terms of social support was the finding that wives' efficacy beliefs in husbands' cardiac capacity were also related to husbands' 6-month cardiovascular functioning (Taylor, Bandura, Ewart, Miller, & DeBusk, 1985).

Although there is not yet direct evidence substantiating the impact of children's efficacy beliefs on health-related behaviors, findings from other areas underscore the potential value of such studies. To cite just one example, Weisz (1986) examined control-related beliefs in children undergoing psychotherapy. Such beliefs, based jointly on impressions of personal competence and perceptions that behaviors affect outcomes, proved to be useful predictors of problem resolution during psychotherapy, but only after the age of 12. These findings suggest the need for a delineation of relations between children's control beliefs and heart-healthy behavior patterns, as well as of the influence of parents' and peers' beliefs about the child's ability to maintain heart-healthy practices. Demonstrations of such linkages would lead naturally to tests of interventions designed to enhance children's efficacy beliefs in realistic and wholesome directions, perhaps by involving them in decisions affecting their own health (Lewis & Lewis, 1983) and providing successful coping and mastery experiences in health-related domains.

Toward Self-Regulatory Competence

A focus on efficacy beliefs leads naturally to consideration of self-regulation versus external management of health options and behaviors.

Just as in other areas of their lives, children need to learn "portable" coping strategies that they can apply across settings and health domains. As they mature, they need to learn how to motivate and reinforce themselves so that they will be able to maintain their own health-promoting behaviors in the absence of external supports.

Given the difficulty or counternormative nature of many health-promoting behaviors, youngsters need to master heart-healthy habits not in the abstract, but with full recognition of the constraints under which they live and the degree of latitude available to them. They need to learn how to match behavioral goals with situational contexts and, perhaps most important, what to do when their efforts are blocked. The types of resistance resources that may be helpful include (a) arranging their own environments to decrease cues that promote unhealthy behaviors; (b) seeking and following prohealth models as antidotes for omnipresent health-risk models; (c) learning health-related trade-offs and other flexible problem-solving strategies that allow, for example, for hanging out with peers at favorite fast-food locales without regularly consuming the typical teenage ration of junk food; and (d) coping with unhealthy transgressions—which will ineluctably occur—as lapses rather than relapses, as useful learning opportunities rather than indicators of failure and futility.

Summary and Conclusion

No matter how compelling the need or cogent the rationale, the potential power of life-style interventions raises concerns about the possibility of negative consequences. Behavior changes may be exaggerated, or their concomitants undesirable. Stringent programs and repetitive behavioral admonitions that begin early in life may engender avoidance or reactance, thereby creating additional barriers rather than pathways to change. A focus on personal responsibilities for health and the dangers of disease may also increase the burden of anxiety and self-doubt already carried by today's youths. In our zeal to improve society's collective cardiovascular health, it is vital to remember that risk-reduction programs are as susceptible as other interventions to unwelcome side effects.

Despite these cautionary statements, the research reviewed in this chapter justifies an optimistic outlook, demonstrating that we have every reason to believe that society can decrease the prevalence of damaging life-styles and strengthen behaviors conducive to health. Even though their effects have been relatively modest thus far (e.g., Walter et al., 1987), risk-reduction programs do indeed work, at least some of the time. The modest track record underscores the fact that there is still much to learn about the

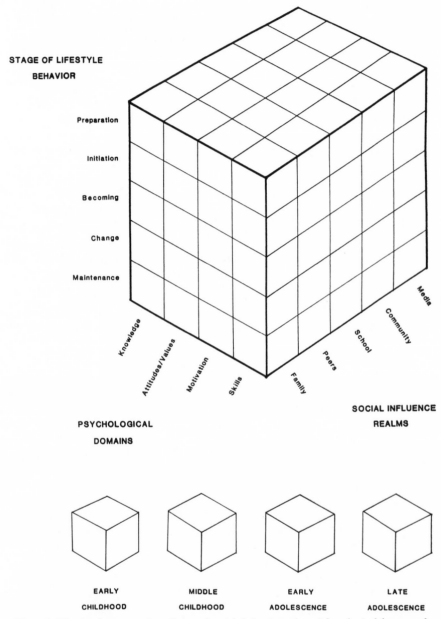

Figure 1. The development of cardiovascular risk behaviors: A social ecological framework. [Adapted from Maddux, J. E., Roberts, M. C., Sledden, E. A., & Wright, L. (1986). Developmental issues in child health psychology. *American Psychologist, 41,* 25–34.]

diverse social factors that contribute to the cardiovascular health of children and adolescents. By way of summary, Figure 1 depicts some of the key ingredients of lifestyle behaviors in youth, highlighting the need to consider specific developmental phases, lifestyle stages, psychological domains, and social influence realms in any prevention or promotion effort. As we have seen throughout this chapter, interpersonal influences may converge or collide, and health and behavior outcomes vary across people, processes, and programs. The field has advanced beyond global efficacy studies or demonstration projects comparing multimodal intervention packages to no-treatment comparison conditions. Needed now are studies addressing and assessing relevant personal, environmental, and treatment factors in the service of optimizing the match between child and program.

References

Albino, J. E. (1984). Prevention by acquiring health-enhancing habits. In M. C. Roberts & L. Peterson (Eds.), *Prevention of problems in childhood: Psychological research and applications* (pp. 200–231). New York: Wiley.

Altman, D. G., Slater, M. D., Albright, C. L., & Maccoby, N. (1987). How an unhealthy product is sold: Cigarette advertising in magazines (1960–1985). *Journal of Communication, 37*, 95–106.

Bachman, E. E., Sines, J. O., Watson, J. A., Lauer, R. M., & Clarke, W. R. (1986). The relations between Type A behavior, clinically relevant behavior, academic achievement, and IQ in children. *Journal of Personality Assessment, 50*, 186–192.

Balding, J. W., & Macgregor, I. D. M. (1987). Health-related behaviour and smoking in young adolescents. *Public Health, 101*, 277–282.

Bandura, A. (1986). *Social foundations of thought and action: A social cognitive theory.* Englewood Cliffs, NJ: Prentice-Hall.

Baranowski, T., Nader, P. R., Dunn, K., & Vanderpool, N. A. (1982). Family self-help: Promoting changes in health behavior. *Journal of Communication, 32*, 161–172.

Bell, C. S., & Levy, S. M. (1984). Public policy and smoking prevention: Implications for research. In J. D. Matarazzo, S. M. Weiss, J. A. Herd, N. E. Miller, & S. M. Weiss (Eds.), *Behavioral health: A handbook of health enhancement and disease prevention* (pp. 775–785). New York: Wiley.

Berenson, G. S. (1986). Evolution of cardiovascular risk factors in early life: Perspectives on causation. In G. S. Berenson (Ed.), *Causation of cardiovascular risk factors in children* (pp. 1–26). New York: Raven.

Bergman, L. R., & Magnusson, D. (1986). Type A behavior: A longitudinal study from childhood to adulthood. *Psychosomatic Medicine, 48*, 134–142.

Botvin, G. J. (1982). Broadening the focus of smoking prevention strategies. In T. J. Coates, A. C. Petersen, & C. Perry (Eds.), *Promoting adolescent health: A dialog on research and practice* (pp. 137–148). New York: Academic Press.

Brandt, E. N., Jr., & McGinnis, J. M. (1985). National Children and Youth Fitness Study: Its contribution to our national objectives. *Public Health Reports, 100*, 1–3.

Brownell, K. D., Greenwood, M. R. C., Stellar, E., & Shrager, E. E. (1986). The effects of repeated cycles of weight loss and regain in rats. *Physiology and Behavior, 38,* 459–464.

Brownell, K. D., & Kaye, F. S. (1982). A school-based behavior modification, nutrition education, and physical activity program for obese children. *American Journal of Clinical Nutrition, 35,* 277–283.

Brownell, K. D., Kelman, J. H., & Stunkard, A. J. (1983). Treatment of obese children with and without their mothers: Changes in weight and blood pressure. *Pediatrics, 71,* 515–523.

Clarke, W. R., Woolson, R. F., & Lauer, R. M. (1986). Changes in ponderosity and blood pressure in childhood: The Muscatine study. *American Journal of Epidemiology, 124,* 195–206.

Coates, T. J., Jeffery, R. W., & Slinkard, L. E. (1981). Heart healthy eating and exercise: Introducing and maintaining changes in health behaviors. *American Journal of Public Health, 71,* 15–23.

Coates, T. J., Perry, C., Killen, J., & Slinkard, L. A. (1981). Primary prevention of cardiovascular disease in children and adolescents. In C. K. Prokop & L. A. Bradley (Eds.), *Medical psychology: Contributions to behavioral medicine* (pp. 157–196). New York: Academic Press.

Coates, T. J., Petersen, A. C., & Perry, C. (1982). Crossing the barriers. In T. J. Coates, A. C. Petersen, & C. Perry (Eds.), *Promoting adolescent health: A dialog on research and practice* (pp. 1–21). New York: Academic Press.

Cohn, L. D., Adler, N. E., & Irwin, C. E. (1987). Body-figure preferences in male and female adolescents. *Journal of Abnormal Psychology, 96,* 276–279.

Cresanta, J. L., Hyg, M. S., Burke, G. L., Downey, A. M., Freedman, D. S., & Berenson, G. S. (1986). Prevention of atherosclerosis in childhood. *Pediatric Clinics of North America, 33,* 835–858.

Desmond, S. M., Price, J. H., Gray, N., & O'Connell, J. K. (1986). The etiology of adolescents' perceptions of their weight. *Journal of Youth and Adolescence, 15,* 461–474.

Dietz, W. H., & Gortmaker, S. L. (1985). Do we fatten our children at the television set? Obesity and television viewing in children and adolescents. *Pediatrics, 75,* 807–812.

Dimsdale, J. E. (1988). A perspective on Type A behavior and coronary disease. *New England Journal of Medicine, 318,* 110–112.

Donovan, J. E., Jessor, R., & Costa, F. M. (1991). Adolescent health behavior and conventionality-unconventionality: An extension of problem-behavior theory. *Health Psychology, 10,* 52–61.

Downey, A. M., Butcher, A. H., Frank, G. C., Webber, L. S., Miner, M. H., & Berenson, G. S. (1987). Development and implementation of a school health promotion program for reduction of cardiovascular risk factors in children and prevention of adult coronary heart disease: "Heart Smart." In B. Hetzel & G. S. Berenson (Eds.), *Cardiovascular risk factors in childhood: Epidemiology and prevention* (pp. 103–121). New York: Elsevier Science.

Drewnowski, A., & Yee, D. K. (1987). Men and body image: Are males satisfied with their body weight? *Psychosomatic Medicine, 49,* 626–634.

Eagleston, J. R., Kirmil-Gray, K., Thoresen, C. E., Wiedenfeld, S. A., Bracke, P., & Arnow, B. (1986). Physical health correlates of Type A behavior in children and adolescents. *Journal of Behavioral Medicine, 9,* 341–362.

Epstein, L. H., Nudelman, S., & Wing, R. R. (1987). Long-term effects of family-based treatment for obesity on nontreated family members. *Behavior Therapy, 2,* 147–152.

Epstein, L. H., Wing, R. R., Koeske, R., Ossip, D., & Beck, S. (1982). A comparison of lifestyle change and programmed aerobic exercise on weight and fitness changes in obese children. *Behavior Therapy, 13,* 651–665.

Epstein, L. H., Wing, R. R., Koeske, R., & Valoski, A. (1987). Long-term effects of family-based treatment of childhood obesity. *Journal of Consulting and Clinical Psychology, 55,* 91–95.

Epstein, L. H., Wing, R. R., & Valoski, A. (1985). Childhood obesity. *Pediatric Clinics of North America, 32*, 363–379.

Epstein, L. H., Wing, R. R., Valoski, A., & Gooding, W. (1987). Long-term effects of parent weight on child weight loss. *Behavior Therapy, 18*, 219–226.

Fielding, J. E. (1987). Smoking and women: Tragedy of the majority. *New England Journal of Medicine, 317*, 1343–1345.

Finch, A. J., Saylor, C. F., & Nelson, W. M. (1987). Assessment of anger in children. In R. J. Prinz (Ed.), *Advances in behavioral assessment of children and families, vol. 3* (pp. 235–265). Greenwich, CT: JAI Press.

Flay, B. R. (1985). Psychosocial approaches to smoking prevention: A review of findings. *Health Psychology, 4*, 449–488.

Flay, B. R., d'Avernas, J. R., Best, J. A., Kersell, M. W., & Ryan, K. B. (1983). Cigarette smoking: Why young people do it and ways of preventing it. In P. J. McGrath & P. Firestone (Eds.), *Pediatric and adolescent behavioral medicine: Issues in treatment* (pp. 132–183). New York: Springer.

Flay, B. R., Ryan, K. B., Best, J. A., Brown, K. S., Kersell, M. W., d'Avernas, J. R., & Zanna, M. P. (1985). Are social-psychological smoking prevention programs effective? The Waterloo study. *Journal of Behavioral Medicine, 8*, 37–59.

Foster, G. D., Wadden, T. A., & Brownell, K. D. (1985). Peer-led program for the treatment and prevention of obesity in the schools. *Journal of Consulting and Clinical Psychology, 53*, 538–540.

Frank, G. C., Webber, L. S., & Berenson, G. S. (1982). Dietary studies of infants and children: The Bogalusa Heart Study. In T. J. Coates, A. C. Petersen, & C. Perry (Eds.), *Promoting adolescent health: A dialog on research and practice* (pp. 329–354). New York: Academic Press.

Frisch, R. E., Wyshak, G., Albright, N. L., Albright, T. E., & Schiff, I. (1986). Lower prevalence of diabetes in female former college athletes compared with nonathletes. *Diabetes, 35*, 1101–1105.

Galst, J. P., & White, M. A. (1976). The unhealthy persuader: The reinforcing value of television and children's purchase-influencing attempts at the supermarket. *Child Development, 47*, 1089–1096.

Garn, S. M., & LaVelle, M. (1985). Two-decade follow-up of fatness in early childhood. *American Journal of Diseases of Children, 139*, 181–185.

Gortmaker, S. L., Dietz, W. H., Sobol, A. M., & Wehler, C. A. (1987). Increasing pediatric obesity in the United States. *American Journal of Diseases of Children, 141*, 535–540.

Graves, T., Meyers, A. W., & Clark, L. (1988). An evaluation of parental problem-solving training in the behavioral treatment of childhood obesity. *Journal of Consulting and Clinical Psychology, 56*, 246–250.

Hamburg, D. A., Elliott, G. R., & Parron, D. L. (1982). *Health and behavior: Frontiers of research in the biobehavioral sciences*. Washington, DC: National Academy Press.

Haynes, S. G., & Matthews, K. A. (1988). Review and methodologic critique of recent studies on Type A behavior and cardiovascular disease. *Annals of Behavioral Medicine, 10*, 47–59.

Hirsch, B. J., Moos, R. H., & Reischl, T. M. (1985). Psychosocial adjustment of adolescent children of a depressed, arthritic, or normal parent. *Journal of Abnormal Psychology, 94*, 154–164.

Hirsch, B. J., & Reischl, T. M. (1985). Social networks and developmental psychopathology: A comparison of adolescent children of a depressed, arthritic, or normal parent. *Journal of Abnormal Psychology, 94*, 272–281.

House, J. S., Landis, K. R., & Umberson, D. (1988). Social relationships and health. *Science, 241*, 540–545.

Israel, A. C., Stolmaker, L., & Andrian, C. A. G. (1985). The effects of training parents in general child management skills on a behavioral weight loss program for children. *Behavior Therapy, 16,* 169–180.

Iverson, D. C., Fielding, J. E., Crow, R. S., & Christenson, G. M. (1985). The promotion of physical activity in the United States population: The status of programs in medical, worksite, community, and school settings. *Public Health Reports, 100,* 212–224.

Jackson, C., & Levine, D. W. (1987). Comparison of the Matthews Youth Test for Health and the Hunter-Wolf A-B Rating Scale: Measures of Type A behavior in children. *Health Psychology, 6,* 255–267.

Jeffery, R. W. (1988). Dietary risk factors and their modification in cardiovascular disease. *Journal of Consulting and Clinical Psychology, 56,* 350–357.

Jeffrey, D. B., McLellarn, R. W., & Fox, D. T. (1982). The development of children's eating habits: The role of television commercials. *Health Education Quarterly, 9,* 174–189.

Jessor, R. (1984). Adolescent development and behavioral health. In J. D. Matarazzo, S. M. Weiss, J. A. Herd, N. E. Miller, & S. M. Weiss (Eds.), *Behavioral health: A handbook of health enhancement and disease prevention* (pp. 69–90). New York: Wiley.

Jessor, R. (1987). Problem-behavior theory, psychosocial development, and adolescent problem drinking. *British Journal of Addiction, 82,* 331–342.

Johnston, L. D. (1986, August). *Testimony before the Subcommittee on Health and the Environment of the Committee on Energy and Commerce, United States House of Representatives, in hearings on cigarette advertising and promotion.* Washington, DC: US Government Printing Office.

Klesges, R. C., Coates, T. J., Brown, G., Sturgeon-Tillisch, J., Moldenhauer-Klesges, L. M., Holzer, B., Woolfrey, J., & Vollmer, J. (1983). Parental influences on children's eating behavior and relative weight. *Journal of Applied Behavior Analysis, 16,* 371–378.

Klesges, R. C., Coates, T. J., Moldenhauer-Klesges, L. M., Holzer, B., Gustavson, J., & Barnes, J. (1984). The FATS: An observational system for assessing physical activity in children and associated parent behavior. *Behavioral Assessment, 6,* 333–345.

Klesges, R. C., Meyers, A. W., Klesges, L. M., & LaVasque, M. E. (1989). Smoking, body weight, and their effects on smoking behavior: A comprehensive review of the literature. *Psychological Bulletin, 106,* 204–230.

Kliewer, W., Lepore, S. J., & Evans, G. W. (1990). The costs of Type B behavior: Females at risk in achievement situations. *Journal of Applied Social Psychology, 20,* 1369–1382.

Krantz, D. S., Contrada, R. J., Hill, D. R., & Friedler, E. (1988). Environmental stress and biobehavioral antecedents of coronary heart disease. *Journal of Consulting and Clinical Psychology, 56,* 333–341.

Leikin, L., Firestone, P., & McGrath, P. (1988). Physical symptom reporting in Type A and Type B children. *Journal of Consulting and Clinical Psychology, 56,* 721–726.

Leventhal, H., Prohaska, T. R., & Hirschman, R. S. (1985). Preventive health behavior across the life span. In J. C. Rosen & L. J. Solomon (Eds.), *Prevention in health psychology* (pp. 191–235). Hanover, NH: University Press of New England.

Lewis, C. E., & Lewis, M. A. (1983). Improving the health of children: Must the children be involved? *Annual Review of Public Health, 4,* 259–283.

MacEvoy, B., Lambert, W. W., Karlberg, P., Karlberg, J., Klackenberg-Larsson, I., & Klackenberg, G. (1988). Early affective antecedents of adult Type A behavior. *Journal of Personality and Social Psychology, 54,* 108–116.

Mallick, M. J. (1983). Health hazards of obesity and weight control in children: A review of the literature. *American Journal of Public Health, 73,* 78–82.

Matthews, K. A., Stoney, C. M., Rakaczky, C. J., & Jamison, W. (1986). Family characteristics and school achievements of Type A children. *Health Psychology, 5,* 453–468.

Matthews, K. A., & Woodall, K. L. (1988). Childhood origins of overt Type A behaviors and cardiovascular reactivity to behavioral stressors. *Annals of Behavioral Medicine, 10,* 71–77.

Mechanic, D. (1983). Adolescent health and illness behavior: Review of the literature and a new hypothesis for the study of stress. *Journal of Human Stress, 7,* 4–13.

Mellin, L. A., Scully, S., & Irwin, C. E. (1986, October). *Disordered eating characteristics in preadolescent girls.* Paper presented at the meeting of the American Dietetic Association, Las Vegas, NV.

Mittelmark, M. B., Murray, D. M., Luepker, R. V., Pechacek, T. F., Pirie, P. L., & Pallonen, U. E. (1987). Predicting experimentation with cigarettes: The Childhood Antecedents of Smoking Study (CASS). *American Journal of Public Health, 77,* 206–208.

Mosbach, P., & Leventhal, H. (1988). Peer group identification and smoking: Implications for intervention. *Journal of Abnormal Psychology, 97,* 238–245.

Murray, D. M., Davis-Hearn, M., Goldman, A. I., Pirie, P., & Luepker, R. V. (1988). Four- and five-year follow-up results from four seventh-grade smoking prevention strategies. *Journal of Behavioral Medicine, 11,* 395–405.

Murray, M., Swan, A. V., Johnson, M. R. D., & Bewley, B. R. (1983). Some factors associated with increased risk of smoking by children. *Journal of Child Psychology and Psychiatry, 24,* 223–232.

Nader, P. R., Sallis, J. F., Patterson, T. L. Abramson, I. S., Rupp, J. W. , Senn, K. L., Atkins, C. J., Roppe, B. E., Morris, J. A., Wallace, J. P., & Vega, W. A. (1989). A family approach to cardiovascular risk reduction: Results from the San Diego Family Health Project. *Health Education Quarterly, 16,* 229–244.

Parker, J. G., & Asher, S. R. (1987). Peer relations and later personal adjustment: Are low-accepted children at risk? *Psychological Bulletin, 102,* 357–389.

Patterson, T. L., Sallis, J. F., Nader, P. R., Kaplan, R. M., Rupp, J. W., Atkins, C. J., & Senn, K. L. (1989). Familial similarities of changes in cognitive, behavioral, and physiological variables in a cardiovascular health promotion program. *Journal of Pediatric Psychology, 14,* 277–292.

Perkins, K. A. (1989). Interactions among coronary heart disease risk factors. *Annals of Behavioral Medicine, 11,* 3–11.

Perry, C. L., Klepp, K., & Shultz, J. M. (1988). Primary prevention of cardiovascular disease: Communitywide strategies for youth. *Journal of Consulting and Clinical Psychology, 56,* 358–364.

Peterson, P. E., Jeffrey, D. B., Bridgwater, C. A., & Dawson, B. (1984). How pronutrition television programming affects children's dietary habits. *Developmental Psychology, 20,* 55–63.

Pirie, P. L., Murray, D. M., & Luepker, R. V. (1988). Smoking prevalence in a cohort of adolescents, including absentees, dropouts, and transfers. *American Journal of Public Health, 78,* 176–178.

Polivy, J., & Herman, C. P. (1987). Diagnosis and treatment of normal eating. *Journal of Consulting and Clinical Psychology, 55,* 635–644.

Pugliese, M. T., Lifshitz, F., Grad, G., Fort, P., & Marks-Katz, M. (1983). Fear of obesity: A cause of short stature and delayed puberty. *New England Journal of Medicine, 309,* 513–518.

Pugliese, M. T., Weyman-Daum, M., Moses, N., & Lifshitz, F. (1987). Parental health beliefs as a cause of nonorganic failure to thrive. *Pediatrics, 80,* 175–182.

Ragland, D. R., & Brand, R. J. (1988). Type A behavior and mortality from coronary heart disease. *New England Journal of Medicine, 318,* 65–69.

Rook, K. S., & Dooley, D. (1985). Applying social support research: Theoretical problems and future directions. *Journal of Social Issues, 41,* 5–28.

Rook, K. S., & Pietromonaco, P. (1987). Close relationships: Ties that heal or ties that bind? In W. H. Jones & D. Perlman (Eds.), *Advances in personal relationships, vol. 1* (pp. 1–35). Greenwich, CT: JAI Press.

Rosen, J. C., & Gross, J. (1987). Prevalence of weight reducing and weight gaining in adolescent girls and boys. *Health Psychology, 6,* 131–147.

Rundall, T. G., & Bruvold, W. H. (1988). A meta-analysis of school-based smoking and alcohol use prevention programs. *Health Education Quarterly, 15,* 317–334.

Shekelle, R. B., Hulley, S. B., Neaton, J. D., Billings, J. H., Borhani, N. O., Gerace, T. A., Jacobs, D. R., Lasser, N. L., Mittlemark, M. B., & Stamler, J. (1985). The MRFIT behavior pattern study: II. Type A behavior and incidence of coronary heart disease. *American Journal of Epidemiology, 122,* 559–570.

Simons-Morton, B. G., Parcel, G. S., & O'Hara, N. M. (1988). Implementing organizational changes to promote healthful diet and physical exercise activity at school. *Health Education Quarterly, 15,* 115–130.

Steinberg, L. (1986). Stability (and instability) of Type A behavior from childhood to young adulthood. *Developmental Psychology, 22,* 393–402.

Strasser, T. (1980). Prevention in childhood of major cardiovascular diseases of adults. In F. Falkner (Ed.), *Prevention in childhood of health problems in adult life.* Geneva: World Health Organization.

Strecher, V. J., DeVellis, B. M., Becker, M. H., & Rosenstock, I. M. (1986). The role of self-efficacy in achieving behavior change. *Health Education Quarterly, 13,* 73–91.

Stunkard, A. J., Sorensen, T. I. A., Hanis, C., Teasdale, T. W., Chakraborty, R., Schull, W. J., & Schulsinger, F. (1986). An adoption study of human obesity. *New England Journal of Medicine, 314,* 193–198.

Sussman, S., Dent, C. W., Mistel-Rauch, J., Johnson, C. A., Hansen, W. B., & Flay, B. R. (1988). Adolescent nonsmokers, triers, and regular smokers' estimates of cigarette smoking prevalence: When do overestimations occur and by whom? *Journal of Applied Social Psychology, 18,* 537–551.

Task Force on Blood Pressure Control in Children. (1987). Report of the second Task Force on Blood Pressure Control in Children—1987. *Pediatrics, 79,* 1–25.

Taylor, C. B., Bandura, A., Ewart, C. K., Miller, N. H., & DeBusk, R. F. (1985). Exercise testing to enhance wives' confidence in their husbands' cardiac capability soon after clinically uncomplicated acute myocardial infarction. *American Journal of Cardiology, 55,* 635–638.

Thoresen, C. E., Eagleston, J. R., Kirmil-Gray, K., & Wiedenfeld, S. A. (1989, March). *Examining anger in low and high Type A children and adolescents.* Poster presented at the meeting of the Society of Behavioral Medicine, San Francisco, CA.

Tye, J. B., Warner, K. E., & Glantz, S. A. (1987). Tobacco advertising and consumption: Evidence of a causal relationship. *Journal of Public Health Policy, 8,* 492–508.

Visintainer, P. F., & Matthews, K. A. (1987). Stability of overt Type A behaviors in children: Results from a two- and five-year longitudinal study. *Child Development, 58,* 1586–1591.

Wagner, P. J., & Curran, P. (1984). Health beliefs and physician identified "worried well." *Health Psychology, 3,* 459–474.

Walter, H. J., Hofman, A., Barrett, L. T., Connelly, P. A., Kost, K. L., Walk, E. H., & Patterson, R. (1987). Primary prevention of cardiovascular disease among children: Three year results of a randomized intervention trial. In B. Hetzel & G. S. Berenson (Eds.), *Cardiovascular risk factors in childhood: Epidemiology and prevention* (pp. 161–181). New York: Elsevier.

Walter, H. J., Hofman, A., Vaughan, R. D., & Wynder, E. L. (1988). Modification of risk factors for coronary heart disease. *New England Journal of Medicine, 318,* 1093–1100.

Weinstein, N. D. (1987). Unrealistic optimism about susceptibility to health problems: Conclusions from a community-wide sample. *Journal of Behavioral Medicine, 10,* 481–500.

Weisz, J. R. (1986). Contingency and control beliefs as predictors of psychotherapy outcomes among children and adolescents. *Journal of Consulting and Clinical Psychology, 54,* 789–795.

Whalen, C. K., & Henker, B. (1980). The social ecology of psychostimulant treatment: A model for conceptual and empirical analysis. In C. K. Whalen & B. Henker (Eds.), *Hyperactive children: The social ecology of identification and treatment* (pp. 3–51). New York: Academic Press.
Whalen, C. K., & Henker, B. (1986). Type A behavior in normal and hyperactive children: Multisource evidence of overlapping constructs. *Child Development, 57,* 688–699.
Whalen, C. K., Henker, B., Hinshaw, S. P., & Granger, D. A. (1989). Externalizing behavior disorders, situational generality, and the Type A behavior pattern. *Child Development, 60,* 1453–1462.

CHAPTER 11

The Role of Social Support in the Modification of Risk Factors for Cardiovascular Disease

Terrence L. Amick and Judith K. Ockene

A strong relationship has been demonstrated between life-style behaviors (e.g., smoking, excessive consumption of foods high in cholesterol, saturated fat and sodium, and lack of exercise) and the development and progression of cardiovascular disease (CVD) (e.g., Kannel, 1983; Page, 1976; Stamler, 1978). A decreased likelihood of developing CVD is related to modification of these risk factors, making such modification an important means for improving an individual's cardiovascular health (Superko, Wood, & Haskell, 1985; Thom & Kannel, 1981).

Life-style behaviors are affected by many factors, including the knowledge, attitudes, and skills, of the individual; his or her social context; and the social support provided within that context (Ockene, Nuttall, Benfari, Hurwitz, & Ockene, 1981). The modification of such behaviors proceeds through several stages before behavior change is eventually maintained (Horn, 1976; Marlatt & Gordon, 1985; Ockene et al., 1981; Prochaska & DiClemente, 1983; Rosen & Shipley, 1983). These stages have been variously labeled by different investigators. Prochaska and DiClemente (1983) define four stages of change: precontemplation, contemplation, action, and maintenance. At each stage different combinations of

TERRENCE L. AMICK • Donahue Institute for Governmental Services, University of Massachusetts, Amherst, Massachusetts 01003.   JUDITH K. OCKENE • Division of Preventive and Behavioral Medicine, University of Massachusetts Medical Center, Worcester, Massachusetts 01605.

Social Support and Cardiovascular Disease, edited by Sally A. Shumaker and Susan M. Czajkowski. Plenum Press, New York, 1994.

factors are related to the individual staying at that stage, moving to the next one, or returning to a previous one (U.S. Department of Health and Human Services [USDHHS], 1989), and different cognitive and behavioral processes are used (Prochaska & DiClemente, 1983). Thus, in order to understand the role that different factors play in the modification of life-style behaviors, they must be considered during each stage of change.

In this chapter we specifically consider the role of social support in the modification of life-style-related risk behaviors for CVD using a framework that integrates social support within a stages-of-change model. This constitutes a useful way to organize concepts regarding the effect of social support on behavior change. Although a number of studies focus on the relationship of support to an individual's ability to make behavioral changes, little work has been done regarding the role of social support during each of the stages of risk factor behavior change.

Modifiable risk factors related to CVD include smoking (e.g., USDHHS, 1989), elevated cholesterol (Kannel, Castelli, & Gordon, 1979; Stamler, 1978), hypertension (Kannel, Dawber, & McGee, 1980), and obesity (Kannel & Gordon, 1974). Sedentary life-style (Kannel & Eaker, 1986; Leon, 1985; Wyndham, 1979), coronary prone behavior (Friedman & Rosenman, 1974; National Heart, Lung and Blood Institute, 1981), and stress (Jenkins, 1983) have also been implicated as affecting CVD. In addition, risk factors have a synergistic effect on the development and progression of CVD, rather than an additive effect when more than one factor is present (Kannel, 1977; Stamler, Wentworth, & Neaton, 1986).

Social Support

Social support has been consistently linked to health outcomes (Broadhead et al., 1983; see reviews by Berkman, 1984; House, Landis, & Umberson, 1988), but its relationship to behavior change has not been as consistently supported (Wilson & Brownell, 1978), and attempts to increase social support to enhance long-term behavior change have produced mixed results (e.g., Brownell, 1982; Lichtenstein, 1982). The lack of consistent findings in this area has been attributed to the lack of a consistent conceptual perspective of social support (Cohen & McKay, 1984). In this chapter we use a definition of social support proposed by Cobb (1976) and expanded by Berkman (1984) and Cohen and Syme (1985). These authors postulate that support involves the following beliefs:

1. That one is cared for and loved and has an opportunity for shared intimacy (emotional support)

2. That one is esteemed and valued (sense of personal worth)
3. That one shares mutual obligations, communication, and companionship with others (sense of belonging)
4. That one has access to information, advice, appraisal, and guidance from others (informational support)
5. That one has access to material or physical assistance (instrumental support)

Three mechanisms have been proposed to account for the effects of social support on health: behavioral, psychological, and physiological (Ganster & Victor, 1988). These mechanisms may have indirect, interactive, or direct effects (Mitchell, Billings, & Moos, 1982). With regard to behavioral mechanisms, social support networks may, for example, influence behavior change by providing appropriate information or encouraging the individual to engage in a healthful behavior, seek assistance, or adhere to treatment regimens (Wallston, Alagna, DeVellis, & DeVellis, 1983). Social support may enhance health via psychological mechanisms by buffering the individual from the negative consequences of stress (Cohen & McKay, 1984; Ockene et al., 1981). This may occur when members of an individual's network redefine a potential stressor as benign; by enhancing the individual's self-esteem, self-efficacy, and perceived social control (Wills, 1985); or by being available to help the individual deal with the stress (Ockene et al., 1981). Finally, persons with high levels of support may have fewer negative physiological responses during stress (e.g., a lowered cardiovascular reactivity to stress) and therefore be buffered against stress (Broadhead et al., 1983). This chapter focuses on the behavioral and, to some extent, psychological mechanisms by which social support may affect risk factor change and, subsequently, health.

Modification of Behavior

Stages of Change

Smoking behavior is used in this section as a means to understand the potential effects of social support on behavior change during each of the stages of change. Other risk factors will be discussed as appropriate.

Several researchers have identified stages through which behavior change proceeds and the processes that occur during each stage. Horn (1976), Rosen and Shipley (1983), and Marlatt and Gordon (1985) present models proposing that several stages are in operation during the process of behavior change. A comprehensive model has been developed by Prochaska and DiClemente (1983, 1988) based on the general psychotherapy literature (Prochaska, 1979) and on data from self-changers (DiClemente & Prochaska, 1982). This model is unique from earlier models in that it identifies an initial stage (termed precontemplation) that precedes the decision-making stage.

The five stages of change are briefly defined for smoking as follows: *precontemplation* is the stage in which the smoker is neither considering quitting nor actively processing smoking and health information. During the *contemplation* stage, the smoker is thinking about quitting and is processing information about the effects of smoking and how to quit. In the *action* or quitting stage, the smoker is no longer smoking and has been without cigarettes for less than 6 months. The *maintenance* stage involves establisl.ment of long-term abstinence (generally over 6 months), whereas *relapse* is the resumption of smoking beyond a temporary slip or lapse after quitting. When relapse occurs, the smoker eventually recycles to any one of the first three stages (DiClemente, Prochaska, & Gilbertini, 1985).

A major feature of the model is its emphasis on the process of behavior change as cyclical rather than linear (see Figure 1). Similar to Marlatt and Gordon's (1980) research on relapse, Prochaska and DiClemente (1983) found that individuals usually pass through the same stage or series of stages several times before a new behavior becomes a permanent part of their lives. In fact, studies of addictive behavior suggest that for some this process of recycling through stages, even numerous times, is the prerequisite for an eventually successful long-term change (Schachter, 1982).

An important implication of a stage model is that interventions may need to be stage specific: An individual in the precontemplation stage may ignore quitting strategies; one ir the contemplation stage may need support to decide to attempt cessation; and the abstainer may need help to develop relapse prevention skills. Different degrees of social support may be more effective or necessary at one stage than another, making it necessaiy to identify and emphasize appropriate support resources and activities in intervention efforts.

There is empirical evidence for some of these support–behavior change connections. For example, Brownell, Heckerman, Westlake, Hayes, and Monti (1978) found that the record-keeping support and reinforcement activities of spouses played a significant role in helping subjects lose weight and keep it off. These subjects were not identified by stage, but if the stages-of-change model is applied, we would deduce that subjects actively losing weight (action stage) would strongly emphasize behavioral activities (e.g., record keeping) and would benefit from support related to their needs and goals at that moment (e.g., reminders of or assistance in record keeping by spouse).

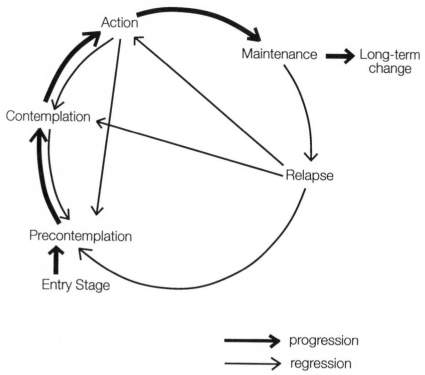

Figure 1. Cyclical model of the stages of change (adapted from Prochaska & DiClemente, 1982).

All support resources may be present or at least available at any one time; however, some support resources may be more important or appropriate than others for a given stage of change. For example, if a person has just learned that he or she has heart disease, an offer of emotional support may be more appropriate than financial support. If this person later determines that he or she may not be able to return to work, then financial support may become more relevant.

Processes of Change

Prochaska and DiClemente (1983) identify 10 processes of change that are used to different degrees during the various stages (Table 1). Certain processes are more likely to be used in some stages than others. For example, a recent ex-smoker is more likely than a precontemplative

Table 1. Processes of Change and Corresponding Examples of Specific Social Support Activities

Process of change	Proximal support	Distal support
Cognitive-Experiential		
Dramatic relief (emotional response to warnings about the consequences of the target behavior)	Warning from physician accompanied by test results showing elevated blood pressure	TV news documentary about cholesterol and heart disease
Consciousness raising (increased levels of awareness of how to change the behavior and of the benefits of changing the behavior)	Feedback from friend relating positive experiences of losing weight	Publicity surrounding Surgeon General's Report on Nutrition and Health
Environmental reevaluation (increased consideration that changing the behavior would improve the environment)	Feedback from nonsmoking adolescent children that secondhand smoke is harmful	News documentary of destructuve nature of alcoholism to family relationships
Self-reevaluation (consideraton of the cognitive dissonance caused by continued indulgence in the behavior)	Encouragement by health care provider to recognize resistance to change by denial or rationalization	Public service ads for assistance towards people who are struggling with a decision to change
Social liberation (increased awareness of changes in social acceptance of the behavior)	Restaurant menus that highlight low-fat entrees	Smoke-free airline advertisements

Behavioral

Counterconditioning (substitution of activities and thoughts other than those associated with the behavior)	Co-worker reminding recent ex-smoker to avoid coffee breaks	Media campaign encouraging substitution of foods low in saturated fat for those regularly used in recipes
Reinforcement management (expectation of reward from others and self when avoiding the behavior)	Spouse who consistently praises person when he/she reponds to a previously stressful situation	Advertisements showing healthy, vibrant people engaging in exercise
Self-liberation (increased self-efficacy—i.e., expectation success—and commitment to overcome and resist the behavior)	A friend who reminds person of past success in quitting smoking	Media recognition of people successfully quitting smoking during the Great American Smokeout
Helping relationships (recognition of the availability of special people who listen to and accept the person, especially with regard to the behavior)	Sensitive response by spouse when person has problems maintaining exercise program	Book or magazine article encouraging people to nurture close relationships
Stimulus control (removal of objects at work or home that trigger the target behavior, or placement of objects that encourage changing the behavior)	Avoidance by co-workers of offering high-fat foods to person concerned with cholesterol	TV public health ad encouraging hypertension treatment compliance

smoker to use the process of stimulus control and remove all reminders of smoking from his or her surroundings to avoid cues to smoke. Certain social support activities provided by people in the smoker's immediate environment (proximal) and by individuals or institutions in his or her more extended environment (distal) can facilitate the use of these processes (Table 1) and in so doing help move the smoker to the next stage of change (Table 2).

Table 3 indicates the relative importance of the different processes of change in each stage. This table shows, for example, that individuals in the precontemplation stage de-emphasize most processes, whereas individ-

*Table 2.   Social Support Activities Suggested
to Facilitate Movement from One Stage to the Next*

Precontemplation
    Encourage person to adopt a more socially acceptable, healthy life-style.
    Provide information to increase awareness of impact of life-style behaviors on health.
Contemplation
    Encourage activities that increase awareness of the problem behavior, its impact on health
        and quality of life, how to change the behavior, and the benefits of changing.
    Give feedback to increase positive affect to avoid effect of negative self-image.
    Direct attention to messages and symbols of greater social acceptance of healthy life-style.
    Encourage efforts to resolve conflicts arising from greater awareness of the problem
        behavior by attempting to change the behavior.
Action
    Encourge focusing on past successes of changing the problem behavior or other trouble-
        some behaviors to increase self-efficacy.
    Provide rewards for avoiding the target behavior and encourage self-rewards.
    Assist in activities that are not compatible with the problem behavior.
    Assist in removing objects in the person's environment that trigger the problem behavior.
    Encourage the person to express feelings regarding the behavior and the consequences of
        changing.
    Encourage the person to view his/her new behavior and changing self-image in a positive
        light.
Maintenance
    Remind the person of his/her prior condition before the problem behavior or encourage
        other activities that he/she might enjoy that are not compatible with the problem
        behavior.
    Remind the person to avoid cues that might trigger a relapse.
    Remind the person of current success in changing.
Relapse
    Help the person avoid getting distressed if relapse occurs.
    Remind the person of the reasons why he/she wanted to change in the first place.
    Avoid situations that might encourage the person to continue the problem behavior.
    Appeal to the person's sensitivity to his/her role as a model to others.
    Remind the person of the availability of special people who can be a resource.

Table 3. Processes of Change Emphasized and De-Emphasized for Each Stage of Change

	Precontemplation	Contemplation	Action	Maintenance	Relapse
Processes emphasized strongly		Consciousness-raising Self-reevaluation Self-efficacy	Self-liberation Reinforcement management Counterconditioning Stimulus control Self-efficacy	Counterconditioning	Self-reevaluation Consciousness-raising
Processes emphasized slightly	Social liberation	Social liberation Dramatic relief	Helping relationships Self-reevaluation	Stimulus control Self-liberation	Stimulus control Environmental reevaluation Helping relationships
Processes de-emphasized slightly	Reinforcement management Consciousness-raising Stimulus control Dramatic relief	Self-liberation Stimulus control	Consciousness-raising	Self-reevaluation	
Processes de-emphasized strongly	Self-liberation Self-reevaluation Counterconditioning Environmental reevaluation		Social liberation	Consciousness-raising	

uals in the action stage are actively engaged in the largest number of processes. It also suggests that more cognitive processes are emphasized in earlier stages (precontemplation and contemplation), whereas more behavioral processes are at work in later stages (action and maintenance).

Social Support and Stages-of-Change Model

The role social support plays in behavioral change will vary depending upon the stage and the change processes in which the individual is engaging. For example, it is likely that a person in the earliest stage (precontemplation) would be more responsive to encouragement to attend a blood cholesterol screening (cognitive-informational) than to a suggestion to reduce the saturated fat level of his or her diet (behavioral).

In the following sections, we describe the processes identified by Prochaska and DiClemente (1983) that are emphasized at each stage of change and identify social support activities and resources likely to affect these processes. The discussion focuses on the role of social support; however, social support may interact with other factors (e.g., gender, personality, cognitive factors, life stage, and health status) to affect behavior change processes differentially.

Precontemplation Stage

Precontemplation has been posited as the initial or entry stage in a cyclical model of behavior change (Prochaska & DiClemente, 1982). Characteristic of precontemplators is a lack of active involvement in processes of change. Of the 10 processes identified by Prochaska and DiClemente (1983), 8 were used significantly less by smokers in the precontemplation stage than in any other stage (see Table 3).

Individuals in the precontemplation stage may feel hopeless about their ability to change a behavior or lack awareness of their own condition or the possible effects of their behavior. Little attention has been given to individuals in this stage, because studies of risk factor modification typically may not include those individuals who are not yet contemplating changes in their behavior. There is little empirical evidence available on how to influence precontemplators to make changes.

Role of Social Support

Peer influence has a significant impact on the establishment, maintenance, and change of behaviors (USDHHS, 1989; Botvin, Eng, & Williams,

1980; Mosbach & Leventhal, 1988); movement toward change is difficult if the peer group supports the behavior. An unhealthy behavior such as smoking is often begun at an early age (O'Donnell, Voss, Clayton, Slatin, & Room, 1976) and most likely is initiated through the influence of parents and friends who smoke (Hundleby & Mercer, 1987). Peer influences are not as strong once the behavior becomes tied to daily life; however, they continue to affect behavior during all phases of life (USDHHS, 1989).

There has been no research to date that specifically looks at the role of social support during the precontemplation stage. It is likely that individuals reevaluate priorities as they enter new stages of life, recognizing the finiteness of life or, at least, the restrictions brought by new physical limitations. Wilcox, Prochaska, Velicer, and DiClemente (1985) found that precontemplators are more likely to move into the contemplation stage when they are faced with health problems. Blazer (1982), in a study of social support among the elderly, found that support plays an important role because of an increase in vulnerability that is perceived to accompany the aging process.

Brod and Hall (1984) suggest that behavior change is stimulated in the earliest stage by vicarious experience, timely information, verbal persuasion, and internal cues. A need for belonging is one of the stronger motivations for precontemplators to move to the next stage for a particular behavior. For example, smokers are finding that smoking is not as acceptable as it once was. An individual's sense of belonging is diminished in an environment in which certain behaviors find little acceptance. This process, termed *social liberation* by Prochaska and DiClemente, indicates that the individual has become aware of the environmental signals that society is less accepting of certain behaviors.

Contemplation Stage

The first stage of change beyond an immotile condition is the contemplation stage. Individuals in this stage range from those who recently have learned that a particular behavior may not be appropriate to those who are actively gathering information on the consequences of their behavior or learning possible ways to change it. It is likely that most contemplators have made some attempt to change the target behavior in the past.

Contemplation is a stage of information gathering, inner reflection, analyzing pros and cons, seeking help, and rationalizing existing behavior in the face of conflicting realities. Contemplators may be more amenable to messages that increase their understanding of the problem behavior, its potential deleterious impact on their lives, and ways to change.

The motivation for changing is largely dependent on the individual's perception of how well his or her personal values will be satisfied (Horn, 1976). Velicer, DiClemente, Prochaska, and Brandenburg (1985), in their research on the decisional balance of contemplators, found that movement (forward or backward) was predicted by the values individuals assign to the negative and positive aspects of the behavior.

Role of Social Support

In the contemplation stage, change is facilitated by the availability of information, social acceptance, and reinforcement of positive self-efficacy. Close network ties may be most important to contemplators as a conduit of information. Family and friends can potentially play a consciousness-raising role, helping to prepare the person to be more receptive to information from both within and outside his or her social network. In this role, family and friends may also define the sources and credibility of information.

Network members who practice healthful behaviors are more likely to reinforce the individual positively than those who do not. Those who model behavior antithetical to health-directed change might impede the individual's progress. Investigators have found that smokers are more likely to quit smoking when they have nonsmoking spouses or other nonsmokers in their environment (Lichtenstein, 1982; Ockene et al., 1981).

The perception of illness severity is the strongest factor distinguishing alcoholics in alcohol treatment from those not in treatment (Bardsley & Beckman, 1988). This suggests that social support might function to encourage individuals to participate in activities that increase their understanding of the nature and severity of their condition (e.g., blood pressure and cholesterol screenings). Support might involve providing appropriate information to the person, notifying him or her of screening opportunities, providing transportation, and encouraging postscreening follow-up.

Contemplators are often confronted by significant others who do not support the change. An unhealthy behavior may be embedded within the structure and activities of the family and not become a source of tension until a family member attempts, or even contemplates, changing. An identity or special role may be assigned to the family member with a problem such as obesity (Rickarby, 1981). In a dysfunctional family the special role may help maintain equilibrium (Frankle, 1985), and any change in that role may be disruptive to the family.

Resistance to change may come from one or more family members or close friends, especially if these individuals indulge in the unhealthy behavior. Elements of the network may intentionally or unintentionally sabotage consciousness-raising by demeaning the credibility of information or its sources, or the efficacy of behavior change methods. They may focus on the contemplator as the source of stress within the family or circle of friends, engendering feelings of guilt or anger.

Action Stage

The action stage occurs when the individual is taking steps to change a behavior. A dieter who has recently reduced caloric intake to a specified level, a smoker who has just quit smoking, or an hypertensive who has begun a program of medication and dietary modifications is considered to be in the action stage. During this stage the greatest number of change processes are used (Prochaska & DiClemente, 1983).

The change processes most strongly emphasized during the action stage include self-liberation, reinforcement management, counterconditioning, and stimulus control (Prochaska & DiClemente, 1983). Perceptions of self-efficacy also play an important role (DiClemente et al., 1985). Positive self-efficacy is based upon past experience; individuals who have made the desired change or a similar change several times in the past have a greater chance of succeeding (Ockene et al., 1981; Schachter, 1982).

During the initial phase of the action stage, behavioral conditioning is particularly relevant (Prochaska & DiClemente, 1983; Brownell, Marlatt, Lichtenstein, & Wilson, 1986). Recent changers are likely to adjust their environment to diminish the old behavior or emphasize the new one. A person reducing serum cholesterol level may substitute a low-fat food for a high-fat one in a favorite recipe, or smokers might remove all smoking paraphernalia from their environment.

Role of Social Support

Several studies demonstrate a positive relationship between social support and modification of such behaviors as excessive eating (Brownell et al., 1978) and smoking (Best, 1980; Colletti & Brownell, 1982; Ockene, Hymowitz, Sexton, & Broste, 1982). Coppotelli and Orleans (1985) and Mermelstein, Cohen, Lichtenstein, Baer, and Kamarck (1986) demonstrate that the availability of social support predicts positive short-term (action) and long-term (maintenance) outcomes for smoking cessation. Families strongly affect the individual family member's ability to control such risk factor behaviors as obesity (Brownell, Kelman, & Stunkard, 1983), and a stable and supportive social network appears to predict greater success at weight reduction (Cooke & Meyers, 1980).

Some studies have attempted to enhance existing social support resources in an effort to increase positive treatment outcomes. Positive short-term effects have been found in some studies. Rosenthal, Allen and Winter (1980) found that women whose husbands are intensively involved in their weight loss program have greater initial weight loss than those whose husbands are less involved, but the difference dissipates over time. The manipulation of artificial social support systems (e.g., short-term treatment groups) has had limited effect. For example, Etringer, Gregory, and Lando (1984) introduced cohesiveness training to two groups of previously unacquainted smokers and found that initial cessation rates were greater than those for two control groups, but that these differences were not maintained.

Moving from contemplation to action, the cognitive processes diminish and the behavioral processes increase (Prochaska & DiClemente, 1983). Receptivity to specific types of social support correspondingly changes. Support activities related to verbal and cognitive processes that influence consciousness-raising presumably have decreased importance, because recent changers have already made a decision to change and thus are less interested in obtaining evidence that the behavior being changed is unhealthy or socially unacceptable. Brownell et al. (1978) observed that mutual monitoring of weight and calories was important in the early stages of change (i.e., action phase) for those attempting weight loss with the help of significant others. These behavioral processes require immediate and constant attention, and support is most helpful on a day-to-day basis.

Prochaska and DiClemente (1983) found helping relationships to be of greatest importance to smokers in the action stage. These smokers responded significantly more positively than did those in other stages to statements such as "I have someone whom I can count on when I'm having problems with smoking." The initial phases of the action stage are inherently stressful and therefore require more help and understanding from significant others.

Maintenance and Relapse Stages

Those who maintain behavior change without relapse for at least 6 months (long-term changers) are considered to be in the maintenance stage (DiClemente & Prochaska, 1985). These individuals use few of the processes of change but are still at risk for relapse. They continue to emphasize some of the behavioral processes that are important during the action stage, but to a lesser degree. Relapsers—individuals who have made a significant change in a risk factor behavior but have not sustained the change and have returned to the problem behavior—will recycle into one of the first three stages, most likely either contemplation or action (DiClemente et al., 1985).

Maintainers who continue to be preoccupied with the negative aspects of the problem behavior continue to see the behavior as an issue, their self-efficacy is lower, and the likelihood of relapse if higher for them than for those who are not so preoccupied (DiClemente et al., 1985). As long-term changers become comfortable with their new behavior, the quantity and intensity of change processes diminishes. High self-efficacy predicts continued successful outcomes for maintainers (Baer, Holt, & Lichtenstein, 1986; DiClemente, 1981).

The variables of greatest importance to maintainers concern those related to relapse avoidance. These include coping skills, adaptation to new behaviors, emotional stability, self-efficacy, motivation, family cooperation, health values, and the presence or absence of others who practice the problem behavior. Negative emotional states (e.g., depression and anxiety) are related to relapse (Cummings, Gordon, & Marlatt, 1980), as is a lack of motivation (Brownell et al., 1986).

Marlatt and Gordon (1985) make a distinction between lapse (a one-time slip) and relapse (a full-blown return to the problem behavior) for addictive behaviors. They suggest that a critical component in determining whether or not a lapse develops into a relapse is the extent to which a negative emotional response is attached to the lapse.

Role of Social Support

The family and social network play important roles in the continued maintenance of life-style changes. For example, long-term maintenance of smoking cessation is strongly related to the number of smoking friends and relatives in the social network (Eisinger, 1971; Mermelstein et al, 1986; West, Graham, Swanson, & Wilkinson, 1977). Emotional stability (Marlatt & Gordon, 1980; Sjoberg & Samsonvitz, 1978), social integration (Umberson, 1987), and family cooperation and support (Brownell, 1982; Gale, Eckhoff, Mogel & Rodnick, 1984; Miller & Sims, 1981; Witschi, Singer, Wu-Lee, & Stare, 1978) influence long-term status for weight reduction, smoking and alcohol cessation, and exercise participation.

There are two roles for social support in relation to maintenance and relapse. The first involves the prevention of relapse; this includes making social support resources available to help minimize interpersonal and environmental stressors, to enhance motivation and commitment, and to promote relapse prevention skills. The second role involves reducing the negative impact of lapses and relapses and increasing self-efficacy to make another change attempt.

As the time since initiating the change increases for maintainers, less importance is allotted to all change processes (DiClemente et al., 1985). This is related to the old behavior being effectively displaced by the new behavior. Therefore, early in the maintenance stage while temptation is high, social resources might be most effectively focused on such behavioral processes as coping techniques and maintaining high expectations for success. Brownell et al. (1978) suggest that the supportive activities most influential in terms of long-term maintenance of weight loss reported by subjects include checking on dietary transgressions and providing potent and immediate reinforcement for appropriate eating behavior. As the behavior becomes more embedded in the individual's life, those support activities that maintain interpersonal stability and self-efficacy might be of greatest assistance.

Conclusion

In this chapter we have considered the role that social support plays in the process of behavior change, using the stages-of-change model as a convenient framework for formulating our approach. Precontemplators are involved in few processes of change but may be encouraged by supportive others to initiate change by the modeling of appropriate behaviors, by the provision of timely information, and by persuasion attempts. Cognitive processes (e.g., consciousness-raising) that are emphasized by contemplators in their decision to make a behavior change may be enhanced by support networks through the provision of information, assistance in decision making, and encouragement that boosts self-confidence.

In the action stage, individuals primarily use behavioral processes and are best supported by network members through timely praise and reinforcement, removal of behavioral stimuli, and encouragement of behaviors incompatible with the problem behavior. Maintainers (long-term changers) are less involved with the processes of change and may be served by support networks that assist in such relapse prevention activities as developing coping skills and adapting to a new behavior. Network members may also be helpful to long-term changers by maintaining emotional stability within the family context and modeling appropriate health behaviors. When lapses occur, support may help the individual avoid guilt or feelings of failure. If relapse occurs, individuals generally recycle into either the contemplation or action stage and emphasize the processes of change characteristic of those stages.

Because there is little evidence to support the value of specific social support activities within specific stages of change, many of the conclusions in this chapter are conjecture. A relationship between social support and behavior change has been observed in many investigations, but little is yet known of the underlying mechanisms at work. Social support measures have been repeatedly correlated with short- and long-term change, but the addition of social support components to standard behavioral change programs has not been found to yield incremental gains in outcome. Future research on social support might include the stages-of-change model as a framework for answering such questions as the following: How is support perceived by individuals at various points along the continuum of change? What is the natural history of support of successful and unsuccessful changers? And do specific support components influence different processes of change?

References

Baer, J. S., Holt, C. S., & Lichtenstein, E. (1986). Self-efficacy and smoking re-examined: Construct validity and clinical utility. *Journal of Consulting and Clinical Psychology, 54,* 846–852.

Bardsley, P. E., & Beckman, L. J. (1988). The health belief model and entry into alcoholism treatment. *International Journal of the Addictions, 23,* 19–28.

Berkman, L. F. (1984). Assessing the physical health effects of social networks and social support. *Annual Review of Public Health, 5,* 413–432.

Best, J. A. (1980). Mass media, self-management, and smoking modification. In P. O. Davidson & S. M. Davidson (Eds.), *Behavioral medicine: Changing health lifestyles* (pp. 371–390). New York: Brunner/Mazel.

Blazer, D. G. (1982). Social support and mortality in an elderly community population. *American Journal of Epidemiology, 115,* 684–694.

Botvin, G. T., Eng, A., & Williams, C. L. (1980). Preventing the onset of cigarette smoking through life skills training. *Preventive Medicine, 9,* 135–143.

Broadhead, W. E., Kaplan, B. H., James, S. A., Wagner, E. H., Schoenbach, V. J., Grimson, R., Heyden, S., Tibblin, G., & Gehlbach, S. H. (1983). The epidemiologic evidence for a relationship between social support and health. *American Journal of Epidemiology, 117,* 521–537.

Brod, M. I., & Hall, S. M. (1984). Joiners and non-joiners in smoking treatment: A comparison of psychosocial variables. *Addictive Behaviors, 9,* 217–221.

Brownell, K. D. (1982). Obesity: Understanding and treating a serious, prevalent, and refractory disorder. *Journal of Consulting and Clinical Psychology, 50,* 820–840.

Brownell, K. D., Heckerman, C. L., Westlake, R. J., Hayes, S. C., & Monti, P. M. (1978). The effect of couples training and partner cooperativeness in the behavioral treatment of obesity. *Behaviour Research and Therapy, 16,* 323–333.

Brownell, K. D., Kelman, J. H., & Stunkard, A. J. (1983). Treatment of obese children with and without their mothers: Changes in weight and blood pressure. *Pediatrics, 71,* 4.

Brownell, K. D., Marlatt, G. A., Lichtenstein, E., & Wilson, G. T. (1986). Understanding and preventing relapse. *American Psychologist, 41,* 765–782.

Cobb, S. (1976). Social support as a moderator of life stress—presidential address. *Psychosomatic Medicine, 38,* 300–314.

Cohen, S., & McKay, G. (1984). Social support, stress and the buffering hypothesis: A theoretical analysis. In A. Baum, S. E. Taylor, & J. E. Singer (Eds.), *Social psychological aspects of health: Handbook of psychology and health, vol. 4*, (pp. 253–267). Hillsdale, NJ: Erlbaum.

Cohen, S., & Syme, S. L. (Eds.). (1985). *Social support and health.* New York: Academic Press.

Colletti, G., & Brownell, K. D. (1982). The physical and emotional benefits of social support: Applications to obesity, smoking, and alcoholism. In M. Hersen, R. M. Eisler, & P. M. Miller (Eds.), *Progress in behavior modification, vol. 13* (pp. 110–179). New York: Academic Press.

Cooke, C. J., & Meyers, A. (1980). The role of predictor variables in the behavioral treatment of obesity. *Behavioral Assessment, 2,* 59–69.

Coppotelli, H. C., & Orleans, C. T. (1985). Spouse support for smoking cessation maintenance by women. *Journal of Consulting and Clinical Psychology, 53,* 455–460.

Cummings, C., Gordon, J. R., & Marlatt, G. A. (1980). Relapse: Prevention and prediction. In W. R. Miller (Ed.), *The addictive disorders: Treatment of alcoholism, drug abuse, smoking, and obesity* (pp. 291–322). New York: Pergamon.

DiClemente, C. C. (1981). Self-efficacy and smoking cessation maintenance: A preliminary report. *Cognitive Therapy and Research, 5,* 175–187.

DiClemente, C. C., & Prochaska, J. O. (1982). Self change and therapy change of smoking behavior: A comparison of processes of change in cessation and maintenance. *Addictive Behaviors, 7,* 133–142.

DiClemente, C. C., & Prochaska, J. O. (1985). Processes and stages of change: Coping and competence in smoking behavior change. In S. Shiffman & T. Wills (Eds.), *Coping and substance use* (pp. 319–344). New York: Academic Press.

DiClemente, C. C., Prochaska, J. O., & Gilbertini, M. (1985). Self-efficacy and the stages of self-change of smoking. *Cognitive Therapy and Research, 9,* 181–200.

Eisinger, R. A. (1971). Psychosocial predictors of smoking recidivism. *Journal of Health and Social Behavior, 12,* 355–362.

Etringer, B. D., Gregory, V. R., & Lando, H. A. (1984). Influence of group cohesion on the behavioral treatment of smoking. *Journal of Consulting and Clinical Psychology, 52,* 1080–1086.

Frankle, R. T. (1985). Obesity, a family matter: Creating new behavior. *Journal of the American Dietetic Association, 85,* 597–602.

Friedman, M., & Rosenman, R. H. (1974). *Type A behavior and your heart.* New York: Ballantine.

Gale, J. B., Eckhoff, W. T., Mogel, S. F., & Rodnick, J. E. (1984). Factors related to adherence to an exercise program for healthy adults. *Medicine and Science in Sports and Exercise, 16,* 544–549.

Ganster, D. C., & Victor, B. (1988). The impact of social support on mental and physical health. *British Journal of Medical Psychology, 61,* 17–36.

Horn, D. A. (1976). A model for the study of personal choice health behavior. *International Journal of Health Education, 19,* 89–98.

House, J. S., Landis, K. R., & Umberson, D. (1988). Social relationships and health. *Science, 241,* 540–545.

Hundleby, J. D., & Mercer, G. W. (1987). Family and friends as social environments and their relationship to young adolescents' use of alcohol, tobacco, and marijuana. *Journal of Marriage and the Family, 49,* 151–164.

Jenkins, C. D. (1983). Psychosocial and behavioral factors. In N. Kaplan & J. Stamler (Eds.), *Prevention of coronary heart disease* (pp. 98–112). Philadelphia: Saunders.

Kannel, W. B. (1977). Importance of hypertension as a major risk factor in cardiovascular disease in hypertension. In J. Genest, E. Koiw, & O. Kuchel (Eds.), *Hypertension: Physiopathology and treatment* (pp. 888–910). New York: McGraw-Hill.

Kannel, W. B. (1983). An overview of the risk factors for cardiovascular disease. In N. M. Kaplan & J. Stamler (Eds.), *Prevention of coronary heart disease* (pp. 20–32). Philadelphia: Saunders.

Kannel, W. B., Castelli, W. P., & Gordon, T. (1979). Cholesterol in the prediction of athero- sclerotic disease: New perspectives based on the Framingham study. *Annals of Internal Medicine, 90*, 85–91.

Kannel, W. B., Dawber, T. R., & McGee, D. L. (1980). Perspectives on systolic hypertension: The Framingham study. *Circulation, 61*, 1179–1182.

Kannel, W. B., & Eaker, E. D. (1986). Psychosocial and other features of coronary heart disease: Insights from the Framingham study. *American Heart Journal, 112*, 1066–1073.

Kannel, W. B., & Gordon, T. (1974). *The Framingham study: An epidemiological investigation of cardiovascular disease, 18 year follow-up*. (DHEW, Public Health Service, Publication No. NIH 74-599). Washington, DC: Government Printing Office.

Leon, A. S. (1985). Physical activity levels and coronary heart disease: Analysis of epidemio- logic and supporting studies. *Medical Clinics of North America, 9*, 3–40.

Lichtenstein, E. (1982). The smoking problem: A behavioral perspective. *Journal of Consulting and Clinical Psychology, 50*, 804–819.

Marlatt, G. A., & Gordon, J. R. (1980). Determinants of relapse: Implications for the maintenance of behavior change. In P. O. Davidson & S. M. Davidson (Eds.), *Behavioral medicine: Changing health lifestyles* (pp. 410–452). New York: Brunner/Mazel.

Marlatt, G. A., & Gordon, J. R. (Eds.). (1985). *Relapse prevention: Maintenance strategies in addictive behavior change*. New York: Guilford.

Mermelstein, R., Cohen, S., Lichtenstein, E., Baer, J. S., & Kamarck, T. (1986). Social support and smoking cessation and maintenance. *Journal of Consulting and Clinical Psychology, 54*, 447–453.

Miller, P. M., & Sims, K. L. (1981). Evaluation and component analysis of a comprehensive weight control program. *International Journal of Obesity, 5*, 57–66.

Mitchell, R. E., Billings, A. G., & Moos, R. H. (1982). Social support and well-being: Implications for prevention programs. *Journal of Primary Prevention, 3*, 77–98.

Mosbach, P., & Leventhal, H. (1988). Peer group identification and smoking: Implications for intervention. *Journal of Abnormal Psychology, 97*, 238–245.

National Heart, Lung and Blood Institute. (1981). Review panel on coronary-prone behavior and coronary heart disease: A critical review. *Circulation, 63*, 1199–1215.

Ockene, J. K., Hymowitz, N., Sexton, M., & Broste, S. K. (1982). Comparison of patterns of smoking behavior change among smokers in the Multiple Risk Factor Intervention Trial (MRFIT). *Preventive Medicine, 11*, 621–638.

Ockene, J. K., Nuttall, R., Benfari, R. C., Hurwitz, I., & Ockene, I. S. (1981). A psychosocial model of smoking cessation and maintenance of cessation. *Preventive Medicine, 10*, 623–638.

O'Donnell, J. A., Voss, H. L., Clayton, R. R., Slatin, G. T., & Room, R. G. W. (1976). Young men and drugs: A nationwide survey (National Institute on Drug Abuse Research Monograph No. 5). Washington, DC: Government Printing Office.

Page, L. B. (1976). Epidemiologic evidence on etiology of human hypertension and its possible prevention. *American Heart Journal, 91*, 527–534.

Prochaska, J. O. (1979). *Systems of psychotherapy: A transtheoretical analysis*. Homewood, IL: Dorsey.

Prochaska, J. O. & DiClemente, C. C. (1982). Transtheoretical therapy: Toward a more integrative model of change. *Psychotherapy: Theory, Research, Practice, 19*, 276–288.

Prochaska, J. O., & DiClemente, C. C. (1983). Stages and processes of self-change of smoking: Toward an integrative model of change. *Journal of Clinical and consulting Psychology, 51*, 390–395.

Prochaska, J. O., & DiClemente, C. C. (1988). Measuring processes of change: Applications to the cessation of smoking. *Journal of Consulting and Clinical Psychology, 56,* 520–528.

Rickarby, G. A. (1981). Psychosocial dynamics in obesity. *Medical Journal of Australia, 2,* 602.

Rosen, T. J., & Shipley, R. H. (1983). A stage analysis of self-initiated smoking reductions. *Addictive Behaviors, 8,* 263–272.

Rosenthal, B., Allen, G. J., & Winter, C. (1980). Husband involvement in the behavioral treatment of overweight women: Initial effects and long-term follow-up. *International Journal of Obesity, 4,* 165–173.

Schachter, S. (1982). Recidivism and self-cure of smoking and obesity. *American Psychologist, 37,* 436–444.

Sjoberg, L., & Samsonvitz, V. (1978). Volitional problems in trying to quit smoking. *Scandinavian Journal of Psychology, 19,* 205–212.

Stamler, J. (1978). Lifestyles, major risk factors, proof and public policy. *Circulation, 58,* 3–19.

Stamler, J. Wentworth, D., & Neaton, J. D. (1986). Prevalence and prognostic significance of hypercholesterolemia in men with hypertension. *American Journal of Medicine, 80*(Suppl. 2A), 33–39.

Superko, H. R., Wood, P. D., & Haskell, W. L. (1985). Coronary heart disease and risk factor modification: Is there a threshold? *American Journal of Medicine, 78,* 826–838.

Thom, T. J., & Kannel, W. B. (1981). Downward trend in cardiovascular mortality. *Annual Review of Medicine, 32,* 427–434.

Umberson, D. (1987). Family status and health behaviors: Social control as a dimension of social integration. *Journal of Health and Social Behavior, 28,* 306–319.

U.S. Department of Health and Human Services. (1989). *Reducing the health consequences of smoking: 25 years of progress. A report of the Surgeon General* (DHHS Publication No. CDC 89-8411). Washington, DC: Government Printing Office.

Velicer, W. F., DiClemente, C. C., Prochaska, J. O., & Brandenburg, N. (1985). A decision balance measure for assessing and predicting smoking status. *Journal of Personality and Social Psychology, 48,* 1279–1289.

Wallston, B. S., Alagna, S. W., DeVellis, B. M., & DeVellis, R. F. (1983). Social support and physical health. *Health Psychology, 2,* 367–391.

West, D. W., Graham, S., Swanson, M., & Wilkinson, G. (1977). Five year follow-up of a smoking withdrawal clinic population. *American Journal of Public Health, 67,* 536–544.

Wilcox, N. S., Prochaska, J. O., Velicer, W. F., & DiClemente, C. C. (1985). Subject characteristics as predictors of self-change in smoking. *Addictive Behaviors, 10,* 407–412.

Wills, T. A. (1985). Supportive functions of interpersonal relationships. In S. Cohen & S. L. Syme (Eds.), *Social support and health* (pp. 61–82). New York: Academic Press.

Wilson, G. T., & Brownell, K. (1978). Behavior therapy for obesity: Including family members in the treatment process. *Behavior Therapy, 9,* 943–945.

Witschi, J. C., Singer, M., Wu-Lee, M., & Stare, F. J. (1978). Family cooperation and effectiveness in a cholesterol-lowering diet. *Journal of the American Dietetic Association, 72,* 384–388.

Wyndham, C. H. (1979). The role of physical activity in the prevention of ischemic heart disease. *South African Medical Journal, 36,* 7–13.

PART V

The Crisis and Rehabilitation Phases of Cardiovascular Disease

CHAPTER 12

Social Support and the Progression and Treatment of Cardiovascular Disease

Larry Gorkin, Michael J. Follick, Dianne L. Wilkin, and Raymond Niaura

The purpose of this chapter is to assess the influence of social support on both the progression and the treatment of cardiovascular disease. This review involves an in-depth discussion of the literature relating specifically to social support and the course of established coronary artery disease (CAD). Less emphasis is placed on the role of support in the etiology of cardiovascular disease among asymptomatic populations. Studies aimed at social support and disease onset or risk factor reduction among populations without cardiac disease are utilized only as relevant to the main thrust of the review.

The term *social support* generally refers to the availability of relationships that convey to an individual the feeling that he or she is cared about, valued, or loved (Sarason, Levine, Basham, & Sarason, 1983). Some of the distinctions that have been drawn between different types of support within social relationships include attachment, social integration, guidance, opportunity for nurturance and reassurance of worth (Weiss, 1974). Most of the literature on social support and cardiovascular disease—including that relied upon primarily in this chapter—refers to support provided by the significant other of the patient or that supplied by health care professionals in medical or postmedical discharge settings.

LARRY GORKIN, MICHAEL J. FOLLICK, and DIANNE L. WILKIN • Institute for Behavioral Medicine, Cranston, Rhode Island 02920.   RAYMOND NIAURA • Division of Behavioral Medicine, Miriam Hospital, Providence, Rhode Island 02906.

Social Support and Cardiovascular Disease, edited by Sally A. Shumaker and Susan M. Czajkowski. Plenum Press, New York, 1994.

Models relating support to health outcomes have long been speculative. Early work in this area proposed support as a buffer against life stress (Cobb, 1976), whereas more recent work has proposed a more active role for support. In the area of recovery from cardiovascular disease, one hypothesized model holds that support modulates distress levels and subsequent cardiac symptoms (Fontana, Kerns, Rosenberg, & Colonese, 1989). In this model, however, these relationships suffer from inadequate internal consistency, instability over time, and a modest amount of variance explained.

This review has six sections: (a) background on the multivariate effects of symptomatic cardiovascular disease, particularly following myocardial infarction (MI), on the patient and social support system; (b) studies of stress, support, and disease progression; (c) epidemiological evidence relating naturally occurring support levels to the progression of cardiovascular disease; (d) the impact of interventions with the patient's family support system; (e) the impact of social support, in terms of secondary prevention interventions conducted by health professions with post-MI patients; and (f) directions for future research.

The following discussion should be viewed not only in terms of the individual with cardiovascular disease, but also in terms of the family life cycle in which the cardiac events occur. The impact of and the response to such events can vary depending on whether, for example, the patient is a primary wage earner with dependent children, a single person at any age, or part of a retirement couple whose children have left home. Whereas individuals at a younger age may be better able to cope with both physical or psychological change than the older adult, the impact upon the family may be far greater for the younger couple. Older men who may be unable or unwilling to return to work and who suddenly become dependent on their families may find it especially difficult to redefine roles and learn to relinquish control (Obier, MacPherson, & Haywood, 1977). Because the majority of symptomatic patients are married males above the age of 40, there are often specific concerns regarding the patient's ability to provide economically for his or her spouse and children, and possibly for his or her parents. It will be argued, accordingly, that the degree of disease progression and recovery will be determined in part by these complex familial patterns and interactions.

Symptomatic Cardiovascular Disease Effects on Patient and Support System

Improvements in coronary care have led to increased survival of acute MI, but patients and families are nonetheless confronted with incontrovertible evidence relating to their own mortality and much uncertainty regarding the future. Major therapeutic interventions (e.g., coronary artery bypass grafting, percutaneous transluminal angioplasty, or more invasive interventions, such as the automatic implantable cardioverter-defibrillator [AICD]) may prove necessary to sustain life. Such interventions, however, may leave patients with compromised ventricular functioning (Packer, 1987) or prone to ventricular tachycardia and fibrillation, precursors of sudden cardiac death. Thus the patient and family members must live with uncertainty regarding the patient's clinical status.

In addition to physical discomfort, post-MI patients and/or patients with malignant arrhythmias often experience deteriorations in both psychological status (e.g., depression, anger, anxiety, hypervigilance, or demanding behavioral styles) and functional status (e.g., unemployment, social isolation; Follick et al., 1988; Mayou, Foster, & Williamson, 1978). Depression may lead to a loss of interest, energy, and an inability to concentrate; sleep, appetitive, and sexual disturbances may emerge. Moreover, many patients (as well as spouses) will fear what they perceive are drastic, permanent, and possibly unrealistic changes that have to be made in their life-styles. Among those patients who experience an uncomplicated MI (i.e., higher ventricular functioning, low rates of arrhythmias, and no ischemia during exercise testing), many will avoid activities because of perceived rather than actual risk (Taylor, Bandura, Ewart, Miller, & DeBusk, 1985).

Deteriorations in psychological and functional status are of primary concern because they often predict subsequent clinical events and can adversely affect the quality of patients' lives. Higher levels of depression, for example, have been associated with increased coronary events among patients undergoing cardiac catheterization (Carney et al., 1988), and with mortality among patients with sustained ventricular tachycardia undergoing electrophysiological stimulation studies (Kennedy, Hofer, & Cohen, 1987). In the post-MI Cardiac Arrhythmia Pilot Study (CAPS), self-reported depression levels predicted mortality or cardiac arrest after adjusting for such measures of disease severity as ejection fraction (EF) and ventricular premature depolarization (VPD) rates (Ahern et al., 1989). Higher levels of depression or anxiety have also predicted lack of short-term improvement as determined by a combination of electrocardiographic and enzyme testing and self-reported pain (Pancheri et al., 1978; Stern, Pascale, & Ackerman, 1977) and a longer latency to return to work (Hlatky et al., 1986).

Shifts in emotional status may also be important because of their relationship to sympathetic nervous system (SNS) activity and subsequent clinical events. Among the survivors of cardiac arrest, acute surges in SNS activity in a predominantly non-MI population may predispose the patient to ventricular fibrillation (Verrier & Lown, 1984; Vlay & Fricchione, 1985). Among post-MI patients, it may be the sustained lack of SNS activity during emotional and physical arousal, as reflected in reduced beat-to-beat heartrate variability, that is important to sudden cardiac death (Kleiger et al., 1987; Rich et al., 1988). In the CAPS study, lack of pulse rate changes from resting baseline in response to psychological challenge was associated with increased mortality or cardiac arrest, even when controlling for severity of disease (Ahern et al., 1989). It may be that the relationship of SNS arousal and concomitant emotional arousal to cardiac-related mortality may depend in part on the presence of cardiovascular disease. These results would be consistent with the emerging pattern suggesting that Type A behavior pattern is predictive of infarct among initially asymptomatic patients (Rosenman, Brand, Sholtz, & Friedman, 1976), but that Type B behavior pattern is predictive of mortality among symptomatic patients (Ahern et al., 1989; Ragland & Brand, 1988).

Many of the emotional strains that affect the patient recovering from an MI, sudden death, or coronary surgery are shared by members of the patient's support system. More than one third of the spouses of post-MI patients, for example, have reported sustained feelings of general anxiety and depression (Skelton & Dominian, 1973) at or near patient levels (Dracup, Guzy, Taylor, & Barry, 1986; Mayou et al., 1978). Moreover, the percentage of spouses experiencing these symptoms is increasing (Thompson & Cordle, 1988). The couple's recreational pursuits may be affected most significantly (Langeluddecke, Tennante, Fulcher, Barid, & Hughes, 1989), including loss of interest in sex (Thompson & Cordle, 1988). The most common reason for decreased sexual activity among convalescing cardiac patients is spousal restraint (Johnston et al., 1978) attributable in part to fears that resumption of sexual activity could cause further harm (Sikorski, 1985).

Such feelings and concerns may result in excessive restrictions being applied to the patient (Taylor et al., 1985). Overly solicitous family members will often assume many of the patient's previously performed routine household tasks. In such cases, the patient may respond with depression and excessive dependency, and spouses in turn may become irritated and impatient with patients' dependent behaviors. Members of the support system who may be forced to take on new roles within the family may harbor feelings of resentment (albeit often unexpressed) toward the patient.

Conversely, use of denial to avoid the emotional impact of an MI is an important consideration to both short- and long-term recovery of patients. A patient's tendency toward denial, in combination with degree of exposure to educational information concerning cardiovascular disease and its treatment, may influence patient outcomes (Shaw, Cohen, Doyle, & Palesky, 1985). Following discharge for an acute MI, "nondeniers" with insufficient information and "deniers" with information overexposure reported poorer medical or social functioning outcomes at 6-month follow-up (Shaw et al., 1985).

Denial also may be manifested by patient delays in seeking medical management, nonadherence to medical recommendations, or by not adopting behaviors consistent with a healthier life-style. Although denial may provide short-term beneficial effects, long-term adverse effects have been demonstrated (Hackett & Cassem, 1974). For example, higher deniers demonstrated fewer signs of cardiac dysfunction during hospitalization and spent fewer days in intensive care than lower deniers, but the high deniers showed less adaptation to disease and had required more days of rehospitalization at a 1-year follow-up (Levine et al., 1987). One rationale for this interaction of denial and time may be that denial serves to minimize stress responses and thereby may decrease one's short-term risk for sudden cardiac death, but results in the avoidance of instrumental responses that increase long-term survival. These instrumental responses may include cardiac rehabilitative efforts as well as a recognition of clinical signs and symptoms of disease.

Implications for patient behavior producing long-term survival or increased quality of life following survival have become even more critical in recent years. In the age of antithrombolytic treatment for a reinfarction, there appears to be a therapeutic "window" of just a few hours in which the agents have their greatest impact in limiting infarct size and ventricular compromise. Thus a delay in the initiation of efforts to identify symptoms of impending infarction will produce dire consequences in a relatively brief period of time.

Infrahuman Investigations

Advantages of the use of animal models to study the influence of social support or social competition on coronary heart disease (CHD) are many, including reliable access to large numbers and the ability to induce systematically both acute ischemic events and long-term atherogenesis, as well as such predictors of sudden cardiac death as ventricular ectopy and compromised ventricular functioning. Limitations of the animal model include the tenuous generalizability from the infrahuman anatomy and social interactions to the human anatomy and human relationships, respectively (Clarkson, Kaplan, Adams, & Manuck, 1987).

The effect of social threat on vulnerability to cardiac disease has recently been investigated using infrahumans (Verrier, Hagestad, & Lown, 1987). Test dogs were altered surgically to simulate the development of coronary stenosis, presented with a dish of food, and allowed to eat a few bites before the dish was removed from reach. A competitor dog was then introduced who attempted to eat the remaining food. This introduction led reliably to aggressive actions by the test dog (e.g., growling, pilo-erection, teeth baring). The provocative animal was then removed. During the immediate recovery period, high rates of S-T segment changes indicative of ischemia on the electrocardiogram were observed. Such ischemic changes are well established as predictors of subsequent clinical events (e.g., Theroux, Waters, Halphen, Debaisieux, & Mizgala, 1979). Although the authors interpreted the paradigm in terms of establishing an angerlike state, the evidence also supports the contention that social provocation and competition can contribute to the deterioration of myocardial function. This argument assumes that social competitiveness is the inverse of social support, although the social support literature has tended to consider social isolation or lack of supportive others (rather than competitiveness) to be the opposite of social support (e.g., Cohen, 1988).

Some support for the competitiveness conceptualization was observed when assessing the influence of social stressors on coronary atherosclerosis among cynomologous monkeys (Kaplan, Manuck, Clarkson, Lusso, & Taub, 1982). These monkeys were chosen because their social interactive patterns and atherosclerotic plaque formations appear to approximate human behavior and human anatomy, respectively. The monkeys were reared in groups of four to six, and dominant and submissive males were categorized in the group hierarchy; these status rankings were found to be 75% to 80% stable over a 2-year period. Kaplan et al. manipulated the degree of social instability (reorganizing group membership or keeping group composition constant). Results indicated that a significant interaction emerged in which dominant monkeys in the unstable environment had significantly greater coronary artery atherosclerosis than submissive cohorts in this environment; in contrast, less atherosclerotic disease was observed among dominant monkeys relative to submissive ones in the relatively stable environment. These results suggest that the continual challenges faced by dominant males in unstable surroundings (e.g., competition for food, water, perch space, and mates) contributed to the atherogenic effect observed. As discussed later in this chapter, these results have implications for the study of the progression of atherosclerotic disease as well (see also Chapter 10).

The degree of maternal support may also influence progression of cardiovascular disease. Among rats, there are strains known to be predisposed to hypertension (SHR) and those predisposed to normal blood pressure (WKY). These differences emerge quite early in life, perhaps in utero (Cierpial, Konarska, & McCarty, 1988). In a randomized trial starting on the day after birth, SHR and WKY litters were reared by either their natural mothers, mothers of the same strain, or mothers of the opposite strain. Results indicated that the SHR litter reared by WKY mothers did not demonstrate the hypertensive effect observed for similar litters reared by natural or same-strain mothers. The authors (Cierpial et al., 1988) attribute these results to nutritional factors (e.g., nursing opportunities, parameters of milk). There is the possibility, though, that differences in SHR and WKY strains may exist in terms of maternal support levels. Consistent with this argument are the results of early experiments in monkeys manipulating the type and degree of maternal comfort (Harlow & Harlow, 1966). Clearly, the absence of maternal support was observed to have profound effects on the social and sexual development of the monkeys. It would be of interest to examine whether the lack of maternal support in infrahumans hastens the onset and progression of coronary artery disease and its sequelae.

Human Evidence

Epidemiological Investigations

The epidemiological literature is divided among those studies that have found network access is important and those that have found that perceived support is the key parameter. In this segment we will explore both, beginning with network support. In a study of psychosocial predictors of survival following an acute MI (Ruberman, Weinblatt, Goldberg, & Chaudhary, 1984), two factors emerged from the 3-year follow-up period as significant: (a) high degree of life stress (e.g., forced retirement, violent crime victim, breakup of marriage); and (b) social isolation status (e.g., marital status, belonging to any social or religious organization, or making visits to others). Results indicated that the combination of high stress and high social isolation produced a fourfold increase in mortality risk, particularly as a result of sudden cardiac death, in comparison to low levels of either factor alone. This interactive effect held for groups both low and high in rates of ventricular ectopy.

In another study of postcoronary patients, marital status (i.e., married, single, divorced, separated, or widowed) was found to discriminate survivors versus nonsurvivors among male and female acute MI patients (Chandra, Szklo, Goldberg, & Tonascia, 1983). Results indicated that for both inpatient and postdischarge survival rates, marital status at the time of the acute MI was associated with increased longevity independent of other factors (e.g., age, gender, smoking history, angina, cardiac complications following qualifying MI, prior history of MI). In a study of hospitalized coronary bypass patients, those who were married and received more frequent spouse visits following surgery took less pain medication and recovered more quickly than their less-supported married counterparts (Kulik & Mahler, 1989). Quality of the marital relationship did not alter these findings.

Results from these correlative studies suggest that differential death rates following emergency admissions to the hospital may occur in part because of the presence or absence of a concerned spouse. The mere presence of someone capable of initiating lifesaving strategies (e.g., initiating cardiopulmonary resuscitation, or phoning for help) may reduce the time to receive cardiac care when faced with a recurrence of clinical events. Alternatively, the postdischarge mortality rates may have occurred because of the lesser preparedness of post-MI patients living alone to care adequately for themselves and, thus, to prevent a recurrent clinical event.

Data congruent with an interpretation based on intimacy in these supportive relationships has been offered recently (Williams et al., 1992). Patients with cardiovascular disease were found to have a threefold higher mortality risk if either unmarried or without a close confidant as compared to patients with a spouse or confidant, after controlling for severity of disease. Perhaps the availability of a confidant provides a feeling of being cared for and security about having someone who would help in times of need.

Perceptions of support provided by a caring individual relate to coronary angiographic findings as well (Seeman & Syme, 1987). Feelings of being loved and beliefs that others would be available in times of need predicted the degree of coronary atherosclerosis better than network support (e.g., marital status, belonging to organizations, number of friends), after controlling for known risk factors of CHD (e.g., serum cholesterol, hypertension, diabetes).

The results from this angiographic study are supported by a recent prospective study conducted as part of the Cardiac Arrhythmia Suppression Trial–1 (CAST–1). This study (Gorkin et al., 1992) was designed to evaluate the influence of several psychosocial variables (e.g., distress, perceived support, social interaction) on mortality, while adjusting for measures of severity of disease (e.g., left ventricular ejection fraction, arrhythmia rates, CHD risk factors). In CAST–1, treatment medications (encainide and flecainide) were powerful multivariate predictors of mortality along with, for example, ejection fraction. In contrast, none of the psychosocial variables emerged significantly in the multivariate model. Accordingly, the mortality analysis conducted was restricted to placebo subjects to eliminate the effect of treatment. Among patients randomized to placebo, the level of perceived social support was a significant multivariate predictor of mortality, adjusting for measures of disease severity. Social support was defined as a 5-point Likert item that assessed perceived availability of instrumental support (e.g., someone to talk to or help with daily chores). The adjusted hazards ratio for a 1-point decrease in the perceived support score, based on a multivariate model, is equal to 1.46.

The relationship of support to disease progression may also be modified by demographic factors. Sex differences, for example, may emerge, as in the study of the effects of social support on diabetic control among men and women with type II diabetes (Kaplan & Hartwell, 1987). Diabetic control was defined as glycosylated hemoglobin (HbA1C). Results indicated that a high level of perceived support was associated with less diabetic control in men, whereas it was associated with greater diabetic control for women. In contrast to the effects of support on women, it may be that forms of support that are satisfactory to men may reinforce patterns of eating, drinking, and exercise that are incompatible with diabetic control. Consistent with this perspective, it was found that husband's food preference, regardless of nutritional content, was the best predictor of meals served in the Family Heart Study (Weidner, Healy, & Matarazzo, 1985).

In certain circumstances, therefore, supportive relationships may actually hinder rehabilitative efforts. In studies involving significant others of patients with chronic low back pain, for example, overly solicitous family members have frequently been associated with greater patient impairment (e.g., Flor, Kerns, & Turk, 1987). Interestingly, male patients in this study with more solicitous spouses reported greater marital satisfaction than patients with less solicitous spouses.

Family Member Support

Cardiac rehabilitation is a social process that can be facilitated or impeded by the attitudes and behaviors of patients as well as those of spouses and other family members. One of the major problems experienced by the post-MI patient is that the family members will often perceive the patient as incapacitated by the clinical event. This perception is strengthened if the family members feel impotent to act in the face of reoccurrence or exacerbation of clinical symptoms. Educating the supportive individual(s) in terms of prognosis and expectations for recovery, as well as providing training in behaviors that will enhance the likelihood of positive outcomes, has been recommended (Dracup et al., 1986). For several reasons, significant others are positioned to shape the behavior of the patient. First, they can monitor the patient's behavior and encourage direct adherence to the prescribed medical, dietary, and psychological regimens. A second means of behavior influence is by role modeling, that is, by engaging themselves in the target behaviors to promote such change. If a spouse changes his or her health habits simultaneously with the patient, the act of mutual engagement and encouragement in health-promoting behaviors may decrease the perceived and actual difficulty of succeeding at behavior change.

Several investigators have examined the role of support specifically in the treatment of hypercholesterolemia, which is based on adherence to drug or diet regimens. It is estimated that 15% to 20% of American adults have cholesterol levels exceeding 240 mg/dL, placing them at increased risk for CHD mortality (Grundy, 1986). Adherence with drugs or dietary treatments is poor; in the Diet-Heart Trial, for example, only 25% of the subjects were judged to be compliant (Mojonnier & Hall, 1968). Moreover, adherence with a low-cholesterol drug treatment has been observed to deteriorate with time (Lipid Research Clinics Programs [LRCP], 1984).

Among the available behavioral strategies, social support interventions may offer the most promise in terms of producing adherence with cholesterol-lowering treatments. Eating habits and lipid changes in response to dietary interventions tend to covary within families (Witschi, Singer, Wu-Lee, & Stare, 1978). Although not targeted explicitly, early efforts at dietary interventions have recognized the importance of including family members, particularly the spouse, in educational efforts to lower cholesterol (Farquhar et al., 1977; Multiple Risk Factor Intervention Trial [MRFIT] Research Group, 1982). Wives of prospective subjects were offered a free lipid analysis when they came in with their husbands. This strategy was based on the belief that interest in the recruitment process and subsequent adherence with dietary modifications would be enhanced by spouse involvement as early as possible (LRCP, 1984).

Of course, the lack of social support among family members may contribute to more adverse outcomes. Stressful life events anteceded hospitalization more often in a group of patients with heart failure living with close relatives than patients, matched for age and gender, living in a nursing home or domiciliary facility (Perlman, Ferguson, Bergun, Isenberg, & Hammarsten, 1971). The authors speculated that emotional life events were more likely to trigger overt heart failure for patients living with relatives than those not living with their relatives.

One context in which support systems are viewed as critical is in the prevention of sudden cardiac death, which is more likely to occur outside the hospital, and often in the home (Simon & Alonzo, 1973). Given that patient survival is inversely related to the length of time between symptom occurrence and the performance of cardiopulmonary resuscitation (CPR), training family members in CPR is a logical intervention. In addition to potential benefits by saving lives, it has been hypothesized (Vlay & Fricchione, 1985) that training family members in CPR would produce psychological benefits to cardiac patients and their families. This hypothesis was tested in a recent study with a mixed group of cardiac patients at varying risk for sudden death and their families. Family members were assigned to one of three groups: CPR training, risk factor reduction education, or no-intervention waiting-list control (Dracup et al., 1986). Patients were mostly married Caucasian males; family members were mostly female Caucasians who were spouses of the cardiac patients. Patients and family members in all three groups were assessed at baseline and at 3- and 6-month follow-ups.

Results indicated that psychological distress levels of family members were not influenced by type of intervention, whereas patients were slightly more anxious than control patients at the 3-month follow-up. Patients in either the CPR or risk factor education group reported poorer adjustment to illness relative to the control group at the 3- and 6-month follow-ups. It is clear, therefore, that the CPR intervention did not produce the desired psychological effects.

The authors suggest several possible reasons for these results. Perhaps the denial that often occurs during the acute MI period was more difficult to maintain because CPR training made the possibility of sudden death more salient. Another contributing factor may have been doubts regarding sufficient training of the spouse to be helpful in case of cardiac arrest. In terms of support factors, perhaps the added sense of responsibility experienced by family members or the increased sense of dependency of patients contributes to these findings. Not addressed during traditional CPR training, adverse outcomes may be generated by the negative feelings experienced by all involved.

Data from our laboratory may address these post hoc explanations regarding the failure of CPR training to produce improvements in emotional status of patients and family members. Follick et al. (1988) studied the impact of a transtelephonic electrocardiographic (ECG) monitor on the quality of life in post-MI patients. This was a prospective randomized trial in which patients were assigned to either a transtelephonic ECG system condition or a standard hospital care condition. Upon experiencing symptoms of acute MI, patients were instructed to forward an ECG strip by phone to be read for the presence of malignant arrhythmic activity.

Patients who received the system reported significantly less concern about physical functioning and symptoms and, over time, reported less depressive affect than those patients assigned to standard hospital care. Moreover, a greater percentage of system patients returned to work by the 9-month follow-up than control patients.

These findings call into question the speculation by Dracup et al. (1986) that CPR training made patient and family member denial more difficult to maintain and sudden death more salient, because the ECG monitoring intervention would be expected to have the same effect. The major distinguishing characteristic between the two studies is the form of support system—a significant other in the Dracup et al. (1986) study and a mechanical device in the Follick et al. (1988) study. Perhaps when responsibility for one's life is seemingly given to another (which is likely to occur when CPR is learned for potential use with a specific individual), feelings of dependency and the burden of responsibility for patients and partners, respectively can lead to resentment on both sides. This hypothesis was supported by Dracup, Taylor, Guzy, and Brecht (1991), who tested the interaction of CPR training for family members and discussion of psychosocial issues following training. The psychological deficits observed among patients whose family members learned CPR were eliminated if the family members were exposed to a one-time nursing discussion of psychological issues following CPR training. At present we are testing a randomized trial of videotapes addressing family issues in CPR (e.g., dependency, loss of identity, fear of actually performing CPR) versus a control dietary videotape on functional and emotional status of patients and partners after the latter have learned CPR. Dependent measures include emotional and functional states of patients and partners, as well as the latters' retention of CPR skills.

Other interventions with family members may prove helpful. As noted previously, a frequent concern of the wife of the MI patient involves her anxiety over her husband's level of activity (Sikorski, 1985). To address this concern directly, a unique social support intervention was conducted with male post-MI patients and their spouses (Taylor et al., 1985). During the patient's exercise tolerance testing (ETT) at week 3, each wife was randomly assigned either to remain in the waiting room, to observe the ETT, or to observe ETT plus perform 3 minutes on the treadmill at her husband's peak workload. Results indicated that at baseline, husbands rated their capacity to handle physical and cardiac stressors significantly higher than did their wives. Furthermore, wives who did not have actual treadmill experience did not significantly alter their ratings post-ETT. In contrast, those wives who experienced the treadmill increased their ratings of their husband's capabilities following ETT. Thus an intervention that increases the confidence of a spouse regarding her partner's capabilities following an MI may have generalized benefits in terms of cardiac recovery and rehabilitation. This hypothesis, however, awaits empirical confirmation in studies that assess actual patient and spouse interactions.

Staff Support

The increasing evidence for a direct relationship between the level of support and clinical outcome from cardiovascular disease has renewed interest in the role played by hospital staff support. Although not often studied, lack of staff social support can impair the health of patients with chronic illness (e.g., end-stage renal disease; Wertzel, Vollrath, Ritz, & Ferner, 1977). Presumably this lack of support may also be found in the care of patients with established cardiac disease, such as class IV congestive heart failure.

In contrast, a study conducted in a cardiac care unit (CCU) points to the positive influence of social support as regards the frequency of ventricular ectopy (Lynch, Thomas, Paskewitz, Katcher, & Weir, 1977). Premature ventricular contraction (PVC) rates were analyzed during human contact involving routine nursing care. Rates of PVCs were also analyzed immediately prior to periods of nursing contact as a baseline control assessment. Results indicated that routine nursing contact was associated with a significant reduction in PVC frequency, particularly among patients with higher rates of PVCs (i.e., more than 3 ectopic beats/minute). These results, although correlational, are impressive given the tremendous degree of natural variability in PVC rates (Pratt et al., 1987).

These data do not point directly to a staff-initiated social support phenomenon, but results are clearly consistent with this interpretation. The routine care periods, it is argued, are more likely to provide reassurance to the patient; nonroutine and emergency care are less likely to reassure the patient, but are conducted as deemed necessary to avoid ventricular tachycardia and subsequent sudden cardiac death.

A crisis intervention program among 539 male survivors of an uncomplicated MI (Frasure-Smith & Prince, 1985) also contained elements of social support as part of its treatment approach. No single theory or approach to stress reduction was tested; instead, nurses with a manageable caseload and access to referral and consultative services constituted the intervention in this prospective randomized design. The experimental treatment consisted of monthly telephone calls involving a psychological distress interview; high stress scores resulted in home visits, and rehospitalization resulted in bedside visits. Control subjects were contacted by phone twice during the study, but these calls did not lead to nurse interventions. These phone assessments were simply for recording purposes.

Results revealed that the intervention program was effective in lowering stress scores by the end of the 1-year follow-up, although there were no differences in rehospitalizations between groups. The striking finding was that experimental patients were 47% less likely to die from ischemic heart disease than were control patients. After 4 months, there was a clear divergence of the two groups with regard to patient mortality (a 70% reduction in mortality). This finding compares favorably with the beneficial effects of beta-blocking medications on mortality incidence (Beta Blocker Heart Attack Trial Research Group, 1982; Norwegian Multicenter Study Group, 1981).

Although not designed originally as a social support study, social support was an important element of the experimental manipulation. In the absence of a specific intervention system, nurses offered help (both functional and emotional) to post-MI patients during periods of physical and psychological trauma. On average, each high stress patient received 5 to 6 hours of home nursing contact. More than half of the visits by the nurse did not result in consultation to other health practitioners; thus it appears that a relationship was established with a competent and caring individual.

Directions for Future Research

Researchers assessing the role of social support in the progression and treatment of CHD have just begun to define the questions to be asked, the paradigms and the measures to be utilized, and the interventions to be evaluated. The evidence reviewed suggests that social support may influence progression of cardiovascular disease via the course of atherosclerotic development and the triggers of sudden cardiac death. These initial findings warrant further systematic investigation to confirm and clarify these relationships.

In terms of the infrahuman literature, Verrier et al. (1987) have introduced a provocative paradigm demonstrating the negative effects of social competition on cardiac function. It would be valuable to investigate the positive influence of support in infrahumans. Perhaps introducing food plus a nonthreatening dog into the Verrier et al. paradigm would raise the threshold for arrhythmias compared to food alone.

Clarkson et al. (1987) provide an infrahuman paradigm in which to study the interaction of social and biological mechanisms in the progression of coronary artery disease. Dominant monkeys show greater aggression, vigilance, and atherosclerotic disease relative to submissive monkeys under conditions of environmental instability and challenge. Because stress-related heart rate increases are related to increased atherosclerosis among monkeys fed a high-cholesterol diet (Manuck, Kaplan, & Clarkson, 1983), this may provide a mechanism to explain the interactive relationships of social status, social stress, aggression, and diet to progression of coronary atherosclerotic disease. The Clarkson et al. (1987) research design could be modified to include monkeys with coronary atherosclerotic disease documented angiographically; these monkeys could then be assigned randomly to either stable or unstable environments. Such a design would enable one to determine the influence of social status, social competition, and dietary cholesterol on the progression of atherosclerotic disease.

In humans, the Frasure-Smith and Prince (1985, 1987) trial of a nursing crisis intervention program with post-MI patients demonstrated an impressive effect on mortality for the intervention. The authors posed competing hypotheses involving reduced sympathetic tone attributable to either the direct effect of support on the vasculature or the indirect effect of increasing adherence to beta-adrenergic blocking medication. Future research could clarify the mechanism involved by obtaining process measures of stress responding (e.g., mental arithmetic as a beta-adrenergic task, down-regulation of beta receptors), and adherence to the medication regimen (e.g., electronic recorders). The implication is that social support is often confounded with other factors (e.g., various treatment modalities, actual medical intervention), preventing an isolation of the effects of social support itself on outcomes. Future studies need to be designed to test social support effects more cleanly.

This review focused on two types of support for symptomatic patients, one involving familial systems and the other involving hospital staff systems. To date there has been no comparative trial of the relative impact of benefits and costs associated with each treatment modality. The promising results in both areas of intervention point to the need for more commensurate comparisons and would also facilitate the testing of the interaction (i.e., of having simultaneous family and staff interventions) on patient outcomes. For example, a study of the impact of physical exercise on class II and III heart failure patients is of recent interest (Sullivan, Higginbotham, & Cobb, 1988). Within such a trial, interventions aimed at increasing patient involvement in the physical regimen could also be tested. Support interventions aimed at spouse participation in exercise and staff interventions triggered by absenteeism from the exercise regimen could be evaluated for their relative contributions to improvements in exercise tolerance, medication adherence, quality of life, hormonal profiles, ventricular functioning, and mortality.

References

Ahern, D. K., Gorkin, L., Anderson, J. L., Tierney, C., Hallstrom, A., & Ewart, C., for the Cardiac Arrhythmia Pilot Study (CAPS) Investigators. (November, 1989). *Biobehavioral variables and mortality or cardiac arrest in the CAPS*. Paper presented at the annual meeting of the American Heart Association, New Orleans.

Beta Blocker Heart Attack Trial Research Group. (1982). A randomized trial of propranolol in patients with acute myocardial infarction: I. Mortality results. *Journal of the American Medical Association, 247*, 1707–1714.

Blumei thal, J. A., Burg, M. M., Barefoot, J., Williams, R. B., Haney, T., & Zimet, G. (1987). Social support, Type A behavior, and coronary artery disease. *Psychosomatic Medicine, 49*, 331–340.

Carney, R. M., Rich, M. W., Freedland, K. E., Saini, J., teVelde, A., Simeone, C., & Clark, K. (1988). Major depressive disorder predicts cardiac events in patients with coronary artery disease. *Psychosomatic Medicine, 50*, 627–633.

Chandra, V., Szklo, M., Goldberg, R., & Tonascia, J. (1983). The impact of marital status on survival after an acute myocardial infarction: A population-based study. *American Journal of Epidemiology, 117*, 320—325.

Cierpial, M. A., Konarska, M., & McCarty, R. (1988). Maternal effects on the development of spontaneous hypertension. *Health Psychology, 7*, 125–135.

Clarkson, T. B., Kaplan, J. R., Adams, D. V. M., & Manuck, S. B. (1987). Psychosocial influences on the pathogenesis of atherosclerosis among nonhuman primates. *Circulation, 76*(Suppl. 1), 29–40.

Cobb, S. (1976). Social support as a moderator of life stress. *Psychosomatic Medicine, 38*, 300–314.

Cohen, S. (1988). Psychosocial models of the role of social support in the etiology of physical disease. *Health Psychology, 7*, 269–297.

Dracup, K., Guzy, P. M., Taylor, S. E., & Barry, J. (1986). Cardiopulmonary resuscitation (CPR) training: Consequences for family members of high-risk cardiac patients. *Archives of Internal Medicine, 146*, 1757–1761.

Dracup, K., Taylor, S. E., Guzy, P. M., & Brecht, M. L. (1991). *Consequences of cardiopulmonary training for family members of cardiac patients*. Final report to National Heart, Lung, and Blood Institute for Grant RO1 HL32171, University of California at Los Angeles.

Farquhar, J. W., Maccoby, N., Wood, P. D., Alexander, J. K., Breitrose, H., Brown, B. W., et al. (1977). Community education for cardiovascular health. *Lancet, 1*, 1192–1195.

Flor, H., Kerns, R. D., & Turk, D. C. (1987). The role of spouse reinforcement, perceived pain, and activity levels of chronic pain patients. *Journal of Psychosomatic Research, 31*, 251–259.

Follick, M. J., Gorkin, L., Smith, T. W., Capone, R. J., Visco, J., & Stablein, D. (1988). Quality of life post-myocardial infarction: Influence of a transtelephonic coronary intervention system. *Health Psychology, 7*, 169–182.

Fontana, A. F., Kerns, R. I., Rosenberg, R. L., & Colonese, K. L. (1989). Support, stress and recovery from coronary heart disease: A longitudinal causal model. *Health Psychology, 8*, 175–193.

Frasure-Smith, N., & Prince, R. (1985). The Ischemic Heart Disease Life Stress Monitoring Program: Impact on mortality. *Psychosomatic Medicine*, 47, 431–445.

Frasure-Smith, N., & Prince, R. (1987). The Ischemic Heart Disease Life Stress Monitoring Program: Possible therapeutic mechanisms. *Psychology and Health*, 1, 273–285.

Gorkin, L, Schron, E. B., Brooks, M. M., Wiklund, I., Kellen, J., Verter, J., Schoenberger, J. A., Pawitan, Y., Morris, M., & Shumaker, S., for the CAST Investigators. (1993). Psychosocial predictors of mortality in the Cardiac Arrhythmia Suppression Trial–1 (CAST–1). *American Journal of Cardiology*, 71, 263–267.

Grundy, S. M. (1986). Cholesterol and coronary heart disease: A new era. *Journal of the American Medical Association*, 256, 2849–2858.

Hackett, T. P., & Cassem, N. H. (1974). Development of a quantitative rating scale to assess denial. *Journal of Psychosomatic Research*, 18, 93–100.

Harlow, H. F., & Harlow, M. K. (1966). Learning to love. *American Scientist*, 54, 244–272.

Hlatky, M. A., Haney, T., Barefoot, J. C., Califf, R. M., Mark, D. B., & Williams, R. B. (1986). Medical, psychological and social correlates of work disability among men with coronary artery disease. *American Journal of Cardiology*, 58, 911–915.

Johnston, B. L., Cantwell, J. D., Watt, E. W., & Fletcher, G. F. (1978). Sexual activity in exercising patients after myocardial infarction and revascularization. *Heart and Lung*, 7, 1026–1031.

Kaplan, J. R., Manuck, S. B., Clarkson, T. B., Lusso, F. M., & Taub, D. M. (1982). Social status, environment and atherosclerosis in cynomolgus monkeys. *Arteriosclerosis*, 2, 359.

Kaplan, R. M., & Hartwell, S. L. (1987). Differential effects of social support and social network on physiological and social outcomes in men and women with type II diabetes mellitus. *Health Psychology*, 6, 387–398.

Kennedy, G. J., Hofer, M. A., & Cohen, D. (1987). Significance of depression and cognitive impairment in patients undergoing programmed stimulation of cardiac arrhythmias. *Psychosomatic Medicine*, 49, 410–421.

Kleiger, R. E., Miller, J. P., Bigger, J. T., Jr., Moss, A. J., & the Multicenter Post-Infarction Research Group. (1987). Decreased heart rate variability, and its association with increased mortality after acute myocardial infarction. *American Journal of Cardiology*, 59, 256–262.

Kulik, J. A., & Mahler, H. I. M. (1989). Social support and recovery from surgery. *Health Psychology*, 8, 221–238.

Langeluddecke, P., Tennant, C., Fulcher, G., Barid, D., & Hughes, C. (1989). Coronary artery bypass surgery impact upon the patient's spouse. *Journal of Psychosomatic Research*, 33, 155–159.

Levine, J., Warrenburg, S., Kerns, R., Schwartz, G., Delaney, R., Fontana, A., et al. (1987). The role of denial in recovery from coronary heart disease. *Psychosomatic Medicine*, 49, 109–117.

Lipid Research Clinics Programs. (1984). The Lipid Research Clinics Coronary Primary Prevention Trial results. *Journal of the American Medical Association*, 251, 351–364.

Lynch, J. J., Thomas, S. A., Paskewitz, D. A., Katcher, A. H., & Weir, L. O. (1977). Human contact and cardiac arrhythmias in a coronary care unit. *Psychosomatic Medicine*, 39, 188–192.

Manuck, S. B., Kaplan, J. R., & Clarkson, T. B. (1983). Behaviorally induced heart rate reactivity and atherosclerosis in cynomolgus monkeys. *Psychosomatic Medicine*, 45, 95–108.

Mayou, R., Foster, A., & Williamson, B. (1978). Psychosocial adjustment in patients one year after myocardial infarction. *Journal of Psychosomatic Research*, 22, 447–453.

Mojonnier, L., & Hall, Y. (1968). The National Diet-Heart Study—assessment of dietary adherence. *Journal of the American Dietetic Association*, 52, 288–292.

Multiple Risk Factor Intervention Trial Research Group. (1982). Multiple Risk Factor Intervention Trial: Risk factor changes and mortality results. *Journal of the American Medical Association, 248,* 1465–1477.

Norwegian Multicenter Study Group. (1981). Timolol-induced reduction in mortality and reinfarction in patients surviving acute myocardial infarction. *New England Journal of Medicine, 304,* 801–807.

Obier, K. M., MacPherson, M., & Haywood, J. L. (1977). Predictive value of psychosocial profiles following acute myocardial infarction. *Journal of the National Medicine Association, 69,* 599–61.

Packer, M. (1987). Prolonging life in patients with congestive heart failure: The next frontier. *Circulation, 75*(Suppl. 4), 1–3.

Pancheri, P., Matteoli, S., Pollizzi, C., Bellaterra, M., Cristofari, M., & Puletti, M. (1978). Infarct as a stress agent: Life history and personality characteristics in improved versus not-improved patients after severe heart attack. *Journal of Human Stress, 4,* 16–42.

Perlman, L. V., Ferguson, S., Bergun, K., Isenberg, E. L., & Hammarsten, J. F. (1971). Precipitation of congestive heart failure: Social and emotional factors. *Annals of Internal Medicine, 75,* 1–7.

Pratt, C. M., Theroux, P., Slymen, D., Riordan-Bennett, A., Morisette, D., Galloway, A., et al. (1987). Spontaneous variability of ventricular arrhythmias in patients at increased risk for sudden death after acute myocardial infarction: Consecutive ambulatory electrocardiographic recordings of 88 patients. *American Journal of Cardiology, 59,* 278–283.

Ragland, D. R., & Brand, R. J. (1988). Type A behavior and mortality from coronary heart disease. *New England Journal of Medicine, 318,* 65–69.

Rich, M. W., Saini, J. S., Kleiger, R. E., Carney, R. M., teVelde, A., & Freedland, K. E. (1988). Correlation of heart rate variability with clinical and angiographic variables and late mortality after coronary angiography. *American Journal of Cardiology, 62,* 714–717.

Rosenman, R. H., Brand, R. J., Sholtz, R. I., & Friedman, M. (1976). Multivariate prediction of coronary heart disease during 8.5 year follow-up of the Western Collaborative Group Study. *American Journal of Cardiology, 37,* 903–910.

Ruberman, W., Weinblatt, E., Goldberg, J. D., & Chaudhary, B. S. (1984). Psychosocial influences on mortality after myocardial infarction. *New England Journal of Medicine, 311,* 552–559.

Sarason, D. G., Levine, H. M., Basham, R. B., & Sarason, B. R. (1983). Assessing social support: The Social Support Questionnaire. *Journal of Personality and Social Psychology, 14,* 127–139.

Seeman, T. E., & Syme, L. (1987). Social networks and coronary artery disease: A comparison of the structure and function of social relations as predictors of disease. *Psychosomatic Medicine, 49,* 341–354.

Shaw, R. E., Cohen, F., Doyle, B., & Palesky, J. (1985). The impact of denial and repressive style on information gain and rehabilitation outcomes in myocardial infarction patients. *Psychosomatic Medicine, 47,* 262–273.

Sikorski, J. M. (1985). Knowledge, concerns, and questions of wives of convalescent coronary artery bypass graft surgery patients. *Journal of Cardiac Rehabilitation, 5,* 74–85.

Simon, A. B., & Alonzo, A. A. (1973). Sudden death in nonhospitalized cardiac patients: An epidemiologic study with implications for intervention techniques. *Archives of Internal Medicine, 132,* 163–170.

Skelton, M., & Dominian, J. (1973). Psychological stress in wives of patients with myocardial infarction. *British Medical Journal, 2,* 101–103.

Stern, M. J., Pascale, L., & Ackerman, A. (1977). Life adjustment post-myocardial infarction. *Archives of Internal Medicine, 137,* 623–633.

Sullivan, M. J., Higginbotham, M. B., & Cobb, F. R. (1988). Exercise training in patients with severe left ventricular dysfunction: Hemodynamic and metabolic effects. *Circulation, 78,* 506–515.

Taylor, C. B., Bandura, A., Ewart, C. K., Miller, N. H., & DeBusk, R. F. (1985). Exercise testing to enhance wives' confidence in their husbands cardiac capability soon after clinically uncomplicated acute myocardial infarction. *American Journal of Cardiology, 55,* 635–638.

Theroux, P., Waters, D. D., Halphen, C., Debaisieux, J.-C., & Mizgala, H. F. (1979). Prognostic value of exercise testing soon after myocardial infarction. *New England Journal of Medicine, 301,* 341–345.

Thompson, D. R., & Cordle, C. J. (1988). Support of wives of myocardial infarction patients. *Journal of Advanced Nursing, 13,* 223–228.

Verrier, R. L., Hagestad, E. L., & Lown, B. (1987). Delayed myocardial ischemia induced by anger. *Circulation, 75,* 249–254.

Verrier, R. L., & Lown, B. (1984). Behavioral stress and cardiac arrhythmias. *Annual Review of Physiology, 46,* 155–176.

Vlay, S. C., & Fricchione, G. L. (1985). Psychosocial aspects of surviving sudden cardiac death. *Clinical Cardiology, 8,* 237–243.

Weidner, G., Healy, A. B., & Matarazzo, J. D. (1985). Family consumption of low fat foods: Stated preference versus actual consumption. *Journal of Applied Social Psychology, 15,* 773–779.

Weiss, R. (1974). The provisions of social relationships. In S. Rubin (Ed.), *Doing unto others* (pp. 17–26). Englewood Cliffs, NJ: Prentice-Hall.

Wertzel, H., Vollrath, D., Ritz, E., & Ferner, H. (1977). Analysis of patient-nurse interaction in hemodialysis units. *Journal of Psychosomatic Research, 21,* 359–366.

Williams, R. B., Barefoot, J. C., Califf, R. M., Haney, T. L., Saunders, W. B., Pryor, D. B., Hlathy, M. A., Siegler, I. C., & Mark, D. B. (1992). Prognostic importance of social and economic resources among medically treated patients with angiographically documented coronary artery disease. *Journal of the American Medical Association, 267,* 520–524.

Witschi, J. C., Singer, M., Wu-Lee, M., & Stare, F. J. (1978). Family cooperation and effectiveness in a cholesterol-lowering diet. *Journal of the American Dietetic Association, 72,* 384–389.

CHAPTER 13

Social Support and Adjustment to Myocardial Infarction, Angioplasty, and Coronary Artery Bypass Surgery

Kathleen Ell and Christine Dunkel-Schetter

Overview

In this chapter we examine social support during three acute cardiac events: myocardial infarction (MI), angioplasty, and coronary artery bypass graft (CABG) surgery. The first event, MI, is life threatening and is characterized by sudden onset as a result of coronary artery thrombosis. Patients are commonly hospitalized for 7 to 10 days, and recovery periods (including participation in cardiac rehabilitation programs) can range up to 6 weeks or longer. Close to one half of the 1.3 million persons experiencing MI each year survive to leave the hospital (Garrity, 1981). Of these, approximately 10% will die during the following year. Subsequently, nonfatal reinfarctions occur at an average annual rate of 3%, and coronary artery disease deaths occur at a rate of 5%, three to four times higher than that of the general population (Kannel, Sorlie, & McNamara, 1979). Myocardial impairment and severity of the underlying disease are the strongest predictors of early mortality (Henning et al., 1979; Sanz, Castaner, Betriu, & Magria, 1982). Three to five percent of patients will undergo CABG surgery within 3 months following an MI (Davidson, 1983).

KATHLEEN ELL • School of Social Work, Hamovitch Social Research Center, University of Southern California, Los Angeles, California 90089-0411. *CHRISTINE DUNKEL-SCHETTER* • Department of Psychology, University of California, Los Angeles, Los Angeles, California 90024-1563.

Social Support and Cardiovascular Disease, edited by Sally A. Shumaker and Susan M. Czajkowski. Plenum Press, New York, 1994.

CABG surgery is a procedure involving the creation of a saphenous vein or mammary artery "bypass" to allow blood to flow around the narrowed or blocked portion of a coronary artery. Patients are hospitalized for about 6 to 7 days, and recovery periods can range up to 6 months. It is estimated that more than 1 million patients have undergone this procedure since its development (Davidson, 1985), and more than 250,000 surgeries are performed yearly in the United States (Politser & Cunico, 1988); approximately 45% of these involve three or more grafts (National Heart, Lung, and Blood Institute [NHLBI], 1988). The number of bypasses performed on a given patient generally ranges from two to five per patient, and approximately 5% to 10% of surgeries are reoperations (Davidson, 1983). For patients with more extensive or specific forms of coronary artery disease (i.e., main artery disease or three-vessel disease), surgery has been shown to prolong life (Hall et al., 1983; NHLBI, 1988). This outcome, however, has not been demonstrated for the majority of patients having undergone the procedure (Detre et al., 1985; Murray & Beller, 1983). Some groups (e.g., patients with stable ischemic heart disease) are no longer viewed as candidates for CABG unless symptoms worsen (CASS Principal Investigators, 1983a). Symptomatic improvement occurs in 70% to 80% of CABG patients (Davidson, 1985; NHLBI, 1988), although 10% to 20% experience a recurrence of symptoms (Murray & Beller, 1983).

Percutaneous transluminal coronary angioplasty (PTCA) is a procedure performed in the cardiac catheterization laboratory with a cardiac surgery team standing by in case an emergency CABG surgery is required. Indicators for the procedure are generally chest pain and angioplasty with blockage or prior MI. It is estimated that 5% to 10% of patients who are candidates for coronary bypass surgery meet recommended selection criteria for having PTCA as an adjustment treatment (Greenspon & Goldberg, 1983). Furthermore, a small proportion of PTCA patients go on to have emergency or elective CABG because the procedure is not successful (Greenspon & Goldberg, 1983). During PTCA, a catheter is introduced into the coronary arteries via an artery in the arm or groin. A second, smaller catheter with a balloon at the end of it is passed through the first one. The balloon tip is then inflated, compressing the atherosclerotic plaque and dilating the soft inner wall of the artery. The procedure widens the coronary artery and thereby increases blood flow to the heart. Patients are usually discharged within 2 days or less and frequently return to normal activities within 1 week following the procedure; however, 20% to 30% of patients require the procedure again within 6 months (Jutzy, Berte, Alderman, Ratts, & Simpson, 1982; Kent et al., 1982). In 1983, 20,000 PTCAs were performed in the United States and predictions estimate that in 1987, this number will have increased to 140,000 (American Heart Association, 1986).

Early results were encouraging as to the value of PTCA in preventing coronary events in selected patients (P. Block, 1985). Comparison of PTCA and CABG outcomes for patients matched demographically and by cardiac condition showed the PTCA group was functioning significantly better 6 and 15 months posttreatment (Raft, McKee, Popio, & Haggerty, 1985). Results from the TIMI-II trial in Boston, however, indicate that MI patients do not need angioplasty if they quickly receive clot-dissolving medications.

A common issue for all three of these patient groups (MI, CABG, PTCA) is their underlying coronary artery disease and the physical, psychological, and social implications of that diagnosis (Davidson, 1983; Doehrman, 1977; Garrity, 1981). Each of these patient groups is aware that their heart is the object of concern, a body organ with considerable symbolic meaning (Goldman & Kimball, 1985; Carr & Powers, 1986). Patients are faced with the threat of both symbolic and actual losses ranging from loss of affection to loss of life. Moreover, patients commonly experience pain in the form of postsurgical discomfort and occasionally angina, significant physical deconditioning from forced inactivity, extended rehabilitation, further treatment decisions, and the threat of recurrence resulting from the ongoing disease process. In the case of CABG or PTCA, many patients have experienced increasing disability over an extended period of time prior to treatment and therefore may experience severe disappointment if blockage or narrowing of the artery occurs again (restenosis) or if angina or chest pain occur following initial treatment (Shaw et al., 1986). Despite many commonalities, however, these three types of cardiac patients each experience distinct events and reactions.

Substantial data indicate that the social and psychological contexts surrounding these acute cardiac episodes influence cardiac outcomes and the overall quality of life of patients and their families (Case, Moss, Case, McDermott & Eberly, 1992; Fletcher, Hunt & Bulpitt, 1987; Folks, Blake, Fleece, Sokol & Freeman, 1986; LaMendola & Pellegrini, 1979; Lloyd & Cawley, 1983; Ruberman, Weinblatt, Goldberg & Chaudhary, 1984; Waltz, 1986b; Williams et al., 1992). Furthermore, social support from both primary network members and professional caregivers is assumed to be an important resource in patients' perceptions of their experiences and in the coping strategies they employ to adapt to the changing life circumstances that result from the event (Caplan, 1976; Dean & Tausing, 1986).

In this chapter we examine the effects of social support as they may influence the patients' recognition of symptoms and their health care–seeking behavior, treatment decision making, hospitalization, and early psychosocial adaptation (approximately 2 to 3 months postdischarge). The experience of the patients' families will be examined in terms of their roles as both support providers to the cardiac patient and recipients of professional caregiver support. Supportive care by health care practitioners will be considered primarily through a review of extant intervention research. Finally, we set a future research agenda.

Symptom Recognition and Health Care-Seeking Behavior

The ability to respond quickly to life-threatening cardiac arrhythmias (irregular heart rhythm) in coronary and intensive care units has resulted in substantial reductions in hospital mortality (Gillum, Feinleib, Margolis, Fabsitz, & Barsch, 1976). Furthermore, there is evidence that the potential effectiveness of medical interventions for limiting the extent of myocardial necrosis is inversely related to the interval between the onset of the ischemic episode and the time the intervention is applied (Turi et al., 1986). The majority of deaths from MI, however, occur before patients reach a hospital (Gillum et al., 1976), and considerable delay between symptom recognition and receipt of medical care has been documented (Davidson, 1979; Gentry, 1975; Hackett & Cassem, 1969).

Some evidence suggests that individuals engage in several stages or processes of symptom recognition and evaluation before initiating contact with the formal medical care system (Berkanovic, Telesky, & Reeder, 1979; Gentry, 1975; Matthews, Siegel, Kuller, Thompson, & Varat, 1983; Safer, Tharps, Jackson, & Leventhal, 1986). It has been proposed that the decision to seek treatment for cardiac symptoms involves three distinct cognitive steps: (a) awareness of the symptoms, (b) an interpretation of their meaning and seriousness, and (c) recognition of the need to obtain medical care (Greene, Moss, & Goldstein, 1974).

Of direct relevance to this discussion is evidence that consultation with members of one's personal social network commonly occurs during symptom appraisal and in decision making prior to seeking health care services (Berkanovic & Telesky, 1982; Coulton & Forst, 1982; Horowitz, 1978; Krantz, 1980; McKinlay, 1973, 1981). Research on the role of others in response to a life-threatening coronary event has been very sparse; however, there is evidence that patients consult laypersons during acute cardiac episodes (Alonzo, 1986; Ell et al., 1993). The extent to which this process is a factor in delay is an important area for study (Alonzo, 1986; Cowie, 1976; Davidson, 1979; Hackett & Cassem, 1969). Research has found that delay is greater when the spouse or others initiate the decision to seek medical care than when the decision is the patient's (Hackett & Cassem, 1969; Moss, Wynar, & Goldstein, 1969). Hackett and Cassem (1969) found further that median delay time was considerably higher when spouses were assisting than when friends or others assisted, perhaps as a result of spouse anxiety. Thus efforts to locate a family member for advice may forestall prompt action, and consultation with others could result in discouraging the seeking of health care or in use of home remedies. A family member, though, could strongly encourage or initiate the decision to seek immediate aid. Physician factors such as denial or misdiagnosis may also be a source of delay in referring to emergent care (Gentry, 1975; Hackett & Cassem, 1969).

Treatment Decision Making

Factors associated with patient's decisions to undergo either CABG or PTCA are a neglected but fertile area for psychosocial study. For example, recent data indicate that CABG may be an overutilized coronary treatment (Graboys, Headley, Lown, Lampert, & Blatt, 1987), especially in view of evidence that survival may not be extended for all patients beyond that of more conservative medical treatments. Moreover, psychosocial outcomes are not optimal for many patients (Gundle, Reeves, Tate, Raft, & McLaurin, 1980; Murray & Beller, 1983). The role of social networks in patients' coronary treatment decisions merits careful examination. For example, the roles of both physicians and family in influencing patients to undergo treatment such as surgery are likely to be critical. Physicians exert influence in their manner of communicating the diagnosis and treatment recommendation; those who provide emotional support as well as information are likely to be the most influential (Dunkel-Schetter, 1984). Encouragement and reassurance by family members (or lack thereof) may exert influence on the patient also, as would their general availability and dependability for assistance during recovery and rehabilitation.

Hospitalization

Hospitalization for CABG, PTCA, or MI is distinguishable by the circumstances preceding hospitalization. Patients having an MI require emergency hospitalization; CABG patients may have either emergency or elective surgery; and PTCA is generally elective. The impact of a scheduled hospitalization for surgery is presumably influenced by treatment expectations and presurgical functional status, such as the extent to which the patient was debilitated by angina or other cardiac symptoms. For example, there is some evidence that postsurgical hospitalization may be less psychologically stressful than waiting for the surgery (Gillis, 1984; Radley & Green, 1986). Emergency hospitalization for any of these procedures has not been researched much with respect to later adjustment, but it is of interest in that these patients are obviously unprepared psychologically.

Admission to a hospital for either a sudden MI or for CABG (and probably for PTCA) is usually a frightening and painful event. Not surprisingly, the vast majority of patients experience significant psychological distress during hospitalization (Acker, 1978). The most common emotional reactions are anxiety and depression (Cay, 1982; Dracup, Meleis, Baker, & Edlefsen, 1984; Michela, 1987; Minckley et al., 1979; Taggart & Carruthers, 1981; Winefield & Martin, 1981–82). Patients undergoing CABG have also been found to be subject to much higher rates of postoperative delirium or psychosis than following other surgical procedures (Rabiner & Willner, 1976; Sveinsson, 1975). The majority of patients experiencing severe psychiatric disturbances recover without specific psychiatric intervention (Rabiner & Willner, 1976), however, and more recent studies suggest that this problem may be occurring less frequently with improved operative technology (Jenkins et al., 1983).

Discharge from Hospital and Early Convalescence

Discharge from the hospital marks a new context for social-psychological distress that continues through early convalescence. Mayou (1984) found that psychosocial assessment at this time period was even more predictive of long-term MI adjustment than hospital assessments. Depression after returning home from the hospital is the most common affective syndrome among MI patients (Davidson, 1983; Garrity, 1981). Depression is also experienced by postsurgical patients; however, patients recuperating from CABG (Davidson, 1983) or PTCA (Shaw et al., 1986) may also display undue optimism that requires repeated emphasis on the need for comprehensive secondary prevention and risk factor modification (Murray & Beller, 1983).

During early convalescence, patients also begin to test their physical capacities and to reformulate perceptions of health status (Bramwell, 1986; Garrity, 1981). For some patients, early negative perceptions persist long after convalescence and are associated with ongoing depression, low morale, and poor functional outcomes (Garrity, 1973a,b). Feelings of uncertainty and ambiguity are major cognitive-emotional problems for the postdischarge MI patient (Garrity, 1981) and for the postsurgical CABG patient as well (Gillis, 1984). Some patients also experience stress as a result of what is perceived to be excessive family surveillance (Bilodeau & Hackett, 1971; Fiske, Coyne, & Smith, 1991).

Research on Early Psychological Adjustment

Adjustment to acute cardiac events can be divided into short- versus long-term responses at about the 2- to 3-month mark. Although the focus of this chapter is on short-term adjustment, research on long-term adjustment is also pertinent. Several general themes emerge from extant research on both short- and long-term psychosocial adjustment of patients having an acute cardiac event. First, the majority of patients with MIs experience fairly rapid psychological recovery and demonstrate little or no long-term psychosocial or affective impairment (Croog & Levine, 1977; Lloyd & Cawley, 1983; Mayou, 1981). There is evidence, however, that approximately one third of MI patients continue to experience debilitating effects in overall psychosocial functioning and quality of life (Mayou, Williamson, & Foster, 1978; Wells et al., 1989) and that an even smaller minority (15% to 20%) experience persistent major depressive symptoms (Ladwig et al., 1992; Schleifer et al., 1989).

The evidence regarding the effects of CABG on psychosocial adjustment is equivocal in part because of such methodological problems as simplistic measures of outcomes, small sample sizes that do not allow for controlling patient presurgical status, and short follow-ups (i.e., 1 year or less; NHLBI, 1988; Wenger, 1986). Some studies document improved overall quality of life following CABG for a majority of patients (CASS Principal Investigators, 1983b; Kornfield, Heller, Frank, Wilson, & Malm, 1982; Folks et al., 1986; Jenkins et al., 1983) especially at the 1-year point; however, it has also been found consistently that a small number of patients report postsurgical deterioration in psychosocial functioning (Gundle et al., 1980; Horgan, Davies, Hunt, Westlake, & Mullerworth, 1984; Zyzanski, Rouse, Stanton, & Jenkins, 1982). Impaired sexual functioning is most commonly reported (Horgan et al., 1984) with some evidence that women are less negatively affected in this area than men (Althof, Coffman, & Levine, 1984). The effects of CABG on employment seem variable and inconclusive or negative (Horgan et al., 1984; Kinchla & Weiss, 1985; NHLBI, 1988). It is estimated that 50% of CABG patients or fewer resume household activities, and that depression decreases but does not disappear after 1 year (NHLBI, 1988). Definitive studies on quality of life after CABG are only now in progress (NHLBI, 1988).

In the cases of MI and CABG, poorer perceived health status, greater symptomatology, lower functional status, and greater premorbid physical and psychosocial impairment are associated with posthospitalization psychosocial impairment and ongoing affective distress (Gundle et al., 1980; Lloyd & Cawley, 1983). Objective measures of cardiac damage and function and of postoperative physical recovery are inconsistently related to the psychosocial adaptation of patients (A. Block, Boyer, & Imes, 1984; Cay, Vetter, Philip, & Dugard, 1972; Croog & Levine, 1977; Horgan et al., 1984).

Substantial evidence indicates that patients' affective and cognitive perceptions of their health status during acute cardiac events are significant predictors of longer-term outcomes (Affleck, Tenne, Croog, & Levine, 1987; Bar-on, 1987; Byrne, 1982; Byrne, Whyte, & Butler, 1981; Croog & Levine, 1977; Garrity & Klein, 1975; Maeland & Havik, 1987; Mayou, 1984; Stanton et al., 1983; Trelawny-Ross & Russell, 1987, Wiklund, Sanne, Vedin, & Wilhelmsson, 1984). Finally, and of major import in a discussion of social network support, a recently growing body of research strongly suggests that adjustment to serious illness (including acute cardiac events) is best understood within the context of primary social relationships, especially marital relationships (Aho, 1977; Bruhn, 1977; Coyne, Ellard, & Smith, 1990; Coyne & Smith, 1991; Davidson, 1979; Dhooper, 1983; Kulik & Mahler, 1984; Litman, 1974; Melamed & Brenner, 1990; New, Ruscio, Priest, Petritsi, & George, 1968; Radley & Green, 1985, 1986; Radley, 1988; Speedling, 1982; Waltz, 1986a,b). In the next section of this chapter, we explore social support during acute coronary events.

Social Support during Acute Coronary Events

In what ways may social support operate during acute coronary events? During this time, patients have access to two primary sources of support: family and friends, and health care professionals. Three types of support would seem applicable: emotional, informational, and instrumental support. The preceding discussion underscores potential avenues of influence of both family and caregivers on patients' affective status and on cognitive appraisals of their situation. Family members' ability to provide support to patients during hospitalization will undoubtedly be influenced by the degree of distress they experience and by their appraisals of the patient's status. Furthermore, family members' ability to obtain informational and emotional social support themselves during this time may be an important factor in their ability to support the patient (Ell & Northern, 1990; Finlayson & McEwen, 1977; Unger & Powell, 1980). Our focus in this section is on the family support issues.

Families' Needs for Support

The lack of extensive research on family responses to patients' acute coronary events is remarkable. Several preliminary studies, however, are heuristic in their identification of stressors experienced by spouses. Noteworthy are a few studies that suggest that spouses were more frequently distressed than patients during acute hospitalization (Mayou, Foster, & Williamson, 1978; Michela, 1987; Speedling, 1982). Speedling (1982) conducted an extensive ethnographic examination of patient and family experiences and reactions in the face of MI in the emergency room, in the admitting area, and in the intensive care unit. He found that during intensive care stays, family members were not only more frequently distressed than patients but also were more pessimistic and fearful of the patient's death and more worried about the future. This may be in part because patients are frequently heavily medicated at this time and are less aware of their circumstances. Speedling (1982), though, proposed that the medical caregiving structure, which is appropriately designed to provide technically sophisticated patient care, has a negative effect on family members. He argued further that restricted family visits, although potentially beneficial to patients, prevent family members from observing and participating in early and subtly manifested aspects of the patient's recovery.

Family visitation and participation in bedside care are areas where further research is merited. For example, data on whether family visits have beneficial effects on patients is conflicting (Fuller & Foster, 1982). This may be mediated by the quality of premorbid family relationships. Male family members have been shown to be less likely to desire to participate in bedside care than female members (Boycoff, 1986). There is also evidence that family members desire strong but supportive nursing management of visitation during intensive care stays (Boycoff, 1986).

Studies also attest to the high degree of distress experienced by family members of coronary patients (e.g., Speedling, 1982). Lack of control of hospital events, lack of opportunities to express distress, lack of information, and inadequate or poor social support for well-meaning friends were reported to be major stressors following CABG in one study (Gillis, 1984). The hospital experiences of spouses of patients with MI in another study were characterized by fear of loss of the spouse, the spouse's health, or financial security; fear of the hospital environment in general; and fear of changes in family roles and personal life goals (Bedsworth & Molen, 1982). High anxiety, depression, and illness coincident with the coronary events also have been found among spouses (M. Stern & Pascale, 1979) and among children of patients who experience an acute coronary event (Dhooper, 1983). Family members also report being stressed by lack of information and express a desire for more information about patients' recommended general activity level (Bramwell, 1986; Thompson & Cordle, 1988) as well as specific information regarding sexual activity (Papadopoulos, Larrimore, Cardin, & Shelley, 1980). Finally, failure to use opportunities to be supportive to family members may result in depriving the practitioner of valuable information about the patient's usual support needs under stress (Speedling, 1982).

Further information on stress and coping in spouses of MI patients is provided by Nyamathi (1987), who interviewed 40 spouses of MI patients within the first year after the hospitalization. During hospitalization, coping focused on reducing the effect of the MI on the husband, family, and self. Almost all of them sought emotional support and help for themselves at some point, although the prevalence of this diminished over time. In general, behavioral coping techniques (e.g., seeking information or problem solving) were preferred over cognitive ones (e.g., distancing or reinterpreting).

Homecoming and the first weeks of convalescence are periods of significant distress for family members of patients with MI and CABG also, especially spouses (Bramwell, 1986; Carter, 1984; Dhooper, 1983; Finlayson & McEwen, 1977; Gillis, 1984; Greenhill & Frater, 1976; Lange-luddecke, Tennant, Fulcker, Barid, & Hughes, 1989; Skelton & Dominian, 1973; Speedling, 1982). Speedling (1982) suggests that problems that remained below the surface during hospitalization become more salient when the family is home and coping without professional help. Conflict around spouse roles in the patient's resumption of activities is reported to be highest during early convalescence (Bramwell, 1986; Gillis, 1984; Wishnie, Hackett, & Cassem, 1977). There is evidence that incongruence between patients' and family members' perceptions of the patient's status is a primary source of conflict and causes affective distress for both patients and family members (Finlayson & McEwen, 1977; Wishnie et al., 1977). Again, at discharge family members are less likely than patients to have been given adequate information regarding recommended physical activity levels for patients (Bramwell, 1986; Gillis, 1984; Rudy, 1980; Taylor, Bandura, Ewart, Miller, & DeBusk, 1985). Furthermore, family members are frequently dissatisfied or distressed by what is perceived to be infrequent outpatient visits and lack of communication with medical staff during the days immediately after discharge (Bramwell, 1986; Mayou, Williamson, & Foster, 1976).

Effects of Family Support

The salutary effects of support from spouses can be inferred from data indicating higher death rates among unmarried hospitalized MI patients (Chandra, Szklo, Goldberg, & Tonascia, 1983) and among post-MI patients reporting high stress in combination with social isolation (Ruberman et al., 1984). In each of these studies, the effect of the social relationship variable was maintained when potentially confounding physical risk factors were controlled. There is also evidence that family support, especially from spouses, during acute episodes enhances patients' psychological well-being during recovery (Ell & Haywood, 1984, 1985–86; Waltz, 1986a,b;

Winefield, 1982) and is an important influence on patients' cognitive restructuring processes (Radley, 1988; Waltz, 1986a,b). Of interest is evidence that having family members touch patients and orient patients frequently to time and place may reduce the manifestations of postoperative psychiatric disturbances (Chatham, 1978). Furthermore, a recent study with male CABG patients found high levels of contact with the spouse during hospitalization was associated with taking fewer pain medications and quicker discharge from ICU and from the hospital compared to patients who had low levels of spousal contact (Kulik & Mahler, 1984). Unmarried patients, however, were between the two groups in outcomes.

There is also evidence that some types of family members' support for patients may not be helpful during hospitalization. For example, visits by family members who had no preparation for the coronary care unit were found to increase patient anxiety (Doerr & Jones, 1979). Speedling (1982) found that advice from family members to patients regarding activity in the unit was frequently in direct conflict with the directions patients received from medical staff. He posited that this dilemma was in large part attributable to failure on the part of health care providers to incorporate family members adequately into the overall care of the patient and to provide the family with sufficient information. Family visits characterized by this form of conflict were stressful for both patients and family members.

The reported conflict between patients and spouses at this time is of concern in light of data suggesting that the presence of conflict is most detrimental to the provision of support from a person's closest relationship (Abbey, Abramis, & Caplan, 1985; Eggert, 1987) and that unmet expectations of support from others increases negative affect (Fiore, Becker, & Coppel, 1983). Indeed, Ell and Haywood (1984) found that unhelpful network support canceled out helpful support during cardiac recovery. In that study, the net number of helpful network members was a stronger predictor of outcomes than the number of either helpful or unhelpful network members.

It would seem that conflicting perceptions about the patient's status that may have developed in the hospital are even more intense at home, and presumably they are acted upon in ways that are distressing for both patients and family members. For example, spouses engage in a process of searching for explanations or causes for the cardiac events (causal attributions), and they evaluate their potential role in influencing patients' posthospitalization behaviors (Bar-on & Dreman, 1987; Bramwell, 1986; Cowie, 1976; Rudy, 1980). Spouses may adopt a supportive role of providing reassurance or understanding, or they may become advocates for changes in life-style and compliance with medical regimens (Aiken, 1975). Lack of adequate and accurate information may lead to spouses' support having negative effects as a result of their assuming an overprotective stance toward patients (Jenkins et al., 1983; Wishnie et al., 1977). Emotional overinvolvement of family at this time may also unduly stress patients (Coyne & DeLongis, 1986; Coyne, Wortman, & Lehman, 1988; Greenhill & Frater, 1976). In contrast, if spouses believe their role to be slight in relation to the patient's life-style changes and health behaviors, patients may be deprived of an important emotional support for their efforts (Aho, 1977). Similarly, incongruent perceptions between patients and spouses of patients' overall health status may result in conflict (New et al., 1968). In an interesting study, congruent causal attributions between post-MI patients and their spouses—regardless of the attributions' content—affected short-term convalescence (Bar-on & Dreman, 1987). Incongruence of the couples' denial pattern was positively related to patient's return to work and functioning during subsequent long-term rehabilitation. Thus, if spouses do not engage in a denial pattern similar to their partners, they may encourage patients to later adopt appropriate secondary prevention health behaviors.

Intervention Research

Taken together, the data reviewed in the preceding sections lend strong support to the proposition that close contact of patients and family members with health care practitioners during acute cardiac episodes provides health professionals with a "window of opportunity" to (a) assess known risk factors for psychosocial impairment, (b) intervene to modify the environments of caregiving, and (c) provide patients and family members with informational and emotional social support. Alternatively, failure to meet these challenges may result in acute care being a dangerous opportunity for negatively affecting patients' and family members' self-perceptions and, ultimately, patient's long-term outcomes (Mumford, Schlesinger, & Glass, 1982). For example, there is evidence that support for smoking cessation is most effective if initiated in the hospital (Sivarajan et al., 1983).

Given the strong justification for employing supportive intervention during acute cardiac episodes, what recommendations to health care practitioners can be made? Most important, what is known about the effectiveness of specific intervention strategies. In general, it can be said that few patients require either extensive psychiatric treatment or elaborate psychosocial intervention (Cay et al., 1972; Lloyd & Cawley, 1983; Mumford et al., 1982). Physicians and nursing staff are advised to provide patients and family members routinely and repeatedly with adequate expert information and with opportunities for safe expression of feelings, fears, and perceptions (Fleming, 1980; Winefield & Katsikitis, 1987). In addition, the distress experienced by both patients and family members during hospitalization and their persistence through early convalescence, in combination with evidence of the salutary effects of social support, provide a strong rationale for developing and testing supportive psychosocial interventions. At present, patients and families are infrequently aware of the psychosocial services that may be available to them (Dhooper, 1983), and the majority of patients make little or no use of such services (Croog, Lipson, & Levine, 1972; Jenkins et al., 1983). Therefore medical staff are advised to integrate psychosocial supportive care provided by other health professionals (e.g., social workers, psychologists, and nurse specialists) routinely into standard medical and surgical treatment protocols (Pozen, Stechmiller, Harris, Smith, & Voigt, 1977; Stewart & Gregor, 1984).

Theories about families suggest that the patient's adjustment to the illness and ability to make future life-style choices will develop within the context of interaction and communication within intimate personal relationships. Indeed, there is evidence of this mutuality among patients and their spouses in coping with cancer (Cassileth et al., 1985; Ell, Nishimoto, Mantell, & Hamovitch, 1988a,b; Coyne, Ellard & Smith, 1990; Gotay, 1984) as well as among cardiac patients (Bar-on & Dreman, 1987; Radley & Green, 1985, 1986; Waltz, 1986a,b). The family context, and most frequently the marital relationship, must be viewed in terms of its structure and content prior to illness and its usual patterns of coping with stress as well as its response to the situational stressors associated with the acute cardiac episode (Croog & Fitzgerald, 1978; Waltz, 1986a,b). This perspective explains findings that family members influence patient's emotional adaptation, acceptance or nonacceptance of the prescribed medical regimen, and behavior during early convalescence.

Routinely providing care to family members is emphasized because evidence indicates that this aspect of care may be most frequently neglected (Ell & Northern, 1990; Sikes & Rodenhauser, 1987) and because family-directed care is assumed to result in direct benefits to patients. Given what is generally known about family coping, intervention will be helpful to most family members when it is directed to easing immediate stressors and enhancing coping responses. Second, identifying family who may be at risk as a result of preillness problem relationships and targeting these families for more extensive psychosocial supportive care is recommended.

To date, the literature consists of frequent calls for supportive psychosocial services and numerous description of model programs (e.g., Bromberg & Donnerstag, 1977; Gardner & Stewart, 1978; Granger, 1974; Gulledge, 1975; Hartly, 1988; Mitchell, 1976). Acute care interventions can be distinguished as being primarily educationally or emotionally directed (or a combination of both); as focused on modifying hospital environments or on posthospital adjustment; as involving professional or self-help auspices; and as being directed to patients, families, or both. Numerous questions remain about how social support influences recovery processes from serious illness. Converging evidence, however, suggests that patients' social support experiences are amenable to professional intervention (Porritt, 1979; Wortman & Conway, 1985). Moreover, although intervention research in acute cardiac care is relatively sparse and in some cases methodologically flawed, results encourage further study.

Supportive Patient Interventions

Preoperative preparation for surgery has been convincingly shown to reduce patients' psychological distress and to speed postoperative recovery by reducing use of analgesics (Andrew, 1970; Egbert, Battit, Welch, & Bartlett, 1964), and length of hospital stay (see Mumford et al., 1982; Reading, 1979, for reviews). In a controlled study, sensory and procedural information preparation, and information plus a coping preparation, were found to reduce psychological distress and the incidence of acute postoperative hypertension among patients having CABG (Anderson, 1987; see also Christopherson & Pfeiffer, 1980). Another interesting study examined the effects of preoperative roommate assignment on preoperative emotions and postoperative recovery in CABG patients (Kulik & Mahler, 1987). Whether the patient's roommate prior to surgery was hospitalized for cardiac surgery had no effects, but if the preoperative roommate was postoperative, CABG patients experienced less anxiety and later ambulated and were discharged quicker than if the roommate had been preoperative. Structured preparation for transfer from intensive care units has also been shown to reduce patient anxiety (Smith, 1976; T. Stern, 1985; Toth, 1980). Despite the advantages of information during hospitalization, it is noteworthy that CABG patients have had difficulty processing and retaining such information (Kinchla & Weiss, 1985), a fact that must be taken into account in cardiac interventions. Information seeking was evident as a coping strategy preoperatively in all CABG patients in one study, however, suggesting that patients want information even if it is hard to digest (King, 1985).

Mended Hearts is a self-help program that is built on a hospital visitation program, where accredited Mended Hearts visitors (recovered patients) visit preoperative and postoperative heart patients in local hospitals. An evaluation of the impact of different elements of the program found that the greatest long-term benefits occur among retired patients who are active in the organization over an extended period of time (Videka, 1979). In that study, the impact of the hospital visits on long-term outcomes was not significant; more recently the visitation program has been extended to include patients with MI and PTCA. Crude measures of the effectiveness of a similar program in Canada suggests that the salutary effects of the pre- and postsurgical visits emerge from patients' exposure to the "living proof" model of successful recovery and from the emotional support provided by the lay helper (Meagher, Gregor, & Stewart, 1987). Also, King (1985) found that for CABG patients it was helpful preoperatively to talk to someone with similar experience as a source of information, but postoperatively family and friends were more helpful.

Descriptions of supportive psychological counseling of patients in the hospital are reported to result in improved recovery (see Garrity, 1981, for a review); however, counseling is generally directed to patients identified as having special needs. Few studies have used controlled research designs or objectively measured specific cardiac outcomes. Three studies are noteworthy for their methodological rigor. In one, 70 patients with a first MI were randomized into a treatment or control group (Gruen, 1975). The treatment consisted of daily psychotherapy during acute hospitalization. Treated patients showed significant favorable differences on intensive care and hospital days; development of arrhythmias and congestive heart failure; nurses' observations of weakness; physician assessment of depression; and self-report of social support, anxiety, and ability to engage in normal activity at a 4-month follow-up.

In the second study, 143 men were randomly assigned to an intensive rehabilitation or a control group (Naismeth, Robinson, Shaw, & MacIntyre, 1979). Treatment patients were first seen on the third day after MI and were subsequently seen periodically in the hospital and at home for a period of 6 months. Patients' wives were seen on several occasions, sometimes alone and sometimes with the patient. Psychological counseling was conducted by a nurse counselor at 6 months after discharge. Treated patients achieved significantly higher scores on social independence; no differences were found for return to work or physical and emotional stability.

Anderson (1987) evaluated the effects of preoperative preparation in male CABG patients on pre- and postoperative outcomes. Control group patients received routine hospital preparation. Two other randomly assigned groups received routine preparation plus detailed information on procedures and sensations. The intervention groups were significantly less anxious and fearful during the time prior to surgery, had a greater belief in their control during recovery, reported less emotional distress post-operatively, and were judged by nurses as having better overall recoveries.

Educational and emotion-focused group treatments are commonly used in the care of post-MI patients, although their effectiveness has not been adequately examined. Indeed, in several studies of group intervention little change in physical or psychological factors was found (Horlick, Cameron, Firor, Bhalerao, & Baltzan, 1984; Ibrahim et al., 1974; Rahe, Word, & Hayes, 1979). Failure to establish significant intervention effects may be a result of providing patients with care regardless of the need for such care.

Targeting Interventions

Despite extensive descriptive data identifying patients at higher risk for poor cardiac outcomes, few interventions have been targeted or tailored to potential high-risk populations (Mumford et al., 1982; Sulman & Ver-haeghe, 1985). The question of whether to screen patients for need and to tailor an intervention to specific patient groups is important. Research indicates that supportive interventions have little effect on patients with little need (Horlick et al., 1984; Naismeth et al., 1979). Furthermore, patients' decision to participate in cardiac groups may be differently influenced by their comfort with whether the cardiac group has a psycho-therapeutic versus an educational format (Hackett, 1978). Finally, some patients may experience iatrogenic effects if they are the recipients of a mismatched intervention.

An example of this latter point was found in the controlled study referred to above (Naismeth et al., 1979). In additional analyses in that study, patients were classified (using the Eysenck Personality Inventory) as neurotic introverts and stable extroverts (Naismeth et al., 1979). Neurotic introverts achieved a much better outcome on all rehabilitation measures than their counterparts in the control groups following the psychological counseling program. No evidence was found that rehabilitation exacer-bated neurosis; however, an impression was gained that for the stable extroverts, the program could have negative effects on established coping strategies.

Recent studies of MI and PTCA patients lend further support to considerations of tailoring educational interventions to patient styles (Cromwell, Butterfield, Brayfield, & Curry, 1977; Shaw, Cohen, Doyle, & Palesky, 1985; Shaw et al., 1986; Weinberger, Schwartz, & Davidson, 1979). These studies have attempted to examine the effects of informational interventions on cardiac outcome among patients with different coping styles (specifically, repressors versus sensitizers). Information is one form of social support that figures prominently in cardiac recovery in the acute phase. In one study, a mismatch between the information intervention and repressive coping style was associated with a higher number of heart alarms among hospitalized MI patients and with patients being rated less cooperative by the staff (Cromwell et al., 1977). Weinberger and colleagues (1979) found that repressors with high levels of cardiac risk information at post-MI discharge reported significantly more medical complications and poorer psychological functioning during the 6 months following discharge than repressors with low levels of risk information. Sensitizers with low levels of risk factor information at discharge reported poorer social functioning (Shaw et al., 1985).

Most recently, mismatch between information and repressive coping style was found to be associated with late medical complications following PTCA (Shaw et al., 1986). In that study sensitizers with a low level of cardiac information and whose PTCA was only moderately successful were at higher risk for restenosis of the artery that had been widened during the treatment. Taken together, these findings suggest that future intervention research should consider various approaches to identifying at-risk patients and to tailoring information and social support in general to patient dispositional characteristics.

Supportive Family Interventions

As already noted, the literature sets forth a strong theoretical and empirical rationale for interventions that influence the support family members naturally provide to patients. Family support has been demonstrated to have potentially salutary or negative effects on patient adjustment; in addition, there is some evidence that spouses perceive the health care practitioner's "bedside manner" and information-giving role to be important to their own psychological well-being (Boycoff, 1986). Interventions therefore may be designed to provide family members with emotional and informational support, or family members can be instructed in specific supportive behaviors that they may direct to patients.

Again, admonitions to practitioners to provide supportive family care are numerous in the literature (Bromberg & Donnerstag, 1977; Davidson, 1979; Ell & Northern, 1990; Gardner & Stewart, 1978; Raymond et al., 1984). Descriptions of such are usually reported to be beneficial to both patients and family members (Pozen et al., 1977). For example, family group conferences conducted one evening a week by nursing staff and a psychiatric clinical specialist are reported to be helpful in reducing family members' anxiety during hospitalization (Holub, Ecklund, & Keenan, 1975), and a drop-in weekly support group for wives of MI patients is reported to be helpful to participants and to provide valuable assessment information to staff (Harding & Morefield, 1976). Rigorous evaluations of family interventions, however, is rare (Thompson & Meddis, 1990).

Several examples illustrate areas for further research. In a preliminary study, 12 patients were randomly assigned to an experimental or control group (Doerr & Jones, 1979). Family members of patients in the treatment group were given an information manual concerning the coronary care unit and an opportunity to ask the nurse questions; control families were given no preparation. Pre- and postvisitation patient assessments using the Spielberger State Anxiety Inventory found patient anxiety declined among those whose families were prepared, whereas patients with unprepared families experienced an increase in state anxiety.

In another study, a treatment and control group—each consisting of 10 male patients undergoing CABG—were examined for postcardiotomy psychosis (Chatham, 1978). All patients received preoperative teaching, and all subjects were maintained on cardiopulmonary bypass for at least 60 minutes. A family member or friend of experimental patients received systematic instruction concerning the functions of the equipment used in the ICU, the postoperative care routine of the patient, and the patient's need for eye contact, frequent touch, and verbal orientation to time, person, and place. Patients in the experimental group were judged during hospitalization by nursing staff to be more oriented to time, person, and place; to be more appropriate and less confused, as demonstrated by speech and behaviors; and to have fewer delusions and longer sleep periods when compared to controls. No differences were found between groups on alertness, agitation, complaints, depression, activity, or anxiety during hospitalization.

It is disturbing that so little intervention research has examined either patient care or family-focused strategies during acute cardiac episodes. Several factors presumably contribute to this gap in the research to date. First, behavioral and social scientists with the requisite research skills are rarely active members of cardiac care teams; as a result, a necessary dialogue between clinicians and researchers is not fostered (Ell, 1985–86). Medical staff and nursing staff are oriented to meeting the demands inherent in providing the technical care that is lifesaving during acute cardiac events.

Furthermore, the structure of intensive care (and, to a great extent, hospital environments in general) excludes specific consideration of family needs and family roles during acute illness episodes. Finally, health care financing mechanisms commonly fail to include coverage for family-oriented care during acute events, and thus there is little administrative support for providing such care (Ell & Northern, 1990; Sikes & Rodenhauser, 1987). It seems that many of the barriers to expanding supportive care during acute cardiac episodes would fall with substantial growth evidence of the utility of such care on cardiac outcomes and on the quality of life of both patients and families.

Research Agenda

Need for Conceptual Frameworks

Perhaps the greatest limitation of past research is its atheoretical nature. The work of Lazarus and colleagues (Lazarus, 1966; Lazarus & Folkman, 1984) is one such framework that might be fruitful for exploring the effects of acute cardiac events. Within this model, stress is defined as a transaction between a person and his or her environment that taxes or exceeds personal resources (Lazarus & Folkman, 1984). Resources include *dispositional factors* (e.g., self-esteem, attitudes, values and beliefs, and personal commitments), *social factors* (e.g., the presence of a social network and its responsiveness to stressful circumstances), and *material resources* (e.g., money and possessions).

When an environmental event or sequence of events is seen as taxing the individual's normal adaptive capacity, the person appraises the circumstances as stressful. Primary or first-order appraisals of stressful events include that they are threatening, challenging, or have already caused harm or loss. Regardless of the specific nature of the stress appraisal, the person must cope in some manner in order to alter the situation (problem-focused coping) and to manage the emotional consequences or distress (emotion-focused coping). Coping is defined as cognitive and behavioral efforts to manage the demands of the situation (Lazarus & Folkman, 1984). For example, a postcoronary bypass patient may attempt to maintain optimism to ward off feelings of depression and may also engage actively in healthy postoperative recovery behavior in order to regain functioning as quickly as possible. Studies on adaptation to acute cardiac events such as myocardial infarction, coronary bypass surgery, or angioplasty can be improved by using a framework such as this to guide research questions and hypotheses, development of measures, and interpretation of results.

Ultimately models that are specific to adaptation to cardiac events may need to be developed, but at this stage of our knowledge, much is to be learned from examining general processes of stress, coping, and adaptation. Conceptual models are needed not only to provide a framework for studying adaptation in cardiac patients, but also for guiding research on social support in this area.

Although effective and well-targeted support attempts are likely to be beneficial to acute cardiac patients, less effective or misdirected efforts are just as likely to have ill effects, to confuse the patients, and complicate the interpersonal situation. One example of this is when a family member is overinvolved in a distressed person's situation (Coyne, Ellard, & Smith, 1990; Coyne & Smith, 1991; Coyne, Wortman, & Lehman, 1988). Other specific behaviors (e.g., cutting off the patient's attempts to communicate distress because it is believed to reflect poor coping, or blaming the patient) have been discussed with respect to cancer (Dunkel-Schetter & Wortman, 1982; Wortman & Dunkel-Schetter, 1979), severe depression (Coyne, 1976; Coates & Wortman, 1980), and negative life events in general (Silver & Wortman, 1980; Wortman & Lehman, 1985). Little consideration of the matter, however, has taken place for heart disease in general or for acute cardiac events specifically. What things do family members and health care providers do that upset or detract from the recovery progress of MI, CABG, and PTCA patients? It is well established that social interaction is a two-edged sword, with possibilities for harm as well as benefit. Thus consideration in future research of the social interactions of coronary patients during the acute phase is necessary.

Very little has been written in the social support literature on the processes by which social support influences health outcomes (see Cohen, 1988; Cohen & Syme, 1985; House, Landis, & Umberson, 1988; Wortman & Dunkel-Schetter, 1982). Considerable epidemiological data exist linking social support to the development of cardiovascular disease (see Chapters 5 and 6), but these studies stop short of explaining the biopsychosocial processes involved. It is widely acknowledged that we must understand social support processes in order to take full advantage of any intervention opportunities or possibilities for application of basic research on social support effects. We need to understand not only the extent to which social support influences recovery from these events in the short term but, most importantly, the process by which any effects occur (House et al., 1988). For example, does support from family and health care providers during the acute phase help recovery rates by reducing physiological arousal and subjective feelings of anxiety? Another hypotheses is that support is most effective when it influences the person to cope in particular ways (e.g., by seeking information). Still a third possibility is that support functions to influence the person's appraisal of his or her cardiac condition; that is, effective and beneficial support might function to alter perceptions of the cardiac condition from one of a threatening and unalterable loss to that of a manageable and challenging situation. In summary, several non–mutually exclusive possibilities exist as the mechanisms by which social support efforts may benefit a cardiac patient during the acute care phase.

Factors Associated with Outcomes
and Avenues for Social Support

One way in which future research on social support and acute cardiac events could be approached is to consider specific factors that have been associated with outcomes for MI, CABG, and PTCA patients as possible avenues for social support influences. Factors associated with outcome can be divided into patient and family factors. One of the most potent variables for both patient and family that may influence outcomes is the patients' and families' perceptions of the situation. For the patient, such perceptions include appraisals of the severity and extent of loss or harm, assessments of risk and future vulnerability, and attributions about the causes and controllability of the situation. Family members' perceptions of the status of the patient as disabled, functional, vulnerable, and so forth are also likely to be relevant. Research could be targeted to determine the supportive efforts that are most likely to influence these appraisal factors, thereby indirectly influencing outcome.

Another factor in determining outcome is the affective responses of both patient and family members. Patients who react to acute cardiac events in particular ways (e.g., with extreme depression) may be targeted for supportive interventions whose goal is to improve the patient's outcome by helping the person to work through or manage his or her emotions. Similarly, extreme emotional reactions on the part of family members may be important factors in outcome. A spouse who is extremely anxious is unlikely to be an effective source of support and is instead likely to be detrimental to the patient. Supportive efforts aimed at helping spouses manage and reduce their anxiety would be another possible way of indirectly influencing medical outcomes (Taylor et al., 1985).

Another set of factors associated with outcomes is patient decision making, adherence, and risk reduction behavior. Each of these has been associated with the outcomes of acute cardiac events. Supportive efforts aimed at improving any of these behaviors would be worth considering as further indirect means of influencing outcomes. As we gain a better idea of which factors influence recovery, they may provide potent avenues for applying social support. This information should also shed light on the processes by which social support works.

Unanswered Research Questions

A plethora of research questions remain unanswered about the role of social support in recovery from acute cardiac events and some research mandates:

1. What types, sources, timing, and qualities of social support most strongly influence cardiac event adjustment?
2. Cardiac programs in acute care involving supportive components must be evaluated scientifically to determine their multiple effects. Do these interventions have negative as well as positive effects for patients and families?
3. Who is most likely to delay seeking care for a cardiac event? To what extent does interpretation, consultation, or a help seeking process increase delay? To what extent do background variables such as ethnicity contribute to delay, and what underlying mechanisms account for ethnic differences?
4. What role do physicians play in influencing patients to undergo risky or unproven treatments?
5. Can families be more involved during hospitalization in observing, learning, and participating in patient care? What benefits, risks, and barriers accompany such efforts?
6. What are the effects of specific supportive behaviors by health care providers in cardiac care on patient recovery?

References

Abbey, A., Abramis, D. J., & Caplan, R. D. (1985). Effects of different sources of social support and social conflict on emotional well-being. *Basic and Applied Psychology*, 6, 111–130.

Acker, J. E. (1978). Psychological aspects of cardiac rehabilitation: Assessment and approach to the patient. *Advances in Cardiology*, 24, 116–119.

Affleck, G., Tennen, H., Croog, S., & Levine, S. (1987). Causal attribution, perceived benefits, and morbidity after a heart attack: An 8-year study. *Journal of Consulting and Clinical Psychology*, 55, 29–35.

Aho, W. R. (1977). Relationship of wives' preventive health orientation to their beliefs about heart disease in husbands. *Public Health Reports*, 92, 65–71.

Aiken, L. H. (1975, August). *Family adjustment following myocardial infarction: Implications for ambulatory medical care*. Paper presented at the annual meeting of the American Sociological Association.

Alonzo, A. A. (1977). The impact of physician consultation on care-seeking during acute episodes of coronary heart disease. *Medical Care*, 15, 34–50.

Alonzo, A. A. (1979). Everyday illness behavior: A situational approach to health status deviations. *Social Science and Medicine*, 13A, 397–404.

Alonzo, A. A. (1980a). Acute illness behavior: A conceptual exploration and specification. *Social Science and Medicine*, 14A, 515–526.

Alonzo, A. A. (1980b). The mobile coronary care unit and the decision to seek medical care during acute episodes of coronary artery disease. *Medical Care*, 18, 297–318.

Alonzo, A. A. (1984). An illness behavior paradigm: A conceptual exploration of a situational-adaptation perspective. *Social Science and Medicine*, 19, 499–509.

Alonzo, A. A. (1986). The impact of the family and lay others on care-seeking during life-threatening episodes of suspected coronary artery disease. *Social Science and Medicine, 22,* 1297–1311.

Althof, S. E., Coffman, C. B., & Levine, S. B. (1984). The effects of coronary bypass surgery on female sexual, psychological, and vocational adaptation. *Journal of Sex and Marital Therapy, 10,* 176–184.

American Heart Association (1986). *1987 heart facts.* Dallas: Author.

Anderson, E. A. (1987). Preoperative preparation for cardiac surgery facilitates recovery, reduces psychological distress, and reduces the incidence of acute postoperative hypertension. *Journal of Consulting and Clinical Psychology, 55,* 513–520.

Andrew, J. (1970). Recovery from surgery, with and without preparatory instruction, for three coping styles. *Journal of Personality and Social Psychology, 15,* 223–226.

Bar-on, D. (1987). Causal attributions and the rehabilitation of myocardial infarction victims. *Journal of Social and Clinical Psychology, 5,* 114–122.

Bar-on, D., & Dreman, S. (1987). When spouses disagree: A predictor of cardiac rehabilitation. *Family Systems Medicine, 5,* 228–237.

Bedsworth, J. A., & Molen, M. T. (1982). Psychological stress in spouses of patients with myocardial infarction. *Heart and Lung, 11,* 450–456.

Berkanovic, E., & Telesky, C. (1982). Social networks, beliefs, and the decision to seek medical care: An analogy of congruent and incongruent patterns. *Medical Care, 20,* 1018–1025.

Berkanovic, E., Telesky, C., & Reeder, S. (1979). Structural and social psychological factors in the decision to seek medical care for symptoms. *Medical Care, 19,* 693–709.

Bilodeau, C. B., & Hackett, T. P. (1971). Issues raised in a group setting by patients recovering from myocardial infarction. *American Journal of Psychiatry, 128,* 105–110.

Block, A. R., Boyer, S. L., & Imes, C. (1984). Personal impact of myocardial infarction: A model for coping with physical disability in middle age. In M. G. Eisenberg & M. A. Jansen (Eds.), *Chronic illness and disability through the life span: Effects on self and family* (pp. 209–221). New York: Springer.

Block, P. C. (1985). Percutaneous transluminal coronary angioplasty: Role in the treatment of coronary artery disease. *Circulation, 72*(Suppl. 5), 161–165.

Bordow, S., & Porritt, D. (1979). An experimental evaluation of crisis intervention. *Social Science and Medicine, 13A,* 251–256.

Boycoff, S. L. (1986). Visitation needs reported by patients with cardiac disease and their families. *Heart and Lung, 15,* 573–578.

Bramwell, L. (1986). Wives' experiences in the support role after husbands' first myocardial infarction. *Heart and Lung, 15,* 578–584.

Bromberg, H., & Donnerstag, E. (1977). Counseling heart patients and their families. *Health and Social Work, 2,* 159–172.

Bruhn, J. G. (1977). Effects of chronic illness on the family. *Journal of Family Practice, 4,* 1057–1060.

Byrne, D. G. (1982). Illness behavior and psychosocial outcome after a heart attack. *British Journal of Clinical Psychology, 21,* 145–146.

Byrne, D. G., Whyte, H. M., & Butler, R. L. (1981). Illness behavior and outcome following myocardial infarction: A prospective study. *Journal of Psychosomatic Research, 25,* 99–107.

Caplan, G. (1976). The family as a support system. In G. Caplan & M. Killilea (Eds.), *Support systems and mutual help* (pp. 19–36). New York: Grune and Stratton.

Carr, J. A., & Powers, M. J. (1986). Stressors associated with coronary bypass surgery. *Nursing Research, 35,* 243–247.

Carter, R. E. (1984). Family reactions and reorganization patterns in myocardial infarction. *Family System Medicine, 2,* 55–64.

Case, R., Moss, A., Case, M., McDermott, M., & Eberly, S. (1992). Living alone after myocardial infarction. *Journal of the American Medical Association, 267*(4), 515–519.

CASS Principal Investigators & Associates. (1983a). Coronary Artery Surgery Study (CASS): A randomized trial of coronary artery bypass surgery survival data. *Circulation, 68,* 939–950.

CASS Principal Investigators & Associates. (1983b). Coronary Artery Surgery Study (CASS): Quality of life of patients randomly assigned to treatment groups. *Circulation, 68,* 951–960.

Cassileth, B. R., Lusk, E. J., Strouse, T. B., Miller, D. S., Brown, L. L., & Cross, P. A. (1985). A psychological analysis of cancer patients and their next-of-kin. *Cancer, 55,* 72–76.

Cay, E. L. (1982). Psychological problems in patients after a myocardial infarction. *Advances in Cardiology, 29,* 108–112.

Cay, E. L., Vetter, N., Philip, A. E., & Dugard, P. (1972). Psychological status during recovery from an acute heart attack. *Journal of Psychosomatic Research, 16,* 425–435.

Chandra, V., Szklo, M., Goldberg, R., & Tonascia, J. (1983). The impact of marital status on survival after an acute myocardial infarction: A population-based study. *American Journal of Epidemiology, 117,* 320–325.

Chatham, M. A. (1978). The effect of family involvement on patients' manifestations of postcardiotomy psychosis. *Heart and Lung, 7,* 995–999.

Christopherson, B., & Pfeiffer, C. (1980). Varying the timing of information to alter preoperative anxiety and postoperative recovery in cardiac surgery patients. *Heart and Lung, 9,* 854–861.

Coates, D., & Wortman, C. B. (1980). Depressive maintenance and interpersonal control. In A. Baum & J. Singer (Eds.), *Advance in environmental psychology, vol. 2* (pp. 149–182). Hillsdale, NJ: Erlbaum.

Cohen, S. (1988). Psychological models of the role of social support in the etiology of physical disease. *Health Psychology, 7,* 269–297.

Cohen, S., & Syme, S. L. (1985). Issues in the study and application of social support. In S. Cohen & L. Syme (Eds.), *Social support and health* (pp. 3–22). New York: Academic Press.

Cooper, R. S., Simmons, B., Castaner, A., Prasad, R., Franklin, C., & Ferlinz, J. (1986). Survival rates and prehospital delay during myocardial infarction among black persons. *American Journal of Cardiology, 57,* 208–211.

Coulton, C., & Frost, A. (1982). Use of social and health services by the elderly. *Journal of Health and Social Behavior, 23,* 330–339.

Cowie, B. (1976). The cardiac patient's perception of his heart attack. *Social Science and Medicine, 10A,* 87–96.

Coyne, J. C., Ellard, J. H., & Smith, D. A. F. (1990). Social support, interdependence, and the dilemmas of helping. In B. R. Sarason, I. G. Sarason, & G. R. Pierce (Eds.), *Social support: An interactional view.* New York: Wiley.

Coyne, J.C., & Smith, D. A. F. (1991). Couples coping with myocardial infarction: A contextual perspective on wives' distress. *Journal of Personality and Social Psychology, 61*(3), 404–412.

Coyne, J. C., & De Longis, A. (1986). Going beyond social support: The role of social relationships in adaptation. *Journal of Consulting and Clinical Psychology, 54,* 454–460.

Coyne, J. C., Wortman, C. B., & Lehman, D. R. (1988). The other side of support: Emotional overinvolvement and miscarried helping. In B. H. Gottlieb (Ed.), *Marshalling social support: Formats, processes, and effects.* Newbury Park, CA: Sage.

Coyne, J. C. (1976). Toward an interactional description of depression. *Psychiatry, 39,* 28–40.

Cromwell, R. L., Butterfield, E. C., Brayfield, F. R., & Curry, J. L. (1977). *Acute myocardial infarction: Reaction and recovery.* St. Louis: Mosby.

Croog, S. H., & Fitzgerald, E. F. (1978). Subjective stress and serious illness of a spouse: Wives of heart patients. *Journal of Health and Social Behavior, 19,* 166–177.

Croog, S. H., & Levine, S. (1977). *The heart patient recovers: Social and psychological factors.* New York: Human Sciences Press.

Croog, S. H., Lipson, A., & Levine, S. (1972). Help patterns in severe illness: The role of kin networks, non-family resources, and institution. *Journal of Marriage and the Family, 34,* 12–23.

Davidson, D. M. (1979). The family and cardiac rehabilitation. *Journal of Family Practice, 8,* 253–261.

Davidson, D. M. (1983). Recovery after cardiac events. In J. S. Spittell, Jr. (Ed.), *Clinical medicine* (pp. 1–20). Philadelphia: Harper and Row.

Davidson, R. H. (1985). Coronary artery bypass surgery and coronary angioplasty. In *Coronary heart disease* (pp. 143–171). New York: Medical Examination Publishing.

Dean, A., & Tausing, M. (1986). Measuring intimate support: The family and confidant relationships. In N. Lin & W. M. Ensel (Eds.), *Social support, life events, and depression* (pp. 117–128). New York: Academic Press.

Detre, K. M., Takaro, T., Hultgren, H., Peduzzi, P., & Study Participants. (1985). Long-term mortality and morbidity results of the Veterans Administration randomized trial of coronary artery bypass surgery. *Circulation, 72,* 84–89.

Dhooper, S. S. (1983). Family coping with the crisis of heart attack. *Social Work in Health Care, 9,* 15–31.

Doehrman, S. R. (1977). Psychosocial aspects of recovery from coronary heart disease: A review. *Social Science and Medicine, 11,* 199–218.

Doerr, B. C., & Jones, J. W. (1979). Effect of family preparation on the state anxiety level of the CCU patient. *Nursing Research, 28,* 315–316.

Dracup, K., Meleis, A., Baker, K., & Edlefsen, P. (1984). Family-focused cardiac rehabilitation: A role supplementation program for cardiac patients and spouses. *Nursing Clinics of North America, 19,* 113–124.

Dunkel-Schetter, C. (1984). Social support and cancer: Findings based on patient interviews and their implications. *Journal of Social Issues, 40,* 77–98.

Dunkel-Schetter, C. & Wortman, C. B. (1982). The interpersonal dynamics of cancer: Problems in social relationships and their impact on the patient. In H. S. Friedman & M. R. DiMatteo (eds.), *Interpersonal issues in health care* (pp. 69–100). New York: Academic Press.

Egbert, L. D., Battit, G. E., Welch, C. E., & Bartlett, M. K. (1964). Reduction of postoperative pain by encouragement and instruction of patients. *New England Journal of Medicine, 270,* 825–827.

Eggert, L. L. (1987). Support in family ties: Stress, coping and adaptation. In T. L. Albrecht, M. B. Adelman, & Associates (Eds.), *Communicating social support* (pp. 80–104). Beverly Hills, CA: Sage.

Ell, K. O. (1985–86). Coping with serious illness: On integrating constructs to enhance clinical research, assessment and intervention. *International Journal of Psychiatry in Medicine, 15,* 335–356.

Ell, K. O., & Haywood, L. J. (1984). Social support and recovery from myocardial infarction: A panel study. *Journal of Social Service Research, 4,* 1–9.

Ell, K. O., & Haywood, L. J. (1985–86). Sociocultural factors in MI recovery: An exploratory study. *International Journal of Psychiatry in Medicine, 15,* 157–175.

Ell, K. O., Nishimoto, R. W., Mantell, J., & Hamovitch, M. B. (1988a). A longitudinal analysis of psychological adaptation among family members of patients with cancer. *Journal of Psychosomatic Research, 32,* 429–438.

Ell, K. O., Nishimoto, R. W., Mantell, J., & Hamovitch, M. B. (1988b). Psychosocial adaptation to cancer: A comparison among patients, spouses and nonspouses. *Family Systems Medicine, 6,* 335–348.

Ell, K. O., & Northern, H. (1990). *Families and health care: Psychosocial practice.* New York: Aldine de Gruyter.

Finlayson, A., & McEwen, J. (1977). *Coronary heart disease and patterns of living.* New York: Prodist.

Fiore, J., Becker, J., & Coppel, D. B. (1983). Social network interactions: A buffer or a stress. *American Journal of Community Psychology, 11,* 423–439.

Fiske, V., Coyne, J. C., & Smith, D. A. (1991). Couples coping with myocardial infarction: An empirical reconsideration of the role of overprotectiveness. *Journal of Family Psychology, 5*(1), 4–20.

Fleming, J. L. (1980). Nonpharmalogical methods for dealing with preoperative anxiety: The use of supportive conversation. In F. Guerra (Ed.), *Emotional and psychological response to anesthesia and surgery.* New York: Grune and Stratton.

Fletcher, A. E., Hunt, B. M., & Bulpitt, C. J. (1987). Evaluation of quality of life in clinical trials of cardiovascular disease. *Journal of Chronic Disease, 40,* 557–566.

Folks, D. G., Blake, D. J., Fleece, L., Sokol, R. S., & Freeman, A. M., III. (1986). Quality of life six months after coronary artery bypass surgery: A preliminary report. *Southern Medical Journal, 79,* 397–399.

Fuller, B. F., & Foster, G. M. (1982). The effects of family/friend visits vs. staff interaction on stress/arousal of surgical intensive care patients. *Heart and Lung, 11,* 457–463.

Gardner, D., & Stewart, S. (1978). Staff involvement with families of patients in critical-care units. *Heart and Lung, 7,* 105–110.

Garrity, T. F. (1973a). Social involvement and activeness as predictors of morale six months after first myocardial infarction. *Social Science and Medicine, 7,* 199–207.

Garrity, T. F. (1973b). Vocational adjustment after first myocardial infarction: Comparative assessment of several variables suggested in the literature. *Social Science and Medicine, 7,* 705–717.

Garrity, T. F. (1981). Behavior adjustment after myocardial infarction: A selective review of recent descriptive, correlational, and intervention research. In S. M. Weiss, J. A. Herd, & B. H. Fox (Eds.), *Perspectives on behavior medicine* (pp. 67–87). New York: Academic Press.

Garrity, T. F., & Klein, R. (1975). Emotional response and clinical severity as early determinants of six month mortality after myocardial infarction. *Heart and Lung, 4,* 730–737.

Gentry, W. D. (1975). Preadmission behavior. In W. D. Gentry & R. B. Williams, Jr. (Eds.), *Psychological aspects of myocardial infarction and coronary care* (pp. 53–62). St. Louis: Mosby.

Gillis, C. L. (1984). Reducing family stress during and after coronary artery bypass surgery. *Nursing Clinics of North America, 19,* 103–111.

Gillum, R. F., Feinleib, M., Margolis, M. D., Fabsitz, M. A., & Barsch, M. D. (1976). Delay in the prehospital phase of acute myocardial infarction: Lack of influence on incidence of sudden death. *Archives of Internal Medicine, 136,* 649–654.

Goldman, L. S., & Kimball, C. P. (1985). Cardiac surgery: Enhancing postoperative outcomes. In A. M. Razin & Associates (Eds.), *Helping cardiac patients: Biobehavioral and psychotherapeutic approaches* (pp. 113–155). San Francisco: Jossey-Bass.

Gotay, C. C. (1984). The experience of cancer during early and advanced stages: The views of patients and their mates. *Social Science and Medicine, 18,* 605–613.

Graboys, T. B., Headley, A., Lown, B., Lampert, S., & Blatt, C. M. (1987). Results of a second-opinion program for coronary artery bypass graft surgery. *Journal of the American Medical Association, 258,* 1611–1614.

Granger, J. W. (1974). Full recovery from myocardial infarction: Psychosocial factors. *Heart and Lung, 3,* 600–610.

Greene, W. A., Moss, A. J., & Goldstein, S. (1974). Delay, denial and death in coronary heart disease. In R. S. Eliot (Ed.), *Stress and the heart.* New York: Plenum.

Greenhill, M. H., & Frater, R. M. B. (1976). Changes in family interrelationships following cardiac surgery. *Archives of the Foundation of Thanatology, 6,* 34–36.

Greenspon, A. J., & Goldberg, S. (1983). What is the role of percutaneous transluminal angioplasty in coronary artery disease? In S. H. Rahimtoola (Ed.), *Controversies in coronary artery disease* (pp. 265–281). Philadelphia: Davis.

Gruen, W. (1975). Effects of brief psychotherapy during the hospitalization period on the recovery process in heart attacks. *Journal of Consulting and Clinical Psychology, 43*, 223–232.

Gulledge, A. D. (1975). The psychological aftermath of a myocardial infarction. In W. D. Gentry & R. B. Williams, Jr. (Eds.), *Psychological aspects of myocardial infarction and coronary care* (pp. 107–123). St. Louis: Mosby.

Gundle, M. J., Reeves, B. R., Tate, S. Raft, D., & McLaurin, L. P. (1980). Psychosocial outcome after coronary artery surgery. *American Journal of Psychiatry, 137*, 1591–1594.

Hackett, T. P. (1978). The use of groups in the rehabilitation of the postcoronary patient. *Advances in Cardiology, 24*, 127–135.

Hackett, T. P., & Cassem, N. H. (1969). Factors contributing to delay in responding to the signs and symptoms of acute myocardial infarction. *American Journal of Cardiology, 24*, 651–658.

Hacket, T. P., & Cassem, N. H. (1973). Psychological rehabilitation of myocardial infarction patients in the acute phase. *Heart and Lung, 2*, 382–388.

Hackett, T. P., & Cassem, N. H. (1975). Psychological intervention in myocardial infarction. In W. D. Gentry & R. B. Williams, Jr. (Eds.), *Psychological aspects of myocardial infarction and coronary care* (pp. 137–149). St. Louis: Mosby.

Hall, R. J., Elayda, M. A., Gray, A., Mathur, V. S., Garcia, E., DeCastro, C. M., Massumi, A., & Cooley, D. A. (1983). Coronary artery bypass: Long term follow-up of 22,284 consecutive patients. *Circulation, 68*(Suppl. 2), 20–26.

Harding, A. L., & Morefield, M. A. (1976). Group intervention for wives of myocardial infarction patients. *Nursing Clinics of North America, 11*, 339–347.

Hartley, L. H. (1988). Physiological mechanisms and behavioral interactions of cardiovascular rehabilitation. In W. A. Gordon, J. A. Herd, & A. Baum (Eds.), *Perspectives on behavioral medicine: Prevention and rehabilitation* (pp. 169–178). San Diego: Academic Press.

Henning, H., Gilpin, E. A., Covell, J. W., Swan, E. A., O'Rourke, R. A., & Ross, J. (1979). Prognosis after acute myocardial infarction: A multivariate analysis of mortality and survival. *Circulation, 59*, 1124–1136.

Holub, D., Eklund, P., & Keenan, P. (1975). Family conferences as an adjunct to total coronary care. *Heart and Lung, 4*, 767–769.

Horgan, D., Davies, B., Hunt, D., Westlake, G. W., & Mullerworth, M. (1984). Psychiatric aspects of coronary artery surgery: A prospective study. *Medical Journal of Australia, 141*, 587–590.

Horlick, L., Cameron, R., Firor, W., Bhalerao, U., & Baltzan, R. (1984). The effects of education and group discussion in the post–myocardial infarction patient. *Journal of Psychosomatic Research, 28*, 485–492.

Horowitz, A. (1978). Family, kin and friend networks in psychiatric help-seeking. *Social Science and Medicine, 12*, 297–304.

House, J. S., Landis, K. R., & Umberson, D. (1988). Social relationships and health. *Science, 241*, 540–545.

Ibrahim, M. A., Feldman, J. G., Sulty, H. A., Stainman, M. G., Young, L. J., & Dean, D. (1974). Management after myocardial infarction: A controlled trial of the effect of group psychotherapy. *International Journal of Psychiatry in Medicine, 5*, 253–268.

Jenkins, C. D., Stanton, B., Savageau, J. A., Ockene, B. S., Denlinger, P., & Klein, M. D. (1983). Coronary artery bypass surgery: Physical, psychological, social and economic outcomes six months later. *Journal of the American medical Association, 250*, 782–788.

Johnson, J. E. (1984). Coping with elective surgery. *Annual Review of Nursing* (pp. 107–132).

Jutzy, K. R., Berte, L. E., Alderman, E. L., Ratts, J., & Simpson, J. B. (1982). Coronary restenosis rates in consecutive patient series one year post successful angioplasty. *Circulation, 66*, 311–331.

Kannel, W. B., Sorlie, P., & McNamara, P. M. (1979). Prognosis after initial myocardial infarction: The Framingham study. *American Journal of Cardiology, 44*, 53–59.

Kent, K. M., Bentivoglio, L. G., Block, P. C., Cowley, M. J., Dorros, G., Gosselin, A. J., Gruntzig, A., Myler, R. K., Simpson, J., Stertzer, S. H., William, D. O., Fisher, L., Gillespie, M., Detre, K., Kelsey, S., Mullin, S. M., & Mock, M. B. (1982). Percussions transluminal coronary angioplasty: Report from the registry of the National Heart, Lung, and Blood Institute. *American Journal of Cardiology, 49*, 2011–2020.

Kinchla, J., & Weiss, T. (1985). Psychologic and social outcomes following coronary artery bypass surgery. *Journal of Cardiopulmonary Rehabilitation, 5*, 274–283.

King, K. B. (1985). Measurement of coping, strategies, concerns, and emotional response in patients undergoing coronary artery bypass grafting. *Heart and Lung, 14*, 579–586.

Kornfield, D. S., Heller, S. S., Frank, K. A., Wilson, S. N., & Malm, J. R. (1982). Psychological and behavioral responses after coronary artery bypass surgery. *Circulation, 66*(Suppl. 3), 24–28.

Krantz, D. S. (1980). Cognitive processes and recovery from heart attack: A review and theoretical analysis. *Journal of Human Stress, 6*, 27–38.

Kulik, J. A., & Mahler, I. M. (1984). Social support and recovery from surgery. *Health Psychology, 311*, 552–559.

Kulik, J. A., & Mahler, I. M. (1987). Effects of preoperative roommate assignment on preoperative anxiety and recovery from coronary-bypass surgery. *Health Psychology, 6*, 525–543.

Ladwig, K. H., Lehmacker, W., Rock, J., Breithhordt, G., Budde, T. H., & Borggrefe, M. (1992). Factors which provoke post-infarction depression: Results from the Post-Infarction Late Potential study (PILP). *Journal of Psychosomatic Research, 36*(8), 723–729.

LaMendola, W. F., & Pellegrini, R. V. (1979). Quality of life and coronary artery bypass surgery patients. *Social Science and Medicine, 13A*, 457–461.

Langeluddecke, P., Tennant, C., Fulcher, G., Barid, D., & Hughes, D. (1989). Coronary artery bypass surgery: Impact upon the patient's spouse. *Journal of Psychosomatic Research, 33*(2), 155–159.

Lazarus, R. S. (1966). *Psychological stress and the coping process*. New York: McGraw-Hill.

Lazarus, R. S., & Folkman, S. (1984). *Stress, appraisal, and coping*. New York: Springer.

Litman, T. J. (1974). The family as a basic unit in health and medical care: A social-behavioral overview. *Social Science and Medicine, 8*, 495–500.

Lloyd, G. G., & Cawley, R. H. (1983). Distress or illness? A study of psychological symptoms after myocardial infarction. *British Journal of Psychiatry, 142*, 120–125.

Maeland, J. G., & Havik, O. E. (1987). Psychological predictors for return to work after a myocardial infarction. *Journal of Psychosomatic Research, 31*, 471–481.

Matthews, K. A., Siegel, J. M., Kuller, L. H., Thompson, M., & Varat, M. (1983). Determinants of decisions to seek medical treatment by patients with acute myocardial infarctions symptoms. *Journal of Personality and Social Psychology, 44*, 1144–1156.

Mayou, R. (1981). Effectiveness of cardiac rehabilitation. *Journal of Psychosomatic Research, 25*, 423–427.

Mayou, R. (1984). Predication of emotional and social outcome after a heart attack. *Journal of Psychosomatic Research, 28*, 17–25.

Mayou, R., Foster, A., & Williamson, B. (1978). The psychological and social effects of myocardial infarction on wives. *British Medical Journal, 1*, 669–701.

Mayou, R., Williamson, B., & Foster, A. (1976). Attitude and advice after myocardial infarction. *British Medical Journal, 1,* 1577–1579.

Mayou, R. A., Williamson, B., & Foster, A. (1978). Outcome two months after myocardial infarction. *Journal of Psychosomatic Research, 22,* 439–445.

McKinlay, J. B. (1973). Social networks, lay consultation and help-making behavior. *Social Forces, 51,* 275–292.

McKinlay, J. B. (1972). Some approaches and problems in the study of the use of services—an overview. *Journal of Health and Social Behavior, 13,* 115–152.

McKinley, J. B. (1981). Social network influences on morbid episodes and the career of help-seeking. In L. Eisenberg & A. Kleinman (Eds.), *The relevance of social science for medicine* (pp. 77–107). Dordrecht, Netherlands: Reidel.

Meagher, D. M., Gregor, F., & Stewart, M. (1987). Dyadic social support for cardiac surgery patients—a Canadian approach. *Social Science and medicine, 25,* 833–837.

Melamed, B. G., & Brenner, G. F. (1990). Social support and chronic medical stress: An interactional-based approach. *Journal of Social and Clinical Psychology, 9*(1), 104–117.

Michela, J. L. (1987). Interpersonal and individual impacts of a husband's heart attach. In A. Baum & J. E. Singer (Eds.), *Handbook of psychology and health: Stress, vol 5* (pp. 255–301). Hillsdale, NJ: Erlbaum.

Minckley, B. B., Burrows, D., Ehrat, K., Harper, L., Jenkin, S. A., Minckley, W. F., Page, B., Schramm, D. E., & Wood, C. (1979). Myocardial infarction stress of transfer inventory: Development of a research tool. *Nursing Research, 28,* 4–20.

Mitchell, M. (1976). Rx for your patient's family. *Supervising Nurse, 7,* 42–43.

Moss, A. J., Wynar, B., & Goldstein, S. (1969). Delay in hospitalization during the acute coronary period. *American Journal of Cardiology, 24,* 659–665.

Moss, A. J., & Goldstein, S. (1970). The pre-hospital phase of acute myocardial infarction. *Circulation, 41,* 737–742.

Mumford, E., Schlesinger, H. J., & Glass, G. V. (1982). The effects of psychological intervention on recovery from surgery and heart attacks: An analysis of the literature. *American Journal of Public Health, 82,* 141–146.

Murray, G. G., & Beller, G. A. (1983). Cardiac rehabilitation following coronary artery bypass surgery. *American Heart Journal, 105,* 1009–1018.

Naismeth, L. D., Robinson, J. F., Shaw, G. B., & MacIntyre, M. J. (1979). Psychological rehabilitation after the first myocardial infarction. *British Medical Journal, 1,* 439–442.

National Heart, Lung and Blood Institute. (1988). Percutaneous transluminal coronary angioplasty: A report from the registry. *American Journal of Cardiology, 49,* 2011– 2020.

New, P. K., Ruscio, A. T., Priest, R. P., Petritsi, D., & George, L. A. (1968). The support structure of heart and stroke patients: A study of the role of significant others is patient rehabilitation. *Social Science and Medicine, 2,* 185–200.

Nyamathi, A. M. (1987). The coping responses of female spouses of patients with myocardial infarction. *Heart and Lung, 16,* 86–92.

Papadopoulos, C., Larrimore, P., Cardin, S., & Shelley, S. I. (1980). Sexual concern and needs of the postcoronary patient's wife. *Archives of Internal Medicine, 140,* 38–41.

Politser, P., & Cunico, E. (1988). *Social-economic factbook for surgery.* Socioeconomic Affairs Department, American College of Surgeons, New York, New York.

Porritt, D. (1979). Social support in crisis: Quantity or quality. *Social Science and Medicine, 13A,* 715–721.

Pozen, M. W., Stechmiller, J. A., Harris, W., Smith, D. D., & Voigt, G. C. (1977). The nurse rehabilitators impact on patients with myocardial infarction. *Medical Care, 15,* 830–837.

Rabiner, C. J., & Willner, A. E. (1976). Psychopathology observed on follow-up after coronary bypass surgery. *Journal of Nervous and Mental Disease, 163,* 295–301.

Radley, A. (1988). *Prospects of heart surgery: Psychological adjustment to coronary bypass grafting*. New York: Springer-Verlag.

Radley, A., & Green, R. (1985). Styles of adjustment to coronary graft surgery. *Social Science Medicine*, *20*, 461–472.

Radley, A., & Green, R. (1986). Bearing illness: Study of couples where the husband awaits coronary graft surgery. *Social Science and Medicine*, *23*, 577–585.

Raft, D., McKee, D. C., Popio, K. A., & Haggerty, J. J. (1985). Life adaptation after percutaneous transluminal coronary angioplasty and coronary artery bypass grafting. *American Journal of Cardiology*, *56*, 395–398.

Rahe, R. H., Ward, H. W., & Hayes, V. (1979). Brief group therapy in myocardial infarction rehabilitation: Three to four year follow-up of a controlled trial. *Psychosomatic Medicine*, *41*, 229–242.

Raymond, M., Conklin, C., Schaeffer, J., Newstadt, G., Matloff, J. M., & Gray, R. J. (1984). Coping with transient intellectual dysfunction after coronary bypass surgery. *Heart and Lung*, *13*, 531–539.

Reading, A. E., (1979). The short term effects of psychological preparation for surgery. *Social Science and Medicine*, *13A*, 641–654.

Ruberman, W., Weinblatt, E., Goldberg, J. D., & Chaudhary, B. S. (1984). Psychosocial influences on mortality after myocardial infarction. *New England Journal of Medicine*, *311*, 552–559.

Rudy, E. B. (1980). Patients' and spouses' causal explanations of a myocardial infarction. *Nursing Research*, *29*, 352–356.

Sanz, G., Castaner, A., Betriu, A., & Magrina, J. (1982). Determinants of prognosis in surveyors of myocardial infarction: A prospective clinical angiographia study. *New England Journal of Medicine*, *306*, 1065–1079.

Safer, M. A., Tharps, Q. J., Jackson, D. R., & Leventhal, H. (1986). Determinants of three states of delays in seeking care of medical clinic. *Medical Care*, *17*, 11–29.

Schaefer, C., Coyne, J. C., & Lazarus, R. S. (1981). The health-related functions of social support. *Journal of Behavioral Medicine*, *4*, 381–406.

Schleifer, S., Macari-Hinson, M., Coyle, D., Slater, W., Kahn, M., Gorlin, R., & Zucker, H. (1989). The nature and course of depression following myocardial infarction. *Archives of Internal Medicine*, *149*, 1785–1789.

Shaw, R. E., Cohen, F., Doyle, B., & Palesky, J. (1985). The impact of denial and repressive style on information gain and rehabilitation outcomes in myocardial infarction patients. *Psychosomatic Medicine*, *47*, 262–273.

Shaw, R. E., Cohen, F., Fishman-Rosen, J., Murphy, M. C., Stertzer, S. H., Clark, D. A., & Myler, R. K. (1986). Psychologic predictors of psychosocial and medical outcomes in patients undergoing coronary angioplasty. *Psychosomatic Medicine*, *48*, 582–597.

Shumaker, S. A., & Brownell, A. (1984). Toward a theory of social support: Closing conceptual gaps. *Journal of Social Issues*, *40*, 11–36.

Sikes, W. W., & Rodenhauser, P. (1987). Rehabilitation programs for myocardial infarction patients: A national survey. *General Hospital Psychiatry*, *9*, 182–186.

Silver, R., & Wortman, C. (1980). Coping with undesirable life events. In J. Garber & M. E. P. Seligman (Eds.), *Human helplessness* (pp. 279–375). New York: Academic Press.

Simon, A. B., Feinleib, M., & Thompson, H. K., Jr. (1972). Components of delay in the prehospital phase of acute myocardial infarction. *American Journal of Cardiology*, *30*, 476–482.

Sivarajan, E. S., Newton, K. M., Almes, M. J., Kempf, T. M., Mansfield, L. W., & Bruce, R. A. (1983). Limited effects of outpatient teaching and counseling after myocardial infarction: A controlled study. *Heart and Lung*, *12*, 65–73.

Skelton, N., & Dominian, J. (1973). Psychological stress in wives of patients with myocardial infarction. *British Medical Journal, 73,* 101–103.

Smith, H. C., Frye, R. L., & Piehler, J. M. (1983). Does coronary bypass surgery have a favorable influence on the quality of life? In S. H. Rahimtoola (Ed.), *Controversies in coronary artery disease* (pp. 253–264). Philadelphia: Davis.

Smith, M. C. (1976). Patient responses to being transferred during hospitalization. *Nursing Research, 25,* 192–196.

Speedling, E. F. (1982). *Heart attack: The family response at home and in the hospital.* New York: Tavistock.

Stanton, B. A., Jenkins, C. D., Denlinger, P., Savageau, J. A., Weintraub, R. M., & Goldstein, R. L. (1983). Predictors of employment status after cardiac surgery. *Journal of the American Medical Association, 249,* 907–911.

Stern, M. J., & Pascale, L. (1979). Psychosocial adaptation post-myocardial infarction: The spouse's dilemma. *Journal of Psychosomatic Research, 23,* 83–87.

Stern, T. A. (1985). The management of depression and anxiety following myocardial infarction. *Mount Sinai Journal of Medicine, 52,* 623–633.

Stewart, M. J., & Gregor, F. M. (1984). Early discharge and return to work following myocardial infarction. *Social Science and Medicine, 18,* 1027–1036.

Sulman, J., & Verhaeghe, G. (1985). Myocardial infarction patients in the acute care hospital: A conceptual framework for social work intervention. *Social Work in Health Care, 11,* 1–20.

Sveinsson, I. S. (1975). Postoperative psychosis after heart surgery. *Journal of Thoracic and Cardiovascular Surgery, 70,* 717–725.

Taggart, P., & Carruthers, M. (1981). Behaviour patterns and emotional stress in the etiology of coronary heart disease: Cardiological and biochemical correlates. In D. Wheatly (Ed.), *Stress and the heart* (pp. 25–37). New York: Raven.

Taylor, C. B., Bandura, A., Ewart, C. K., Miller, N. H., & DeBusk, R. F. (1985). Exercise testing to enhance wives' confidence in their husbands' cardial capacity soon after clinically uncomplicated acute myocardial infarction. *American Journal of Cardiology, 55,* 635–638.

Thompson, D. R., & Cordle, C. J. (1988). Support of wives of myocardial infarction patients. *Journal of Advanced Nursing, 13*(2), 223–228.

Thompson, D. R., & Meddis, R. (1990). Wives' responses to counseling early after myocardial infarction. *Journal of Psychosomatic Research, 34*(3), 249–258.

Toth, J. C. (1980). Effect of structured preparation for transfer on patient anxiety on leaving the coronary care unit. *Nursing Research, 29,* 28–34.

Trelawny-Ross, C., & Russell, O. (1987). Social and psychological responses to myocardial infarction: Multiple determinants of outcome at six months. *Journal of Psychosomatic Research, 31,* 125–130.

Turi, Z. G., Stone, P. H., Muller, J. E., Parker, C., Rude, R. E., Raabe, D. E., Jaffe, A. S., Hartwell, T. D., Robertson, T. L., Braunwald, E., & Milis Study Group. (1986). Implication for acute intervention related to time of hospital arrival in acute myocardial infarction. *American Journal of Cardiology, 58,* 203–209.

Unger, D. G., & Powell, D. R. (1980). Supporting families under stress: The role of social networks. *Family Relations, 29,* 566–575.

Videka, L. M. (1979). Psychosocial adaptation in a medical self-help group. In M. A. Lieberman (Ed.), *Self-help group for coping with crisis* (pp. 362–386). San Francisco: Jossey-Bass.

Waltz, M. (1986a). Marital context and post-infarction quality of life: Is it social support or something more? *Social Science and Medicine, 22,* 791–805.

Waltz, M. (1986b). Type A, social context, and adaptation to serious illness: A longitudinal investigation of the role of the family in recovery from myocardial infarction. In T. H.

Schmidt, T. M. Dembroski, & G. Blumchen (Eds.), *Biological and psychological factors in cardiovascular disease*. New York: Springer-Verlag.

Weinberger, D. A., Schwartz, G. E., & Davidson, J. R. (1979). Low anxious, high anxious and depressive coping styles: Psychomatic patterns and behavioral physiological responses to stress. *Journal of Abnormal Psychology, 88,* 369–380.

Wells, K., Stewart, A., Hays, R., Burnam, A., Rogers, W., Daniels, M., Berry, S., Greenfield, S., & Ware, J. (1989). The functioning and well-being of depressed patients: Results from the medical outcomes study. *Journal of the American Medical Association, 262*(7), 914–919.

Wenger, N. K. (1986). Quality of life concerns in the rehabilitation of patients with cardiovascular disease. *Bibliotheca Cardiolosica, 40,* 109–128.

Wiklund, I., Sanne, H., Vedin, A., & Wilhelmsson, C. (1984). Psychosocial outcome one year after a first myocardial infarction. *Journal of Psychosomatic Research, 28,* 309–321.

Williams, R., Barefoot, J., Califf, R., Haney, T., Saunders, W., Pryor, D., Hlatky, M., Siegler, I., & Mark, D. (1992). Prognostic importance of social and economic resources among medically treated patients with angiographically documented coronary artery disease. *Journal of the American Medical Association, 267*(4), 520–524.

Winefield, H. R. (1982). Male social support and recovery after myocardial infarction. *Australian Journal of Psychology, 34,* 45–52.

Winefield, H. R., & Katsikitis, M. (1987). Medical professional support and cardiac rehabilitation of males and females. *Journal of Psychosomatic Research, 31,* 567–573.

Winefield, H. R., & Martin, C. J. (1981–82). Measurement and prediction of recovery after myocardial infarction. *International Journal of Psychiatry in Medicine, 11,* 145–154.

Wishnie, H. A., Hackett, T. P., & Cassem, N. H. (1977). Psychological hazards of convalescence following myocardial infarction. In R. H. Moos (Ed.), *Coping with physical illness.* New York: Plenum.

Wortman, C. B., & Conway, T. L. (1985). The role of social support in adaptation and recovery from physical illness. In S. Cohen & S. L. Syme (Eds.), *Social support and health.* New York: Academic Press.

Wortman, C. B., & Dunkel-Schetter, C. (1979). Interpersonal relationships and cancer: A theoretical analysis. *Journal of Social Issues, 35,* 120–155.

Wortman, C. B., & Dunkel-Schetter, C. (1987). Conceptual and methodological issues in the study of social support. In A. Baum, S. Taylor, & J. E. Singer (Eds.), *Handbook of psychology and health, vol. 5* (pp. 63–108). Hillsdale, NJ: Erlbaum.

Wortman, C. B., & Lehman, D. R. (1985). Reactions to victims of life crises: Support attempts that fail. In I. G. Sarason & B. R. Sarason (Eds.), *Social support: Theory, research, and application* (pp. 469–489). Dordrecht, Netherlands: Martinus Nijhoff.

Zyzanski, S. J., Rouse, B. A., Stanton, B. A., & Jenkins, C. D. (1982). Employment changes among patients following coronary bypass surgery: Social, medical, and psychological correlates. *Public Health Reports, 97,* 558–565.

CHAPTER 14

Cardiac Rehabilitation
The Role of Social Support in Recovery and Compliance

Kathleen Dracup

Recovery from a myocardial infarction or cardiac surgery is often accompanied by a host of psychological and physical problems (Bigos, 1981; Jenkins, Stanton, Savageau, Denlinger, & Klein, 1983; Magni et al., 1987; Stern, Pascale, & Ackerman, 1977). The consequences of a cardiac event include energy loss, recurring chest pain, dependence on others, and tension in social and sexual relationships. As patients begin to understand the ramifications of chronic heart disease and experience the emotions related to that understanding, enrollment in a structured, outpatient cardiac rehabilitation program can provide them with information, guidance, and support.

Despite the popularity of cardiac rehabilitation programs, their effectiveness remains controversial, and the mechanisms by which they achieve their outcomes have not been clearly delineated. In this chapter I present evidence suggesting that enhanced social support is a powerful but relatively untested component of all cardiac rehabilitation programs. The purpose of this discussion is to review the data related to these rehabilitation programs in the context of what is known about the effects of social support on the health outcomes, psychosocial adaptation, and

KATHLEEN DRACUP • School of Nursing, University of California, Los Angeles, Los Angeles, California 90024.

Social Support and Cardiovascular Disease, edited by Sally A. Shumaker and Susan M. Czajkowski. Plenum Press, New York, 1994.

compliance of patients in the immediate period following hospitalization for cardiac disease.

The Need for Cardiac Rehabilitation Programs

The diagnosis of coronary heart disease has a profound impact on an individual's self-image and sense of well-being. This impact may be heightened when hospitalization is required. Whether the patient is recovering from an acute coronary event (myocardial infarction or out-of-hospital cardiac arrest) or from a surgical procedure (e.g., coronary artery bypass graft surgery, coronary valve replacement, or cardiac transplantation), recovery is often characterized by depression, anxiety, changes in self-image, and loss of self-esteem (Bigos, 1981; Cassem & Hackett, 1971; Waltz, 1986). Long-term emotional distress, family turmoil, and occupational problems occur in a significant number of patients (Finkelmeier, Kenwood, & Summers, 1984; Garrity & Klein, 1975; Stern et al., 1977; Jenkins et al., 1983).

The most difficult time period in the recovery process is the first month following discharge from the hospital (see Croog, Levine, & Lurie, 1968; Doehrman, 1977, for reviews of this research). Emotional distress, particularly depression, tends to peak after hospital discharge, rather than during hospitalization as one might expect. Several mechanisms can be posed to explain this trajectory. First, patients with cardiac disease frequently use denial as a defense mechanism to ward off anxiety. Most observers of acute-phase coronary patients find denial to be ubiquitous (Razin, 1982). The usefulness of this defense mechanism was documented by Hackett, Cassem, and Wishnie (1968), who found that patients who used denial in the coronary care unit were less anxious and experienced less morbidity and mortality on follow-up than patients who did not use denial. The return to the familiar surroundings of home, however, can seriously erode denial as a defense mechanism. Decisions about return to work, social commitments, and daily schedules must be made; the losses associated with a cardiac event—financial, social, and personal—can no longer be ignored once the patient returns home.

Family tensions also increase during the immediate posthospitalization phase, with oversolicitation on the part of family members being the most frequently cited source of conflict by patients (Jenkins et al., 1983; Wishnie, Hackett, & Cassem, 1971). Spouses have identified these early days as the most difficult and frightening time in the recovery process (Gillis, 1984). They feel responsible for the patient's welfare and are unsure if they will know what to do if an emergency occurs. Conflict over activity limitations often characterize family interactions, with patients desiring to test their capabilities and family members fearing that such tests will have disastrous consequences (Gillis, 1984).

One strategy used to bridge the gap between hospitalization and return to routine activity and work is enrollment in a formal outpatient cardiac rehabilitation program. Such programs proliferated across the United States in the 1980s. They are designed, among other things, to reduce the incidence of dysfunctional emotional responses to chronic heart disease and to promote required life-style changes.

Cardiac Rehabilitation

The first formal cardiac rehabilitation programs were developed in the United States in the early 1970s. Although designed to enhance the entire recovery process of patients with coronary artery disease, the focus was almost entirely on physical conditioning. Rehabilitation was translated into monitored exercise sessions in which guidance was provided regarding the degree of physical exertion that could be undertaken safely. This past decade has seen a more multidisciplinary approach to cardiac rehabilitation with the addition of psychologists, nutritionists, social workers, and vocational counselors to the original triad of physicians, nurses, and physical therapists (Sivarajan & Newton, 1984).

Goals and Program Components

The aim of all cardiac rehabilitation programs is the return to an enjoyable and productive life for patients with heart disease. Because such patients have a progressive chronic disease, the goal is not cure but rather improvement of function based on relief from physical symptoms, a decrease in the severity of the illness, and a delimitation of disease progression. This goal is achieved in a multimodal intervention program that includes the following:

1. *Exercise therapy or physical training* aimed at improving aerobic capacity and submaximal exercise ability. The effects are measured by increases in ejection fraction and contractile function of the left ventricle, decreased cardiographic ST-segment depression at maximal exercise, reduction in body fat, increases in circulating high-density lipoprotein concentrations, reductions in serum triglycer-

ide values, and increases in glucose utilization (Barnard, Guzy, Rosenberg, & O'Brien, 1983; Conn, Williams, & Wallace, 1982; Greenland & Chu, 1988)

2. *Psychological counseling* directed toward reducing the emotional sequelae of cardiac events and improving stress management (Dracup, 1985)

3. *Nutritional counseling* directed toward improving dietary habits, as demonstrated by reduced serum cholesterol levels (Vermueulen, Lie, & Durrer, 1983)

4. *Education about coronary heart disease and cardiac risk factors* designed to enhance patient compliance (Dracup, Meleis, Clark, Clyburn, Shields, & Staley, 1984; Haynes, 1984)

5. *Vocational counseling* to facilitate return to work

The first phase of a cardiac rehabilitation program is initiated in the hospital, as soon as the patient's condition becomes stable. Passive exercises, at a level of 1 to 2 metabolic equivalents (METs), are conducted to prevent the negative effects of bed rest. One MET is equal to 3.5 ml O_2/kg body weight/minute, with lying quietly being approximately equal to 1 MET of energy expenditure. The passive exercises of this phase involve a nurse or physical therapist moving the patients' arms and legs in standard exercises several times a day. In addition, information about the hospital routine and the disease process is provided to the patient and family to reduce their anxiety.

The second phase is also in-hospital and spans the period between discharge from the critical care unit and return to home. Activities (walking, bathing, etc.) are encouraged at a 3 MET level, and the patient and family members begin a formal educational process (usually conducted by nursing staff) to prepare them for hospital discharge. The third phase begins with the patient's return home. Patients are given an exercise prescription based on the results of exercise testing. As soon as it is considered appropriate, they attend three weekly exercise sessions that involve exercise at a 4 to 8 MET level. These exercise sessions are combined with formal or informal education and counseling to achieve the necessary behavioral changes required by cardiac risk factor reduction and to restore self-esteem. The usual duration of this phase is 8 to 12 weeks.

Finally, the fourth phase involves a lifetime program of regular exercise and risk factor modification that begins with patients' return to work. For the 60% to 70% of individuals who never return to work following their heart attack or coronary artery bypass surgery (CASS Principal Investigators, 1983), this last phase begins with the patients' graduation from a third-phase program. A minority of patients elect to continue in a nonmonitored, outpatient fourth-phase program to provide structure to their exercise sessions (Berra, 1981; Pashkow, Schafer, & Pashkow, 1986). Such programs are based in community centers (e.g., YMCAs) or in hospitals as an extension of third-phase outpatient cardiac rehabilitation programs.

Availability of Cardiac Rehabilitation Programs

The proportion of patients who are able to participate in a cardiac rehabilitation program is currently unknown. The following factors affect participation in such programs.

Medical Contraindications

Patients who are at high risk for sudden death or who have physical conditions that might be exacerbated by exercise are excluded from participation in cardiac rehabilitation programs. Examples include patients with unstable angina pectoris, severe aortic stenosis, uncontrolled systemic or pulmonic hypertension, recurrent malignant ventricular tachyarrhythmias, acute myocarditis, and acute thrombophlebitis (Wenger, 1981).

Geographic Availability

Because most outpatient programs require participants to attend exercise sessions three times a week, patients who live in rural areas or in communities with few or no free-standing rehabilitation programs are excluded by virtue of the distance required to attend such programs.

Financial Constraints

Private insurance companies and Medicare reimburse up to 80% of the cost of participating in cardiac rehabilitation programs (through the third phase). Few insurance carriers reimburse patients beyond 12 weeks, regardless of the perceived benefit or need. Because Medicaid and other safety-net government programs do not provide for any cardiac rehabilitation services, the poor rarely have access to such programs.

In summary, many patients who are at high risk for cardiac invalidism because of the severity of their medical illness or because of psychosocial sequelae of a cardiac event are deprived of cardiac rehabilitation services. This reality unfortunately means that those patients who are most isolated during recovery because of their socioeconomic status or medical condition (i.e., they are unemployed, have few social resources, and/or have severe medical complications) are denied access to a cardiac rehabilitation program.

Social Support and Cardiac Rehabilitation

Social support has been defined as an interpersonal transaction involving one or more of the following: emotional concern (liking, love, empathy); instrumental aid (goods or services); information and advice; and/or appraisal support or affirmation of self-worth (House, 1981). It is broadly viewed as the resources provided by one's social network, with family, friends, coworkers, health professionals, and community resources all included in that network. These resources provide individuals with a sense of intimacy and belonging, social integration, opportunities for nurturance, and tangible support. Appropriate social support facilitates one's view of oneself as part of a group with certain behavioral expectations and sociocultural norms. This view can lead to an enhanced personal identity and sense of security in the "grand scheme of things." It can also provide the individual with an increased sense of worth and importance.

Models of Social Support

Social support has been viewed from a variety of perspectives. Many investigators and theorists have attempted to clarify its content and functions. Its qualitative and quantitative dimensions have been explored as they relate to a social network—the numbers of people in it, its density, and the role of real versus expected support. Finally, the mechanisms or sequence of steps involved in social support have been studied to elucidate the nature of the process and the variables that affect it.

Although social support is clearly a complex phenomenon that requires multiple approaches, part of the source of the conceptual confusion surrounding it lies in the variety of theories used by investigators to explain their research findings (see Tilden, 1985, for a review). For example, attachment theory, with its emphasis on the social nature of human beings and the need for human contact derived from the initial mother-child bond, has been used to explain the nature and function of social support. Epidemiologists have used ecological theories of host resistance and vulnerability to examine the effect of social support on health. Sociologists have used social exchange theory and interactionist role theory to study the interdependence and reciprocity involved in the provision of social support. Last but not least, theories of stress, coping, and adaptation have been used to explain the effects of social support on well-being.

Using a stress framework, many investigators have attempted to elucidate the nature of the association between social support and well-being. Two models have been proposed. The direct effects model suggests that social support is beneficial during nonstressful as well as stressful times. The second model proposes that support is related to well-being only for persons under stress. This is termed the buffering model, because it posits that support buffers or protects persons from the potentially pathogenic influence of stressful events. Evidence has been found for both models (Cohen & Wills, 1985).

Social Support and Cardiac Disease

Although the specific mechanisms are still under investigation, it appears that social support can buffer the effects of a stressful event (e.g., an illness) by enabling the individual to perceive the event as less stressful, by facilitating the coping efforts of the individual, or by lessening the degree of reactance of the individual to the stressful event (House, 1981). There is strong empirical evidence suggesting that social support buffers the stress experienced by cardiac patients in the immediate recovery period and that it directly and positively affects patients' long-term adjustment, psychological well-being, and health outcomes. Appropriate social support positively influences self-esteem, perceptions of health, mood, and adjustment to coronary heart disease (Waltz, 1986).

Ultimately, these positive outcomes are reflected in reduced mortality rates for patients who experience significant social support. For example, investigators who conducted interviews with 2,320 male survivors of acute myocardial infarction found that patients classified as being socially isolated and having a high degree of life stress had more than four times the risk of death than men with low levels of isolation and stress (Ruberman, Weinblatt, Goldberg, & Chaudhary, 1984). These findings are similar to those of other investigators who have identified an inverse relationship between social support and mortality in chronically ill populations (Berkman, Leo-Summers, & Horowitz, 1992; Berkman & Syme, 1979; Case, Moss, Case, McDermott, & Eberly, 1992; Revenson, Wollman, & Felton, 1983).

Social Support within Cardiac Rehabilitation

Cardiac rehabilitation programs have an important social support component. Health professionals working in these programs provide participants with information about the disease and recovery process, as well as offer emotional support. Group exercise sessions provide patients with an opportunity to expand their social networks to individuals who are experiencing similar recovery issues.

The four dimensions of social support described by House (1981) are clearly provided in the context of a well-designed cardiac rehabilitation program:

1. *Emotional support* is provided by both staff and fellow participants on an ongoing basis. In effective programs, an emotional climate is established in which individuals feel free to express their feelings and fears without self-consciousness.
2. Rehabilitation program staff provide *instrumental support* as they help patients obtain appropriate community and government services (e.g., disability payments and access to appropriate community services).
3. In educational sessions designed to augment the exercise prescription, professional staff and fellow participants provide patients with *information* about the disease process and the life-style changes required.
4. Finally, patients share similar experiences and reactions related to the recovery process. As described by Yalom (1985), the consequent sense of universality has the potential of increasing the participants' *sense of self-worth*, which is often severely shaken by an acute coronary event. The patient's realization that the majority of persons who experience a heart attack or surgery share the same fears and emotional turmoil can be a powerful source of support and affirmation during this period of psychological disequilibrium.

Unfortunately, social support is such an integral component of any formal cardiac rehabilitation program that, to date, researchers have not distinguished its contribution to rehabilitation outcomes from that of other components (e.g., increasing exercise capacity). For example, when positive changes have been documented in participants' self-concepts and affective states following participation in a rehabilitation program, researchers have credited the improved functional status and decreased symptomatology that occur with physical conditioning (Prosser et al., 1978), rather than examining the role of social support in achieving these outcomes. Little or no attempt has been made to evaluate the role of social support in the rehabilitative process.

Interestingly, researchers in both social support and cardiac rehabilitation have focused on the same categories of outcome variables: morbidity and mortality, psychosocial adjustment, and compliance with the medical regimen. This fact strengthens the argument that enhanced social support is an integral component of a rehabilitation program and a major cause of the positive health outcomes documented in the cardiac rehabilitation literature. It is imperative that these two literatures come closer together and that researchers working in cardiac rehabilitation begin to draw on the established methodologies and measurement techniques used in the social support literature. In this way, the contributions that each area of research can make to the other will be enhanced.

Mechanisms of Social Support

Social support potentially operates to enhance health outcomes in a cardiac rehabilitation program through a variety of mechanisms. These include social persuasion, modeling, enhanced self-esteem, and increased feelings of mastery (Antonucci et al., this volume). Their role in the recovery process is schematically presented in Figure 1.

The role of social support in enhancing the efficacy of *persuasive messages* has been demonstrated for such positive health care practices as seat belt use, exercise, nutrition, and medical and dental care (Hubbard, Muhlenkamp, & Brown, 1984; Langlie, 1977; Mechanic & Cleary, 1980). In all cardiac rehabilitation programs participants are persuaded to reduce cardiac risk factors. Using both formal and informal education and counseling sessions, rehabilitation staff target cigarette smoking, obesity, sedentary life-styles, high-fat dietary intake, and stress as important risk factors to be modified during the recovery process (Sivarajan & Newton, 1984). The provision of social support by rehabilitation staff and other patients can be a powerful force for changing cardiac risk factors and

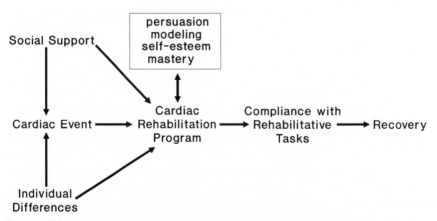

Figure 1. Relationship of social support and participation in a cardiac rehabilitation program to recovery following myocardial infarction or cardiac surgery.

serves to augment the written material provided by the nursing and medical staff.

A second social support mechanism is that of *role modeling*. Through group sessions with other cardiac patients, individuals have the opportunity to learn what is required of them through imitation, even in the absence of directly experienced reinforcements (Bandura, 1971). The structure of a rehabilitation program encourages patients who are several months away from their cardiac events to participate in exercise and group discussions with patients who have been discharged recently from the hospital. By engaging in appropriate strategies for risk factor reduction, more senior patients model the necessary rehabilitative behaviors for patients who are new to the program.

Although to date no studies have been conducted in a cardiac rehabilitation setting to tease out the differential effects of social support provided by program staff, families, or other patients, there are some intriguing data to suggest that fellow patients provide a more powerful form of support than family members. In comparing the effects of social support groups that met for 10 weekly sessions as part of the cardiac rehabilitation program, patients who met together with two staff members were more compliant on follow-up than patients who met with spouses attending the groups (Dracup, Meleis, Clark, et al., 1984). In explaining these results, the investigators described a feeling of competition that occurred in the patient-only group regarding cardiac risk factors. For example, some patients brought in histograms of their weight loss and decreasing cholesterol levels to the patient group sessions. In contrast, the patient-spouse groups focused less on cardiac risk factor changes and more on the emotional status of the family.

A third dynamic is the effect of perceived social support on the *self-esteem* of rehabilitation patients. Most theorists agree that self-esteem is a learned phenomenon involving a lifelong process (Crouch & Straub, 1983; Stanwyck, 1983). Basic self-esteem is the relatively enduring foundation that is formed through early life experiences, whereas functional self-esteem is developed across the life span through ongoing evaluations that are derived from interactions with others. Functional self-esteem substantially exceeds basic self-esteem; that is, an individual's self-concept depends more on the multiple interactions that occur after childhood than on early family experiences (Crouch & Straub, 1983), and it is this aspect of the cardiac patient's self-concept that is threatened by hospitalization and treatment. Patients are forced by the exigencies of the disease to reexamine and, at times, reorder their life goals (Dracup, 1985; Stern, Gorman, & Kaslow, 1983). During this period of values clarification, many patients are vulnerable to feelings of confusion and lowered self-worth. The instrumental, informational, and emotional support offered within the context of an ongoing rehabilitation program can be a powerful source of reassurance and can increase the individual's own sense of self-regard (Cobb, 1976).

Finally, a dynamic that is related to increasing feelings of self-worth is the *sense of mastery* or control that patients acquire through a program of physical conditioning. As symptoms decrease and patients feel increasing confidence in their ability to perform physical activity, self-esteem and feelings of self-efficacy are enhanced. The importance of this mechanism is supported by studies conducted in both normal and cardiac populations. In the former, subjects who participated in experimental trials of cardiovascular conditioning reported increased psychological well-being and, in some cases, increased self-confidence (Folkins, 1976; Folkins, Lynch, & Gardner, 1972; Goldwater & Collis, 1985). Similar results have been reported in trials involving patients with documented myocardial infarctions (McPherson et al., 1967; Prosser et al., 1978; Stern & Cleary, 1981).

Appropriate social support can enhance the feelings of mastery patients develop in a physical conditioning program. The importance of enlisting spousal support was highlighted in a unique social support intervention study conducted with male post-MI patients (Taylor, Bandura, Ewart, Miller, & DeBusk, 1985). During the patients' exercise tolerance test at the third week following hospital discharge, each of the patients' wives was randomly assigned either to remain in the waiting room, to observe the exercise test, or to observe the exercise test plus walk for three minutes on the treadmill at the husband's peak workload. Wives' final ratings of confidence in their husbands' physical and cardiac capability were significantly higher in the group that walked on the treadmill compared to the other two groups.

Furthermore, spouses' and patients' perceptions of the patients' cardiac capability after treadmill testing at 3 weeks was the most consistent predictor of patients' cardiovascular functioning at 11 and 26 weeks, whether measured in terms of peak heart rate or maximal workload during exercise testing. Therefore, an intervention that increased the confidence of a spouse regarding her partner's capabilities following a heart attack led to increased benefits in terms of patients' physical functioning. Although not performed within a cardiac rehabilitation program, this intervention highlights the importance of wives' perceptions of their partners' physical and cardiac capabilities and suggests the potential benefit of including spouses in selected exercise sessions as part of the rehabilitation protocol.

As suggested by the above findings, the view of one's family and friends regarding a cardiac patient's ability to tolerate physical activity can have a profound influence on the patient's sense of self-efficacy. In almost all cases, a cardiac event threatens an individual's sense of robustness. Whether the patient continues to feel frail and vulnerable to another cardiac event depends in part on the view that other people hold of his or her physical capabilities. As noted by Pearlin and Aneshensel (1986), a natural product of social interactions is the acquisition of norms—shared ways of defining situations and of prescribing or approving modes of action and reaction. The norms of membership in reference groups can reinforce the perception of a situation as threatening or help to define a situation as undeserving of concern. The norms of all cardiac rehabilitation programs emphasize health promotion and physical fitness. By virtue of the patient selection criteria, patients considered to be too ill to tolerate any form of exercise are excluded from such programs. Therefore the membership group is composed of cardiac patients who can justifiably trivialize the effects of heart disease on their ability to maintain a reasonable level of physical fitness.

Effects on Psychosocial Adaptation, Morbidity, and Mortality

A number of investigators have found that a lack of social and community ties is associated with an overall increase in mortality in both patients with cardiac disease and those without identified disease (Berkman & Syme, 1979; Blazer, 1982; Chandra, Szklo, Goldberg, & Tonascia, 1983; Ruberman, Weinblatt, Goldberg, & Chaudhary, 1984). If a major component of cardiac rehabilitation programs is the increase in social support available to the patient recovering from a cardiac event and the expansion of his or her social network, one would expect that such programs would have a positive effect on morbidity and mortality. Although no such relationship has been documented in the nine randomized clinical trials conducted to date, using both fatal and nonfatal myocardial infarctions as end points (American Association of Cardiovascular and Pulmonary Rehabilitation [AACPR], 1986; Greenland & Chu, 1988), these results are confounded by a high patient dropout rate (approximately 50% to 60% within the first year of study in most of the trials) and by small sample sizes. In seven of the nine trials, rehabilitation was defined as exercise or physical training; exercise or physical training was included as one component of a multifactorial rehabilitation strategy in the other two trials. In all nine trials, subjects met the usual criteria for inclusion in a cardiac rehabilitation program, including documented atherosclerotic heart disease. When the nine studies were pooled using meta-analytic techniques (AACPR, 1986), there was a significant difference in mortality attributed to participation in a cardiac rehabilitation program. The control patients ($n = 1,675$) had a mortality rate of 14.2% on follow-up, whereas the experimental patients ($n = 1,671$) had a mean mortality rate of 9.6% (follow-up occurred over a range of 20 to 108 months, with the mean being 45.5 months). The rate of nonfatal recurrent myocardial infarctions, however, was almost identical for the two groups over the same period of follow-up (10.5% in the experimental and 10.1% in the control group).

Even given these results, it is currently impossible to identify the contribution of social support to the reduction in mortality that was found using this meta-analytical approach. A complex interaction undoubtedly exists between the physiological and psychological changes affected by exercise and social support. One approach to teasing out this interaction is found in studies comparing standard group rehabilitation programs with medically directed at-home rehabilitation programs. Because home exercise programs are by definition carried out individually by patients without the support and companionship of other cardiac patients, they exclude the social support component provided in formal cardiac rehabilitation programs. In two studies (DeBusk, Haskell, Miller, Berra, & Taylor, 1985; Heath, Maloney, & Fure, 1987), however, only one used reinfarction rates as an end point. In this study, DeBusk and colleagues (1985) found no significant difference in nonfatal reinfarction rates between the two groups over the period of 26 weeks following an event. The reinfarction rates were 3% or less in both groups, with no cardiac deaths occurring in either group. Unfortunately, the low fatal and nonfatal reinfarction rates in most patients who are candidates for cardiac rehabilitation (i.e., without significant medical complications) make any assessment of the relationship between the social support and exercise components of cardiac rehabilitation on morbidity and mortality quite difficult to identify.

A second approach to differentiating the effects of exercise and social support has been taken by investigators who have compared the additive effects of a weekly support group within a standard cardiac rehabilitation program or who have compared exercise therapy to a group counseling intervention. In the first instance, cardiac rehabilitation patients who were randomly assigned to weekly support groups reported increased feelings of self-esteem and decreased feelings of anxiety and depression compared to patients who participated in cardiac rehabilitation programs without a specific social support group (Dracup, Meleis, Baker, & Edlefson, 1984; Dracup, Meleis, Clark, et al., 1984). Unfortunately, the small sample size ($n = 55$) prevented a meaningful comparison of morbidity and mortality data, although patients in the control group had a higher number of rehospitalizations at 6 months follow-up than patients in the social support groups.

In the second instance, investigators compared the effects of exercise therapy and group counseling on functional status, psychosocial function, morbidity, and mortality (Stern et al., 1983). Each intervention lasted 12 weeks, with evaluations carried out up to 1 year. Exercise substantially increased mean work capacity, decreased fatigue, lessened anxiety and depression, and promoted independence and sociability. Counseling substantially reduced depression and promoted a sense of friendliness and independence. Changes between groups diminished over time; the control group reported no substantial change on any measured factor. Although the exercise group reported fewer major cardiovascular sequelae, sample size ($n = 106$) again restricted comparisons of morbidity and mortality.

In discussing the results of the exercise–counseling comparison, Stern and colleagues note that exercise should increase performance levels on treadmill testing and that a decrease in anxiety and depression would follow as an indirect effect of the sense of well-being generated by exercise. Group counseling emphasizes learning positive qualities about oneself and experimenting with new behavior. It should also improve participants' sense of self-worth and thereby decrease anxiety and depression. Thus once again we are reminded that part of the problem of identifying the potential role of social support in cardiac rehabilitation programs is that both exercise and social support affect the same outcome variables.

Effects on Compliance

Although patients are strongly motivated at the time of hospital discharge to make behavioral changes to enhance their health, long-term adherence to exercise and nutrition guidelines, as well as abstinence from cigarette smoking, present formidable challenges. Cardiac rehabilitation program staff target these behaviors for change in the immediate recovery period and attempt to provide patients with strategies to maintain these changes following discharge from the program.

Two questions can be posed about the relationship of social support and compliance. First, does the social support delivered within the context of a cardiac rehabilitation program affect the ultimate compliance of cardiac patients to the medical regimen? Second, does social support affect the compliance of patients to the cardiac rehabilitation program itself?

With regard to the first question, published evidence suggests that patients who receive social support from family and friends are more likely to comply with risk factor modification behaviors (Gianetti, Reynolds, & Rign, 1985; Haynes, 1976). Positive interpersonal relationships may facilitate such appropriate health behaviors as complying with medical regimens (Brownell & Shumaker, 1984). It could then be assumed that patients who participate in a cardiac rehabilitation program would be more likely to maintain long-term compliance than nonparticipants. Amazingly, no studies have been conducted to date comparing the long-term adherence of cardiac rehabilitation participants and nonparticipants, and therefore the answer to this question remains unknown.

Regarding the second question, data suggest that social support enhances compliance to the rehabilitation program. Specifically, spousal support has been consistently identified as a critical predictor of program adherence (Andrew et al., 1979). One of the most commonly espoused methods for enhancing regular involvement in cardiac rehabilitation is the building of social relationships among participants and staff (Sivarajan & Newton, 1984). Peer support received both inside and outside an exercise program is an important determinant of attendance (Wankel, 1984).

Data from healthy populations also indicate that adherence to an exercise regimen is superior when patients participate in a group (rather than individual) exercise program, presumably because of the enhanced motivation provided through peer support (Massie & Shephard, 1971). This finding has been challenged by a group of studies in which home exercise was compared to group rehabilitation (DeBusk et al., 1985; Heath et al., 1987; Stevens & Hanson, 1987). Compliance with exercise prescriptions and functional status were similar in both groups in all three studies. These results are not definitive, however, because social support was provided to the home exercise groups in other ways, a fact that confounds the results. For example, DeBusk and colleagues arranged for nurses to call the patients in the home program to discuss their exercise program and to transmit a 1-minute electrocardiogram during exercise over the telephone twice weekly. According to the investigators, "patient satisfaction was closely related to the extent of contact with the professional staff, especially the nurse" (DeBusk et al., 1985, pp. 255–256).

In summary, although the long-term effects of social support offered within the context of a cardiac rehabilitation program are unknown in relation to patient compliance, the enhanced social support provided in a structured cardiac rehabilitation program seems to increase patient adherence to the medical regimen in the immediate posthospitalization phase. The importance of enlisting the support of family members, particularly spouses, is once more underscored. These findings are consistent with the bulk of social support research in the area of compliance.

The Dark Side of Social Support

The average length of time it takes someone who experiences sudden chest pain of cardiac origin to arrive at an emergency room is 4 hours (Alonzo, 1986; Moss & Goldstein, 1970). If that individual is with a friend or colleague from work when he or she has symptoms, the delay time drops to 2 hours. But if the individual is with a family member, the delay time *increases* to 12 hours (Hackett & Cassem, 1969). In a survey of 40 wives of first-time post-MI patients, 18 of the 40 (45%) evaluated the cardiac symptoms as non–heart related and discouraged their spouses from seeking medical care. When queried by the investigator, the wives said that they felt that the victim was not having a heart attack "because he was young, healthy, or physically active; because his symptoms were minor, such as indigestion; or because his parents had lived to an old age without any evidence of heart disease" (Nyamathi, 1988, p. 70). Clearly not all social support yields positive results.

As part of our growing understanding of the nature and role of social support, researchers have given up their unquestioning enthusiasm for social support and begun to acknowledge its darker side. If the wrong kind of support is given or the timing of the support does not match the need, it may actually exacerbate stress and/or impede recovery (Jacobson, 1986; Wortman, 1984). Social support can have negative consequences when family members allow, or even encourage, a cardiac patient to deny the meaning of symptoms. If the patient is grappling with the realities of chronic cardiac disease but a family member is using denial, social support may take the form of the family's minimizing the patient's sense of loss. Admonitions to "cheer up" are usually ineffective and lead patients to a further sense of social isolation.

At the other end of the continuum, the physical and emotional recovery of patients following an acute coronary event may be impeded by the medically unwarranted concerns of family members. For example, Lewis (1966) found that men who reported a change in their family members' attitudes toward them since the onset of their congestive heart failure were less likely to return to work than were those who perceived no change. Preferential treatment shown to patients by family members in the early stages of chronicity can increase patient disability (Hyman, 1971; Mechanic & Volkart, 1960). The associated protectiveness and socialization to the sick role provided by family members who incorrectly perceive the newly diagnosed cardiac patient as a physical invalid can greatly impede recovery. Thus family members must walk the narrow line between lack of concern (or active support of denial as a defense mechanism) and over-involvement. Cardiac rehabilitation program staff can provide important guidance in this regard.

Summary and Recommendations

Social support is a valuable resource to the patient recovering from an acute coronary event. Unfortunately, this resource can be critically threatened by the experiences surrounding the diagnosis and treatment of coronary heart disease. Hospitalization removes the patient from his or her usual network of social support; these same sources also feel stress in their own lives and have less to give. Cardiac rehabilitation programs, which theoretically begin when the patient is hospitalized and are available as long as the patient seeks the support and structure of an outpatient program, provide one means to increase the social support available to the individual recovering from an acute coronary event.

Many questions remain: What kind of social support can be provided by a cardiac rehabilitation program that cannot be provided by family and friends? Are there particular types of support that are needed by the cardiac patient in the immediate posthospitalization period? If so, are these types more acceptable from a cardiac rehabilitation staff than from family and friends? How do individual differences (sociodemographic characteristics, medical status, etc.) alter each patient's need for social support in cardiac rehabilitation? Do group exercise sessions provide sufficient social support for participants, or would other social support interventions enhance rehabilitation outcomes? How can family members be incorporated into the rehabilitation program in an economical and time-efficient manner? If they are incorporated, what difference does it make in ultimate patient outcome?

Although substantive research has been done in the two areas of social support and cardiac rehabilitation, almost nothing is known about how cardiac rehabilitation does or does not capitalize on social support to enhance physical function and psychosocial adaptation. The evaluation of the effectiveness of interventions designed to increase social support within cardiac rehabilitation programs has been hampered by a number of methodological and logistical problems. Most problematic is the difficulty in differentiating the effects of social support on patient outcomes from the other interventions provided within a cardiac rehabilitation program. For example, physical conditioning leads to certain neuroendocrine and psychological responses, some of which are similar to those documented following social support interventions. With few exceptions, researchers have not attempted to identify the contributions of the different interventions to patient outcome.

One approach to identifying the specific mechanisms by which social support is enhanced within cardiac rehabilitation programs and to distinguishing the effects of exercise from those of social support on various patient outcomes lies in the design of appropriate experimental trials that vary these two independent variables. For example, interventions designed to alter the amount of social support received within a standard cardiac rehabilitation program (exercise alone, group exercise, group exercise combined with sessions with program staff, group exercise combined with patient social support groups, etc.) could be compared experimentally to identify any differential effects on physical and psychosocial outcomes. A second approach lies in the variety of multivariate statistical approaches currently available to the researcher. The contribution and interaction of various levels of exercise and social support on patient outcome could be assessed using standard discriminant analysis and multiple regression techniques.

Despite the difficulties inherent in identifying the relationship of social support to rehabilitation outcomes, cardiac rehabilitation programs provide an important setting to test many of the tenets of social support theory. Future research needs to focus on identifying the specific mechanisms by which social support is enhanced within structured cardiac rehabilitation programs. Once identified, interventions that capitalize on these processes can be developed and tested.

ACKNOWLEDGMENTS. The writing of this chapter was supported in part by a grant from the National Heart, Lung, and Blood Institute (BEM R201 HL 32171).

References

Alonzo, A. A. (1986). The impact of the family and lay others on care-seeking during life-threatening episodes of suspected coronary artery disease. *Social Science and Medicine*, 22, 1297–1311.

American Association of Cardiovascular and Pulmonary Rehabilitation. (1986). *Cardiac rehabilitation services: A scientific evaluation*. New York: Author.

Andrew, G. M., Oldridge, N. B., Parker, J. O., Cunningham, D. A., Rechnitzer, P. A., Jones, N. L., Buck, C., Kavanagh, T., Shephard, R. J., Sutton, J. R., & McDonald, W. (1979). Reasons for dropout from exercise programs in post-coronary patients. *Medical Science in Sports and Exercise*, 11, 376–378.

Bandura, A. (1971). *A social learning theory*. Morristown, NJ: General Learning.

Barnard, R. J., Guzy, P. M., Rosenberg, J. M., & O'Brien, L. T. (1983). Effects of an intensive exercise and nutrition program on patients with coronary artery disease: Five-year follow-up. *Journal of Cardiac Rehabilitation*, 3, 183–190.

Berkman, L. F., Leo-Summers, L., & Horowitz, R. I. (1992). Emotional support and survival after myocardial infarction. *Annals of Internal Medicine*, 117, 1003–1009.

Berkman, L., & Syme, L. (1979). Social networks, host resistance, and mortality: A nine-year follow-up study of Alameda County residents. *American Journal of Epidemiology*, 2, 186–204.

Berra, K. (1981). YMCArdiac therapy: A community based program for persons with coronary artery disease. *Journal of Cardiac Rehabilitation*, 1, 354.

Bigos, K. M. (1981). Behavioral adaptation during the acute phase of a myocardial infarction. *Western Journal of Nursing Research*, 3, 150–171.

Blazer, D. G. (1982). Social support and mortality in an elderly community population. *American Journal of Epidemiology*, 115, 684–694.

Brownell, A., & Shumaker, S. A. (1984). Social support: An introduction to a complex phenomenon. *Journal of Social Issues, 40*(4), 1–9.

Case, R. B., Moss, A. J., Case, N., McDermott, M., & Eberly, S. (1992). Living alone after myocardial infarction: Impact on prognosis. *JAMA, 267,* 515–519.

CASS Principal Investigators. (1983). Coronary Artery Surgery Study (CASS): A randomized trial of coronary artery bypass surgery: Quality of life in patients randomly assigned to treatment groups. *Circulation, 68,* 951–960.

Cassem, N. H., & Hackett, T. P. (1971). Psychiatric consultation in a coronary care unit. *Annals of Internal Medicine, 75*(1), 9–14.

Chandra, V., Szklo, M., Goldberg, R., & Tonascia, J. (1983). The impact of marital status on survival after an acute myocardial infarction: A population-based study. *American Journal of Epidemiology, 117,* 320–325.

Cobb, S. (1976). Social support as a moderator of life stress. *Psychosomatic Medicine, 38,* 300–314.

Cohen, S., & Wills, T. A. (1985). Stress, social support, and the buffering hypothesis. *Psychological Bulletin, 98,* 310–357.

Conn, E. H., Williams, R. S., & Wallace, A. G. (1982). Exercise responses before and after physical conditioning in patients with severely depressed left ventricular function. *American Journal of Cardiology, 49,* 296–300.

Croog, S. H., Levine, S., & Lurie, Z. (1968). The heart patient and the recovery process: a review of the literature on social and psychological factors. *Social Science and Medicine, 2,* 111–164.

Crouch, M. A., & Straub, V. (1983). Enhancement of self-esteem in adults. *Family and Community Health, 6*(2), 76–78.

DeBusk, R. F., Haskell, W. L., Miller, N. H., Berra, K., & Taylor, C. B. (1985). Medically directed at-home rehabilitation soon after clinically uncomplicated acute myocardial infarction: A new model for patient care. *American Journal of Cardiology, 55,* 251–257.

Doehrman, S. R. (1977). Psycho-social aspects of recovery from coronary heart disease: A review. *Social Science and Medicine, 11,* 199–218.

Dracup, K. (1985). A controlled trial of couples group counseling in cardiac rehabilitation. *Journal of Cardiopulmonary Rehabilitation, 5,* 436–442.

Dracup, K., Meleis, A., Clark, S., Clyburn, A., Shields, L., & Staley, M. (1984). Group counseling in cardiac rehabilitation: Effect on patient compliance. *Patient Education and Counseling, 6,* 169–177.

Dracup, K., Meleis, A., Baker, C., & Edlefson, P. (1984). Family-focused cardiac rehabilitation: A role supplementation program for cardiac patients and spouses. *Nursing Clinics of North America, 19,* 113–124.

Finkelmeier, B. A., Kenwood, N. J., & Summers, C. (1984). Psychologic ramifications of survival from sudden cardiac death. *Critical Care Quarterly, 7,* 71–79.

Folkins, C. H., Lynch, S., & Gardner, M. M. (1972). Psychological fitness as a function of physical fitness. *Archives of Internal Medicine, 53,* 503–508.

Folkins, C. H. (1976). Effects of physical training on mood. *Journal of Clinical Psychology, 32,* 385–388.

Garrity, T. F., & Klein, R. F. (1975). Emotional response and clinical severity as early determinants of six-month mortality after myocardial infarction. *Heart and Lung, 4,* 730–734.

Gianetti, V. J., Reynolds, J., & Rign, T. (1985). Factors which differentiate smokers from ex-smokers among cardiovascular patients: A discriminant analysis. *Social Science and Medicine, 20,* 241–245.

Gillis, C. L. (1984). Reducing family stress during and after coronary artery bypass surgery. *Nursing Clinics of North America, 19,* 103–112.

Goldwater, B. C., & Collis, M. L. (1985). Psychologic effects of cardiovascular conditioning: A controlled experiment. *Psychosomatic Medicine, 47,* 174–181.

Greenland, P., & Chu, J. S. (1988). Efficacy of cardiac rehabilitation services: With emphasis on patients after myocardial infarction. *Annals of Internal Medicine, 109,* 650–663.

Hackett, T. P., & Cassem, N. H. (1969). Factors contributing to delay in responding to the signs and symptoms of acute myocardial infarction. *American Journal of Cardiology, 24,* 651–656.

Hackett, T. P., Cassem, N. H., & Wishnie, H. A. (1968). The coronary care unit: An appraisal of its psychological hazards. *New England Journal of Medicine, 279,* 1365–1370.

Haynes, R. B. (1976). A crit.cal review of the "determinants" of patient compliance with therapeutic regimens. In D. L. Sackett & R. B. Haynes (Eds.), *Compliance with therapeutic regimens.* Baltimore: Johns Hopkins University Press.

Haynes, R. B. (1984). Compliance with health advice: An overview with special reference to exercise programs. *Journal of Cardiac Rehabilitation, 4,* 120–123.

Heath, G. W., Maloney, P. M., & Fure, C. W. (1987). Group exercise versus home exercise in coronary artery bypass graft patients: Effects on physical activity habits. *Journal of Cardiopulmonary Rehabilitation, 7,* 190–195.

House, J. S. (1981). *Work stress and social support.* Reading, MA: Addison-Wesley.

Hubbard, P., Muhlenkamp, A. F., & Brown, N. (1984). The relationship between social support and self-care practices. *Nursing Research, 33,* 266–270.

Hyman, M. D. (1971). Disability and patients' perceptions of preferential treatment: Some preliminary findings. *Journal of Chronic Disease, 24,* 329–342.

Jacobson, D. E. (1986). Types and timing of social support. *Journal of Health and Social Behavior, 27,* 250–264.

Jenkins, C. D., Stanton, B., Savageau, J. A., Denlinger, P., & Klein, M. D. (1983). Coronary artery bypass surgery: Physical, psychological, social, and economic outcomes six months later. *Journal of the American Medical Association, 250,* 782–788.

Langlie, J. K. (1977). Social networks, health beliefs, and preventive health behavior. *Journal of Health and Social Behavior, 18,* 244–260.

Lewis, C. E. (1966). Factors influencing the return to work of men with congestive heart failure. *Journal of Chronic Disease, 19,* 1203–1204.

Massie, J. F., & Shephard, R. J. (1971). Physiological and psychological effects of training: A comparison of individual and gymnasium programs, with a characterization of the exercise "dropout." *Medical Science in Sports and Exercise, 3,* 110–117.

Magni, G., Unger, H. P., Valfre, C., Polesel, E., Cesari, F., Rizzardo, R., Paruzzolo, P., & Gallucci, V. (1987). Psychosocial outcome one year after heart surgery: A prospective study. *Archives of Internal Medicine, 147,* 473–477.

McPherson, P. D., Paivio, A., Yuhasz, M. S., Rechnitzer, P. A., Pickard, H. A., & Lefcoe, N. M. (1967). Psychological effect of an exercise program for post-infarct and normal adult men. *Journal of Sports Medicine, 7,* 95–102.

Mechanic, D., & Cleary, P. D. (1980). Factors associated with the maintenance of positive health behavior. *Preventive Medicine, 9,* 805–814.

Mechanic, D., & Volkart, E. A. (1960). Illness behavior and medical diagnoses. *Journal of Health and Human Behavior, 1,* 86–94.

Moss, A. J., & Goldstein, S. (1970). The pre-hospital phase of acute myocardial infarction. *Circulation, 41,* 737.

Nyamathi, A M. (1988). Perceptions of factors influencing the coping of wives of myocardial infarction patients. *Journal of Cardiovascular Nursing, 2,* 65–76.

Pashkow, F., Schafer, M., & Pashkow, P. (1986). Heartwatchers: Low-cost, community-based cardiac rehabilitation. *Journal of Cardiopulmonary Rehabilitation, 6,* 469–473.

Pearlin, L. I., & Aneshensel, C. S. (1986). Coping and social supports: Their functions and applications. In L. Aiken & D. Mechanic (Eds.), *Application of social science to clinical medicine and health policy.* New Brunswick, NJ: Rutgers University Press.

Pickard, H. A., & Lefcoe, N. M. (1967). Psychological effect of an exercise program for post-infarct and normal adult men. *Journal of Sports Medicine, 7,* 95–102.

Prosser, G., Carson, P., Gelson, A., Tucker, H., Neopsytou, M., Phillips, R., & Simpson, T. (1978). Assessing the psychological effects of an exercise training programme for patients following myocardial infarction: A pilot study. *British Journal of Medical Psychology, 51,* 95–192.

Razin, A. M. (1982). Psychosocial intervention in coronary artery disease: A review. *Psychosomatic Medicine, 44,* 363–387.

Revenson, T. A., Wollman, C. A., & Felton, B. J. (1983). Social supports as stress buffers for adult cancer patients. *Psychosomatic Medicine, 45*(4), 321–331.

Ruberman, W., Weinblatt, E., Goldberg, J. D., & Chaudhary, B. S. (1984). Psychosocial influences on mortality after myocardial infarction. *New England Journal of Medicine, 311,* 552–559.

Sivarajan, E. S., & Newton, K. M. (1984). Exercise, education, and counseling for patients with coronary artery disease. *Clinics in Sports Medicine, 3,* 349–369.

Stanwyck, D. J. (1983). Self-esteem through the life span. *Family and Community Health, 6*(2), 11–28.

Stern, M. J., & Cleary, P. (1981). National exercise and heart disease project: Psychosocial changes observed during a low-level exercise program. *Archives of Internal Medicine, 141,* 1463–1467.

Stern, M. J., Gorman, P. A., & Kaslow, L. (1983). The group counseling vs. exercise therapy study. *Archives of Internal Medicine, 143,* 1719 –1725.

Stern, M. J., Pascale, L., & Ackerman, A. (1977). Life adjustment postmyocardial infarction. *Archives of Internal Medicine, 137,* 1680–1685.

Taylor, C. B., Bandura, A., Ewart, C. K., Miller, N. H., & DeBusk, R. F. (1985). Exercise testing to enhance wives' confidence in their husbands' cardiac capability soon after clinically uncomplicated acute myocardial infarction. *American Journal of Cardiology, 55,* 635–638.

Tilden, V. P. (1985). Issues of conceptualization and measurement of social support in the construction of nursing theory. *Research in Nursing and Health, 8,* 199–206.

Vermueulen, A., Lie, K. I., & Durrer, D. (1983). Effects of cardiac rehabilitation after acute myocardial infarction: Changes in coronary risk factors and long-term prognosis. *American Heart Journal, 105,* 798–801.

Waltz, M. (1986). Marital context and post-infarction quality of life: Is it social support or something more? *Social Science and Medicine, 22,* 791–805.

Wankel, L. M. (1984). Decision-making and social support strategies for increasing exercise involvement. *Journal of Cardiac Rehabilitation, 4,* 124–135.

Wenger, N. K. (1981). *Coronary care—rehabilitation of the patient with symptomatic coronary atherosclerotic heart disease.* Prepared for the Coronary Care Committee, Council on Clinical Cardiology and the Committee on Medical Education, American Heart Association, Dallas, 70-002-F.

Wishnie, H. A., Hackett, T. P., & Cassem, N. H. (1971). Psychological hazards of convalescence following myocardial infarction. *Journal of the American Medical Association, 215,* 1292–1296.

Wortman, C. B. (1984). Social support and the cancer patient. *Cancer, 53*(Suppl. 10), 2339–2360.

Yalom, I. D. (1985). *The theory and practice of group psychotherapy* (3rd ed.). New York: Basic Books.

Index